# Medical Ethics and Medical Law

## For the MLA and Medical Exams

# CRASH COURSE

SERIES EDITOR
## Philip Xiu
MA (Cantab), MB BChir, MRCP, MRCGP, MScClinEd, FHEA, MAcadMEd, RCPathME
Honorary Senior Lecturer
Leeds University School of Medicine
Leeds, United Kingdom

FACULTY ADVISORS
## Pirashanthie Vivekananda-Schmidt
C Psychol, MA (Ed), DPhil, PFHEA, AFBPsS, Occ Psy
Professor of Medical Education
School of Medicine and Population Health, The University of Sheffield
Sheffield, United Kingdom

## Richard J. Cooper
BSc (Hons), LLB, MA, PhD
Professor of Public Health and Social Pharmacy
Senior University Teacher, School of Medicine and Population Health
The University of Sheffield
Sheffield, United Kingdom

# Medical Ethics and Medical Law
## For the MLA and Medical Exams

## William Brooks
BMedSci (Hons), MBChB (Hons), MEd, MRCGP, FHEA
General Practitioner and Honorary Clinical Teacher
School of Medicine and Population Health, The University of Sheffield
Specialist Advisor, Primary and Community Care, CQC
Sheffield, United Kingdom

## India Mayhook-Walker
iBSc, DPMSA, MBChB (Hons)
Foundation Doctor in Jersey General Hospital
States of Jersey

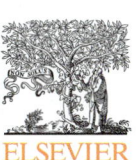

ELSEVIER

---

### Notice

---

ISBN: 978-0-443-24603-6

*Content Strategist:* Trinity Hutton
*Content Project Manager:* Tapajyoti Chaudhuri
*Design:* Miles Hitchen
*Marketing Manager:* Deborah J. Watkins

Printed in India

Last digit is the print number: 9  8  7  6  5  4  3  2  1

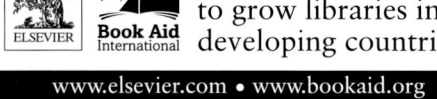

Working together
to grow libraries in
developing countries

www.elsevier.com • www.bookaid.org

# Series editor's foreword

With great honour and pride, we present the latest edition of the Crash Course series. This series has traversed a journey of nearly a quarter century, stemming from the vision of Dr Dan Horton-Szar, and his legacy continues to walk with us on this pathway of knowledge.

The series has been popular with students worldwide, selling over **1 million copies** and being translated into more than **eight languages**, reinforcing our commitment to global learning. We remain extremely grateful for your unwavering trust. The series has once again been refreshed and fully upgraded in accordance with the rapidly changing medical guidelines, ensuring the content is comprehensive, accurate and fully up to date.

This latest series continues our tradition of integrating clinical practice with basic medical sciences, tailored meticulously for today's medical undergraduate curriculum. A central highlight of this instalment is our emphasis on high-yield examination content designed specifically for the Medical Licensing Assessment (MLA) curriculum.

We have also revised all self-assessment questions to align with the single best answer format in line with the latest MLA examination style.

Utilizing student feedback, we have strived to maintain the core principles of this series: delivering precise and readable text that brings together depth and clarity. The authors are experienced junior doctors who successfully navigated these examinations recently, ensuring practical and tested guidance. A team of expert faculty advisors from across the United Kingdom ensures the content's accuracy, making it resilient and reliable.

As we turn a new chapter with the latest edition, we honour the past, cherish the present and embrace the promise of the future. We wish you every success in your journey of learning and growth and hope that this series adds value to your life, both as students and as future medical professionals.

**Philip Xiu**

# Authors

Well done for getting this far. Your up-to-date biomedical knowledge and clinical skills are essential to your current and future practice with patients and colleagues, but you will need more than these to succeed. Medical ethics and medical law underpin all branches of clinical practice: they inform and reflect the attitudes and behaviours that are consistent with the socio-cultural context of the profession. Similar to medical science, ethics and the law also evolve and change over time—sometimes in response to research and often in response to events. This volume incorporates actual cases that are seminal determinants of current practice in the United Kingdom.

We have gratefully built on the foundations laid by a previous Elsevier title, *Medical Ethics and Sociology*, revising, refocusing and revitalizing with extensive new content to help you towards the Medical Licensing Assessment and life beyond. Enjoy this book and make good use of it: wishing you every success.

# Notes on language

Languages are always in a state of flux to a greater or lesser degree. Terminology in some of the areas discussed is currently unsettled, particularly around transgender. We aim to write respectfully and with balance: our intention is to provide useful and engaging educational content to support your developing practice and that of your fellow readers.

# Notes on contributions

William Brooks largely wrote Chapters 2, 3 and 5. India Mayhook-Walker largely wrote Chapters 1 and 4.

### William Brooks

Medical ethics and medical law are integral to the practice of medicine. While they are both rewarding subjects, they can prove frustrating at sometimes. The law might seem dry and dull, while at times ethical arguments can generate many bad options and seemingly no right ones. I hope that this book will prove useful during these moments and inspire you.

It has been a great privilege to be involved in the writing of the new edition of this book, especially having been taught as a medical student at Sheffield by Professor Pirashanthie

Vivekananda-Schmidt and Dr Richard J. Cooper, and as a student on the Apothecaries' Diploma in the Philosophy of Medicine by Dr Andrew Papanikitas, the author of the previous edition.

**India Mayhook-Walker**

# Faculty advisors

'Ars longa, vita brevis, occasio praeceps, experimentum periculosum, judicium difficile.' This Latin aphorism can be translated as 'life is short, the art (craft/skill) long, opportunity fleeting, experimenting can be perilous, judgement difficult'.

The aphorism summarizes the complexities and uncertainties surrounding life and the practice of medicine. Medicine may have a scientific and evidence-based foundation, but the practice and daily decisions can be difficult and complex. We hope that this book will support you with your daily choices in the workplace and Good Medical Practice.

**Pirashanthie Vivekananda-Schmidt**

# Series editor's acknowledgements

We would like to express our sincere gratitude to those who have provided their support and expertise in preparing this latest edition of the Crash Course series. Our resident doctor contributors' participation in crafting the manuscript has been indispensable. Their first-hand experience and current medical knowledge have infused realism and practicality into our content.

Our faculty editors deserve a special note of thanks. They have extensively validated the correctness of the information, ensuring that the content is not just accurate but also contemporaneous, credible and aligns with the latest medical standards.

We extend our heartfelt thanks to our publisher, Elsevier. Their staff have demonstrated an unwavering commitment to quality, maintaining the high standards set since the first edition. Their insights have routinely enriched the content and process alike.

Our Commissioning Editor, Jeremy Bowes, deserves a special mention for his consistent support and guiding hand throughout the development process. His directions and advice have bettered this edition and spurred us on our quest for excellence.

We are greatly indebted to Alex Mortimer for her wisdom, practical insights and valuable guidance. A big thank you to our Content Strategists, Trinity Hutton and Jennifer Dooley, who need special acknowledgement for meticulously outlining the direction and scope of the content. They have managed to mix details with a strategic plan, keeping our readers in mind.

Lastly, much gratitude is owed to our Content Product Managers, Taranpreet Kaur, Ayan Dhar, Shivani Pal and Tapajyoti Chaudhuri, who have juggled the numerous day-to-day tasks with utmost dedication and perseverance. Despite the ever-approaching deadlines, they have shown remarkable patience and steadfast determination, ensuring that each step of the book's development was accomplished seamlessly.

In conclusion, we sincerely thank each of these wonderful people for their outstanding contributions and support, without which this work would not have been achieved. Their passion, commitment and collaborative effort have helped us bring this edition together.

**Philip Xiu**

# Contents

# Introduction 1

Medical ethics and law have always developed hand in hand with medicine itself. There are perennial questions around how doctors should behave and what treatments should or should not be permitted. Hippocrates' famous oath is one of the oldest and best-known examples of this and forbids doctors from poisoning patients, performing abortions and practising surgery, while requiring doctors to keep patient confidentiality. The potential for medical practice to cause serious harm is clear from the 20th century examples, including the Tuskegee syphilis experiments, Nazi and Imperial Japanese medical experimentation and exterminations and unauthorized removal and retention of organs in the National Health Service (NHS).

This chapter provides an introduction to the English legal system and key ethical theories. There are regional variations in medical law within the four nations of the United Kingdom due to devolution of certain powers to the Scottish Parliament, Welsh Assembly and the Northern Irish Assembly, and you should refer to appropriate guidance depending on your location. Some examples at the time of writing are: Scotland requires witnesses for consent to certain procedures; the *Mental Capacity Act (2005)* does not apply in Scotland (the equivalent is the *Adults with Incapacity Act,* 2000) and involuntary admission criteria for patients with serious mental illness are different between England and Wales. Where there is a significant difference in law, it is noted in a box. Subsequent chapters will examine ethics and law as applied to specific issues and situations.

## WHAT IS MEDICAL ETHICS?

Ethics is the realm of philosophy dealing with right and wrong actions and conduct and what ought or ought not to be done. It is sometimes called moral philosophy. Medical ethics is the study of right and wrong actions or morals within medicine. Ethics deals with the critical evaluation of assumptions and arguments. It is distinguished from:

- Law and professional codes of practice, which rely on the interpretation of preexisting legal and professional rules.
- Religious teaching or theological arguments, which derive from one or more sources of religious scripture or custom.
- Sociological or psychological explanations for why we behave in certain ways, which do not necessarily indicate if the behaviour is good or bad.
- The discussion of moral decision-making within medicine in a historical or anthropological light. This does not necessarily answer the question, 'what is the right thing to do at this point in time?'

All the disciplines above may contribute to the study of medical ethics or overlap with it.

There is no uniform concept of ethics held by doctors, with Campbell and Higgs (1982) describing three different concepts:

1. Professional etiquette: the accepted conventions of a social role.
2. Synonymous with 'morals or morality'.
3. Moral philosophy: the critical study of morality.

In the past, many medical schools did not formally teach ethics. It was thought the student would be able to learn what was considered right and wrong by observing senior doctors *and by doing as they did*. The explicit teaching of ethics aims to foster *an ability to make rational, moral decisions*—rather than to simply do things as they have been done before. The importance for students, in professional life and in exams, is that it is not just the conclusion you reach that is important. Rather it is also the strength and coherence of the arguments leading you to your conclusion which are important.

---

**ETHICS**

How you reach your conclusion is just as important as the conclusion that you reach. You should be able to explain and justify your professional decisions and actions.

---

## WHAT IS MEDICAL LAW?

Like everyone else, doctors and medical students are subject to the laws of society. The law has several functions, including:

- To maintain civil order.
- To resolve disputes without resorting to use of force.
- To establish and define standards of acceptable behaviour.
- To maintain those standards and punish 'offences'.
- To provide rules enabling trade and business.
- To provide fair recompense for injury.
- To do justice and put right wrongs.

There are two types of law: civil and criminal. Medical law encompasses both civil and criminal law. The body of statutes and common law provide the legal framework for the practice of medicine. It exists to protect both doctors and patients and to adjudicate in the most severe disputes (Fig. 1.1).

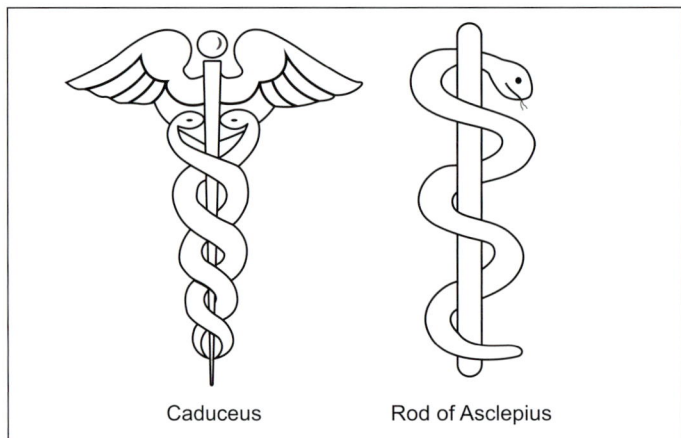

**Fig. 1.1** The Caduceus, symbol of the god Hermes and the Rod of Asclepius, symbol of the legendary physician.

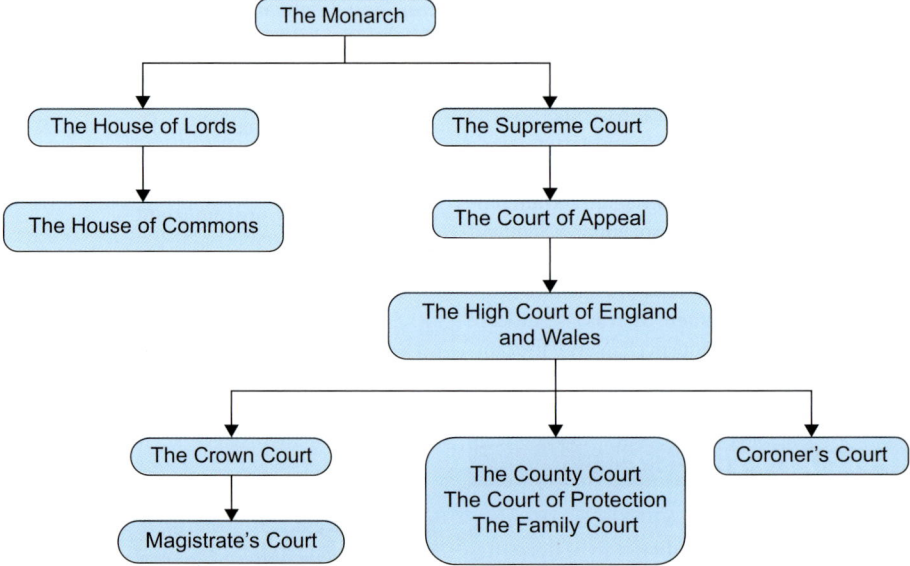

**Fig. 1.2** The structure of the UK legislative and judicial systems. The devolved legislatures of Wales, Scotland and Northern Ireland all answer to Parliament. In Scotland and Northern Ireland, the structure of the courts is slightly different. The decisions of higher courts are binding on lower courts; this is known as precedence.

## THE UK LEGAL SYSTEM

Unlike many other jurisdictions, where law is imposed from a single constitutional source, the English and UK legal systems have developed organically since before the Norman Conquest in 1066. The legal system is intrinsically linked with the system of government although the courts are independent. Britain means England, Wales and Scotland; the UK means Britain and Northern Ireland. Fig. 1.2 shows the structure of the legislative and judicial systems.

The monarch is the source of the entire constitutional system and is politically neutral by convention. All ministers and judges are ultimately appointed by the monarch, as is any government, and all laws only come into force with the monarch's assent. Until 2008 the highest court of appeal was the Law Lords, based in the House of Lords. Since then the Supreme Court has been established which is independent of Parliament. However, the courts are still subject to Parliamentary supremacy; they may not overturn Parliamentary law, and Parliament may create new legislation to overrule a judicial ruling. The key principles are that Parliament

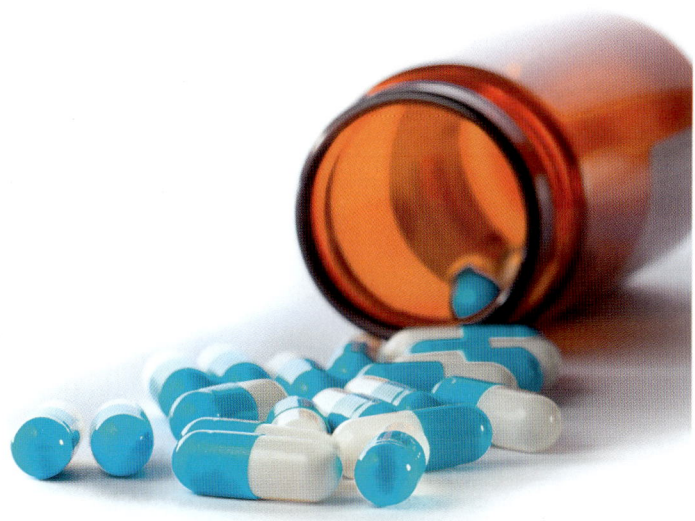

**Fig. 1.3** A negligence claim relies on there being a duty of care, a breach in the duty of care and harm being caused by the breach.

(or the Crown in Parliament) is supreme and that no Parliament may bind its successors. Within the English legal system there are two *sources* of law: parliamentary law and the common law.

- Parliament creates law by Acts of Parliament (also called Statutes); these are termed primary legislation and can further allow secondary legislation to be made by authorized others.
- The courts develop the common law through decisions made by judges acting in accordance with precedence, which is often known as *Case Law*. The courts do not make new laws.

## Case law

The courts are able to interpret statutes but not overturn them. In contrast, Parliament can overrule judge-made decisions. Parliament can 'change' the law, especially on controversial matters. English Common Law is built on case law—the body of decided judgements from which legal principles have been established. These principles are applied in subsequent cases unless the facts of the new case are different or a compelling case for change can be made. 'Precedent' is the term describing the binding power of previous decisions of the court on subsequent similar cases. As shown in Fig. 1.2, the judicial hierarchy determines what decision is binding on what court. Decisions in 'higher' courts are binding on 'lower' courts: decisions in the High Court are binding on Magistrates' and Coroners' Courts and usually followed in High Court decisions. Judgements from the Supreme Court are binding on the Court of Appeal, and judgements from both are

**Table 1.1** Some of the main differences between the civil and criminal court

| Civil cases | Criminal cases |
|---|---|
| Disputes between individuals or organizations | Involves the allegation of lawbreaking |
| Claims brought by claimant | Case is brought by a prosecutor |
| On the balance of probabilities | Beyond reasonable doubt |
| Normally tried by a judge | Trial by jury for more serious offences |
| Remedied by compensation and/or injunctions | Punishments include fines and imprisonment |
| Heard in the County Court, High Court and Court of Appeal | Heard in the Magistrates' Court, Crown Court and Court of Appeal |

binding on all lower courts. The Supreme Court may very rarely reverse a decision of its own. Since the *Human Rights Act 1998*, cases founded on the European Convention on Human Rights may have a final appeal to the European Court of Human Rights (ECHR). Several recent cases of relevance to UK medical law and ethics have found their way to the ECHR (Fig. 1.3).

Court cases are either heard in the civil or criminal division of the justice system. Table 1.1 shows the key differences between the two. A civil case arises from a conflict between two or more people and aims to fairly compensate the injured person(s).

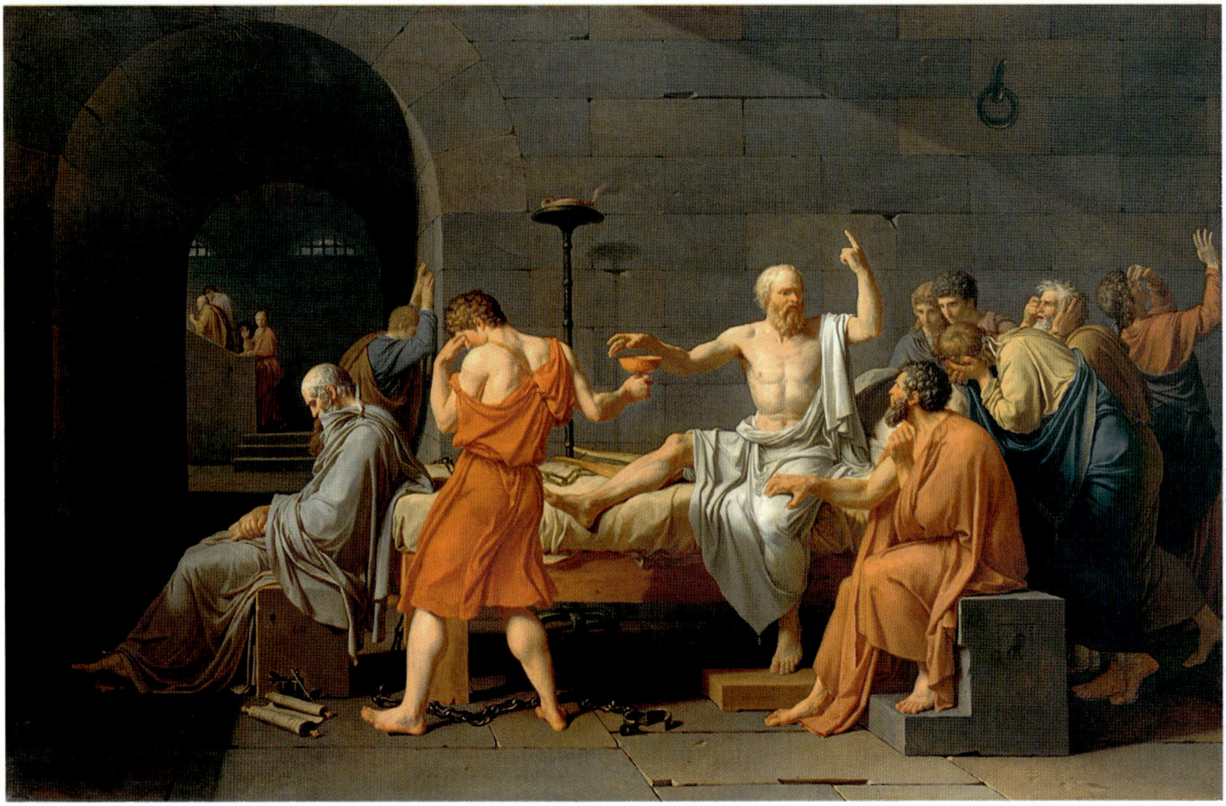

**Fig. 1.4** Ethical arguments can have serious consequences, as Socrates found out. He was ordered to commit suicide for 'corrupting the youth of Athens'. (*The Death of Socrates* by Jacques-Louis David (1787). Available in the Public Domain.)

A criminal case examines whether someone has broken the law of the state and whether they should receive punishment. A major difference between the two is that in criminal cases the prosecution must demonstrate beyond all reasonable doubt (i.e. be certain) that the accused has broken the law in order to secure a conviction. To be decisive in a civil case, the burden of proof is 'the balance of probabilities', that is, one side needs to demonstrate their facts are more likely and arguments are more persuasive than the other. Most medical law cases are brought within the civil justice system rather than the criminal. There are many branches of civil law, including property, tax and family law. Most medicolegal cases are brought under tort law, often regarding negligence. However, healthcare professionals can be charged with criminal offences, including battery and assault (Fig. 1.4).

**HINTS AND TIPS**

*Remember*: Higher court decisions are more influential than lower court decisions, but changes to the law are made by Parliament in the United Kingdom.

## Statute law

Parliament may create law in two ways. First, it may pass primary legislation as Acts of Parliament. Second, it may create secondary legislation, such as Statutory Instruments, which in turn permit Regulations, Orders and Rules to be created by government ministers and others under the authority granted in Acts of Parliament. These allow for changes and additions to be made more easily. Although the courts may interpret statutes, they may neither amend nor reverse them, and only Parliament may do so. Key Acts of Parliament relating to health legislation include:

- *National Health Service Act* 2006
- *National Health Service (Wales) Act* 2006
- *National Health Service (Consequential Provisions) Act* 2006
- *Health and Social Care Act* 2012 and *Health and Social Care Act* 2008
- *Abortion Act* 1967
- *Human Fertilisation and Embryology Act* 2008
- *Medical Act* 1983
- *Public Health (Control of Disease) Act* 1984
- *Coronavirus Act* 2020

Many Acts delegate the detail of how they are implemented to a minister, local authority or other official. When there are concerns that these powers have been used unreasonably, an application may be made in the courts for judicial review. However, a successful challenge needs to demonstrate that, for example, a ministerial decision is clearly unreasonable or in conflict with other laws. Health legislation is a complex area that has required frequent amendments in order to keep policies inline with evolving circumstances. However, much of the health legislation made since 1977 has been summarized within four Acts of Parliament:

- *National Health Service Act 2006*
- *National Health Service (Wales) Act 2006*
- *National Health Service (Consequential Provisions) Act 2006*
- *Health and Social Care Act 2012*

In particular, the legal duty of care owed by doctors to patients in NHS is statutory and not contractual, following the *NHS Act 2006*.

## Legal rights and the Human Rights Act

After the Second World War, there was an emphasis on protecting human rights, and the European Convention on Human Rights was established in 1950. The United Kingdom ratified the convention in 1951, and it came into force in 1953. To adjudicate claims related to the convention, a court of judges was set up in Strasbourg: the ECHR. In 1998 the UK government introduced the Human Rights Act, which enshrined the convention rights into law. This makes such rights enforceable against public authorities, including hospitals. Some convention rights are absolute, meaning signatory countries have an obligation to protect them. Others are qualified rights, which means that other duties of the state may supersede them. For examples of important medicolegal cases considered by the ECHR, see the discussion of *H.L. v. The United Kingdom* (2004) and *Christine Goodwin v. The United Kingdom* (2002) in Chapter 3 and *Pretty v. The United Kingdom* (2002) in Chapter 4. Some of the Articles that are important to medical law include:

**Article 2: Right to life (Absolute Right)**
Everyone's right to life shall be protected by law. The Article also mandates an obligation to investigate deaths under the state.

- This Article might be used to challenge a 'Do not attempt resuscitation' order placed against a patient's wishes.
- It might be used to challenge the withholding or withdrawal of lifesaving or life-sustaining treatment.

**Article 3: Prohibition of torture, inhuman and degrading treatment (Absolute Right)**
No one shall be subjected to torture or inhuman or degrading treatment or punishment.

- This could be used to challenge poor-quality treatment or failure to provide treatment within a certain time. Consider—does waiting 18 months for a hip replacement constitute degrading treatment? Does waiting for 24 hours on a trolley in an emergency department constitute degrading treatment?
- It has been argued, unsuccessfully so far in the United Kingdom, that laws prohibiting the assisted suicide/euthanasia of terminally ill patients constitute inhuman or degrading treatment.

**Article 8: Right to respect for private and family life (Qualified Right)**
Everyone has the right to respect for their private and family life, their home and their correspondence:

- *R (on the application of Tracey) v. Cambridge University Hospital NHS Trust* (2014) was argued on the basis of Article 8 (see Chapter 4).

**Article 9: Freedom of thought, conscience and religion (Qualified Right)**
Everyone has the right to their religious and cultural beliefs:

- How might this affect the rights of others? For example, where a doctor or nurse does not wish to provide information about or take part in contraception services because they believe this is morally wrong.

**Article 12: Right to marry and found a family (Qualified Right)**
Individuals of marriageable age have the right to marry and find a family according to the national laws governing the exercise of that right.

**Article 14: Right to protection from discrimination (Qualified Right)**
Individuals should be able to enjoy their rights free from unlawful discrimination on the basis of sex, race, religion, political opinion, and so on.

- This Article could be used to challenge inequities in access to fertility treatment on the basis of, for example, sexual orientation or geographical location.

## Medical negligence

Doctors may sometimes fall foul of the criminal law, but the majority of cases against doctors are medical negligence cases heard in the civil courts under tort law. Three key components are required for medical negligence cases to succeed: (1) a duty of care must have existed, (2) the duty of care must have been breached and (3) the breach must have caused the harm in question. The concept of duty of care itself is complex, and this section is limited to explaining it in the context of medical negligence.

## Duty of care

It must be shown that the defendant (the person or authority accused of negligence) owed the claimant (the injured party or the person accusing the defendant) a duty of care:

- The duty of care of a general practitioner (GP) crystallizes when the patient registers with that GP and then consults with the GP on the occasion in question.
- The duty of care of a hospital doctor crystallizes when the patient is formally accepted into hospital.

The ethical obligation to benefit another person using one's medical expertise can be complex to evaluate depending on the context and the specific factors. English law does not oblige doctors to give emergency treatment outside of the above situations except when:

- A patient presents to an emergency department.
- A GP is requested to provide emergency/immediately necessary treatment to a person in their practice area.

By contrast, in France or Australia, 'Good Samaritan' laws oblige doctors to stop and assist anyone who is taken ill or injured.

## Breach of the duty of care

There must be a standard of care that could be expected from the defendant. The standard of care doctors are expected to reach was asserted by the case *Bolam v. Friern Hospital Management Committee* (1957). The standard of care was set as that of 'the ordinary skilled man exercising and professing to have that special skill'. This standard has become known as the Bolam Test—it is applicable to all aspects of treatment, diagnosis and disclosure of information or risks to patients. This standard was modified in *Bolitho v. City and Hackney Health Authority* (1997), where it was held that a court must also find the medical opinion to be 'reasonable' and 'responsible'. The claimant must show that the defendant did not reach a reasonable standard of care.

## Causation

The claimant must show that the breach of the duty of care caused the damage they claim to have suffered; the test used to prove causation is often referred to as the '*but for*' test. It says the claimant must demonstrate that *but for* the defendant's negligence, the claimant would not have suffered the harm in respect of which they seek damages. For example, in *Barnett v. Chelsea and Kensington Hospital Management Committee* (1969), a casualty officer refused to attend a night watchman who was vomiting after drinking tea and who later died from arsenic poisoning. Although there was a breach of duty, the claim still failed because even if he had received treatment the man would have died anyway, and there was, therefore, no causation.

**Damages or harm**: Damage must have occurred to the claimant for compensation to be awarded. The purpose of bringing an action is to usually gain compensation; if no damages have occurred, there is little point in bringing an action.

### HINTS AND TIPS

*Remember*: To succeed, a medical negligence case must demonstrate there was a duty of care, there was a breach of that duty and the breach caused harm to the patient.

As well as being subject to the law, doctors are also subject to professional regulation. In the United Kingdom, the General Medical Council (GMC) issues guidance on what it considers to be the ethical duties of doctors. Core guidance covers truth-telling, confidentiality and good medical practice in general (General Medical Council, 2023). The professional duties set down by the GMC have been described as quasi-legal (Fulford et al., 2002). This is because the duties are *enforced*. Failure to adhere to the GMC code of practice can mean removal from the register of licenced doctors. Being 'struck off' means you can no longer work as a doctor in the United Kingdom and are unlikely to find work as a doctor in Europe or elsewhere in the world. Professionalism and regulation are discussed in Chapter 2.

## ETHICAL ARGUMENTS

Like any other form of academic writing and argument, ethics has a particular way of being proposed. Ethical arguments must be valid and justifiable, as well as logical and relevant to the point in hand. Here is an example of a classic logical proposition: *Socrates is a man. All men are mortal. Socrates is mortal.* You can see that for the proposition *Socrates is mortal*, to be valid, it must agree with the first two statements. While you do not need to worry about the formal rules of logic, you should ensure your writing has the same logical coherence.

Logical fallacies such as the straw man argument, where you present the weakest possible version of the opposing argument, should be avoided. For discussion of the slippery slope argument, see Chapter 5 (Euthanasia). These general principles are normally used in conjunction with an ethical theory to make your argument.

## ETHICAL THEORIES

Ethical theories attempt to provide a framework for addressing the problem of how human beings should behave with one another in the world. There are three key theories which have historically dominated medical ethics teaching: *Utilitarianism, Deontology* and *Virtue Ethics*. More recent frameworks attempt to reconcile different theories and values. Many students and doctors are familiar with the four principles of biomedical ethics

(Beauchamp & Childress, 2013). 'Values-Based Practice' or 'Values in Medicine' has recently gained prominence in psychiatry and general practice and is taught on some undergraduate medical degrees. Rights-based approaches to ethics are often used in public debates, particularly around the availability of healthcare services.

Why bother with these theories? Can we not rely on some 'Golden principle', such as 'Do unto others as you would have them do unto you'? Perhaps such a principle is sufficient to help guide our moral decisions on a day-to-day basis. But often it falters on the ethical dilemmas where there is no obvious path to take or where individuals have greatly differing concepts of what is acceptable. Philosophers and ethicists often devise thought experiments to highlight these differences, and this book includes thought experiments for the readers to consider. In addition, we need to provide reasons why any approach is right and why others might be wrong. The purpose of ethical theory is to help us to think more clearly about ethical problems.

---

**CASE 1.1 THOUGHT EXPERIMENT: THE TROLLEY PROBLEM**

You are walking by a railway line that splits into two tracks. One track has three workers on it, and the other has 20 children playing. There is an out-of-control train coming down the tracks, and it is currently on course to hit the children. You can pull a lever to shift the tracks, saving the children but causing the train to hit the workers instead. What do you do? (Fig. 1.5).

Foot, P. (1967). The problem of abortion and the doctrine of the double effect. *Oxford Review*, 5, 5–15.

---

# Utilitarianism

Utilitarianism is the most well-known branch of consequentialism, an ethical theory that holds the outcomes or consequences of an action that are the most important part in determining the morality of an action. To the utilitarian, it is the *principle of utility* that determines the morally correct action, which causes the greatest utility. This is sometimes summed up as 'the greatest good for the greatest number' but not always. The principle of good simply holds that we ought to produce the maximum amount of good.

What then is 'utility'? The founders of Utilitarianism, Jeremy Bentham (1748–1832: Fig. 1.6) and John Stuart Mill (1806–73: Fig. 1.7), thought that utility was pleasure or happiness. Others have considered utility to include values such as friendship, knowledge, health and beauty. Still others believe the concept of utility is best applied to the satisfaction of preferences rather than any intrinsic values.

The advantages of utilitarianism are that:

- It fits with two strong intuitions, that is
  - Morality is about promotion of well-being.
  - We should maximize well-being.
- It is a single principle that tries to deal with appropriateness of other principles, such as the principle of *always* telling the truth or of *always* acting to prevent suffering.
- It incorporates a principle of equality: each person's happiness is equal.

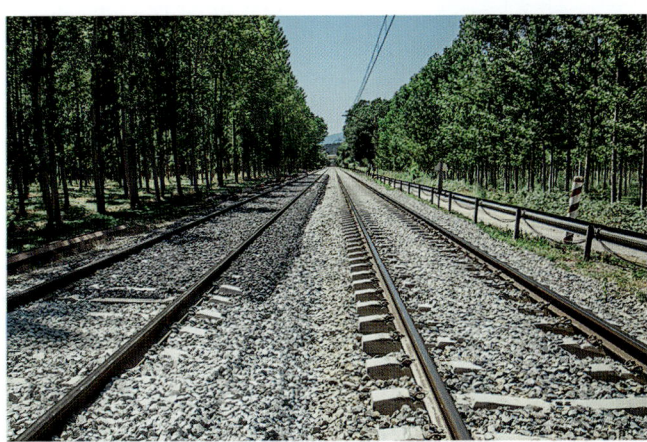

**Fig. 1.5** What medical ethics applications can you think of for the trolley problem?

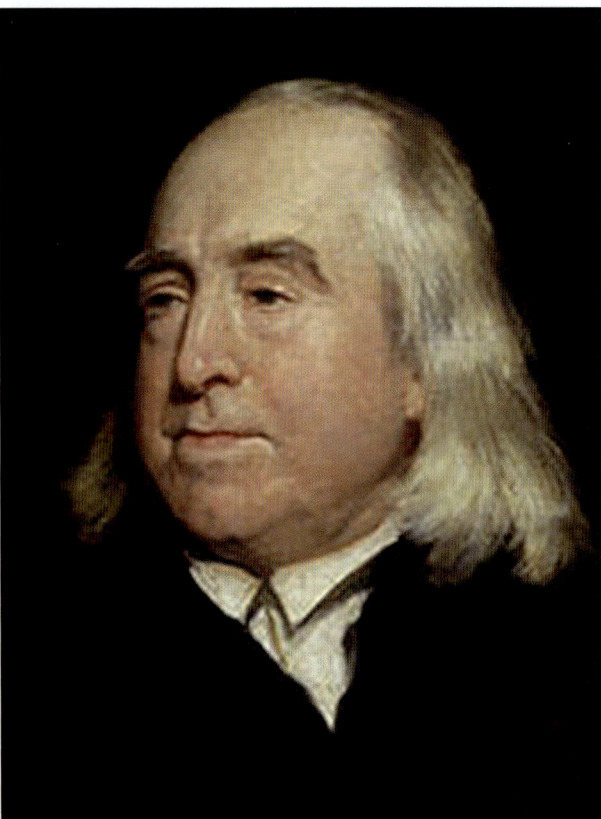

**Fig. 1.6** Jeremy Bentham (1748–1832), one of the founders of utilitarianism.

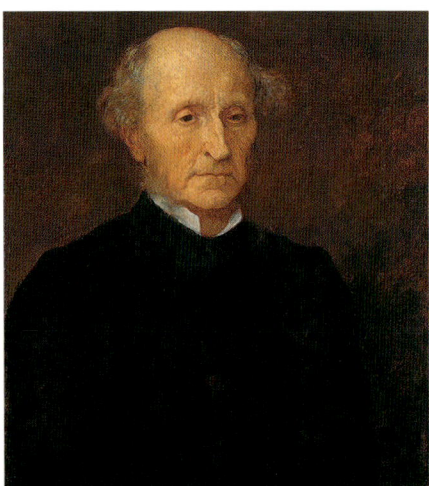

**Fig. 1.7** John Stuart Mill (1806–73). (Courtesy National Portrait Gallery, London.)

- It can be extended to the animal kingdom: some utilitarians have argued that the capacity to suffer (and feel pain) means our treatment of animals also ought to be subject to moral scrutiny.

The disadvantages of utilitarianism are that:

- There are problems dealing with intuitively immoral actions: is it right to kill one patient in order to harvest their organs and perhaps save five lives?
- Utilitarianism demands too much: In always asking us to do the *best* action, everyone is expected to be both heroic and saintly. For example, it could be argued that 'maximizing utility' demands that not only should we donate blood and bone marrow as often as we can but also that we may well be morally obliged to donate one of our kidneys as well.
- The equality principle is overly impersonal in demanding that we treat the well-being of our friends and family as equivalent to that of strangers.
- In principle, a small increase in pleasure for the majority will override a vast degree of pain for a minority; this is also known as the repugnant conclusion.
- It is impossible to know what all the consequences of an action will be before the action is done.

Bentham believed law and morality could be made rational by a scientific study of human nature. He thought humans were governed by two factors: 'pleasure and pain', and that it was in their nature to seek pleasure and avoid pain. For Bentham, laws were only 'good' if they maximized pleasure and minimized pain for the majority of people. The 'scientific' foundation of utilitarianism comes from the requirement to do 'happiness sums'. Bentham thought it was possible to classify how good an action is by measuring how much pleasure or pain was brought about by that action. He called this process 'felicific calculus'.

Mill differed from Bentham in two important ways:

1. He thought cultural and spiritual pleasures should be sought in preference to physical pleasures.
2. He thought people should ordinarily stick to moral rules rather than calculate the balance of utility for each ethical problem.

Even though Mill advocated moral rules, he is still a utilitarian because he held that these moral rules should be calculated using the principle of utility. This is known as *rule utilitarianism*. For example, lying in general might produce less utility than telling the truth. Therefore there is a rule that says, 'Do not lie!' However, we could imagine a scenario where telling a particular lie might produce more utility than telling the truth would. The rule utilitarian would still tell the truth. Other utilitarians, known as *act utilitarians*, would appeal directly to the principle of utility and lie (Fig. 1.8).

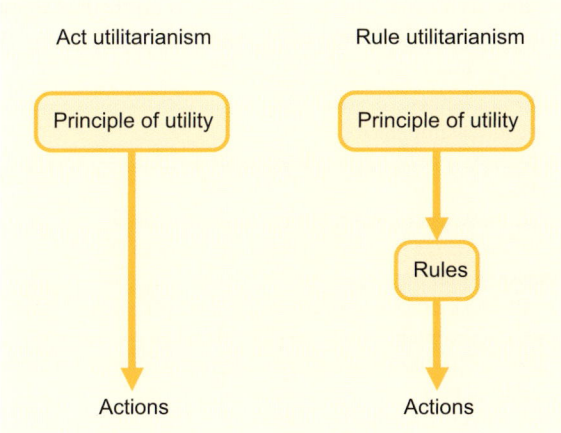

**Fig. 1.8** Act versus rule utilitarianism. In 'act utilitarianism', the principle of utility is directly used to guide actions. In 'rule utilitarianism', the principle of utility is used to formulate general rules which in turn are used to guide actions.

---

**CASE 1.2 THOUGHT EXPERIMENT: THE UNWILLING ORGAN DONOR**

You are a doctor and a utilitarian. In your waiting room there are six patients. One needs a heart transplant, another a liver, another a kidney, the fourth needs a new lung and the fifth needs a kidney and a cornea. The sixth patient is entirely healthy apart from his broken arm.

　　The five patients needing transplants come to you and propose that they kill the sixth patient and that you transplant his organs into them as they all have large families and he has no relatives or friends. They argue this would cause more benefit to more people and would only harm one person. What do you do?

---

## Deontology

Deontology covers those theories emphasizing moral *duties* and *rules* rather than consequences (from the Greek *deon*, meaning 'duty'). Where utilitarianism focuses on the consequences of an action, deontology focuses on the action itself. The most well-known deontological theory is that of Immanuel Kant (1724–1804), often referred to as Kantian ethics. He believed that:

- Morality was not dependent on how much happiness resulted from particular actions.
- Morality was something humans imposed on themselves because they are *rational beings*.
- God was not necessary for moral law (although Kant was a Christian himself).

　　Kant argued that we can find out which moral rules to obey by using our powers of reason. He said by seeing whether our desires

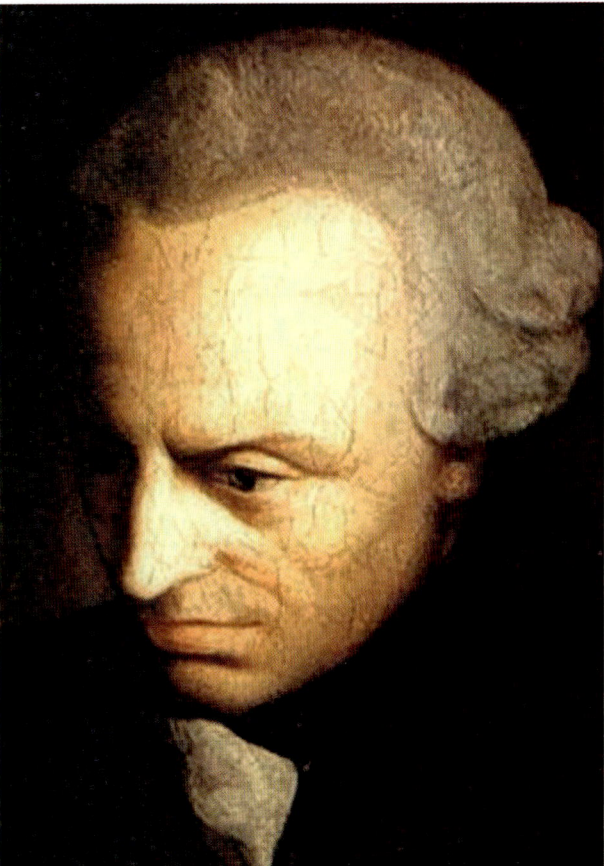

**Fig. 1.9** The German philosopher Immanuel Kant (1724–1804).

can be applied universally, we can tell whether or not they follow rational moral principles. This 'universalisability' test is called the 'categorical imperative'. It states, act only on that maxim through which you can at the same time will that it should become a universal law. This means we should behave in such a way that we can imagine everyone can behave (Figs 1.9–1.13).

　　For example, if our 'maxim' or 'desire' is to 'steal other people's things when we want them', we need to consider whether or not this maxim could be held for everyone. Kant said that if everyone stole things whenever they wanted, the whole notion of theft and personal property would collapse; if this happens, the concept of 'stealing' becomes illogical. The same holds for the idea of lying. Telling a lie only 'works' if people generally tell the truth. If everyone lied whenever it might benefit them, a general belief in truth-telling would collapse and lying would itself become pointless. Therefore Kant said that moral law obliges us not to steal and not to lie. Kant also said that because humans are rational beings, we should never treat people *simply as a means but always at the*

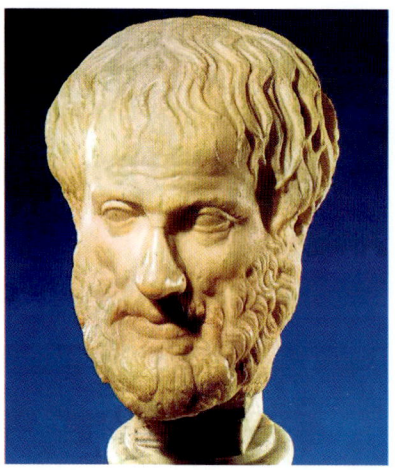

**Fig. 1.10** The Greek philosopher Aristotle (384–322 BCE).

*same time as an end.* The emphasis here is on the fact that all people are equal and deserve equal respect.

The advantages of Kantian deontology are:

- It has a simplicity of structure: moral rules must pass the 'categorical imperative'.
- It places a special responsibility on individuals for their actions.
- It addresses factors other than consequences, such as motives, which intuitively seem important in moral decision-making.
- It allows a certain degree of choice; if more than one option is morally acceptable, then the individual can choose which to carry out (unlike utilitarianism where the *best* option *must* be selected).

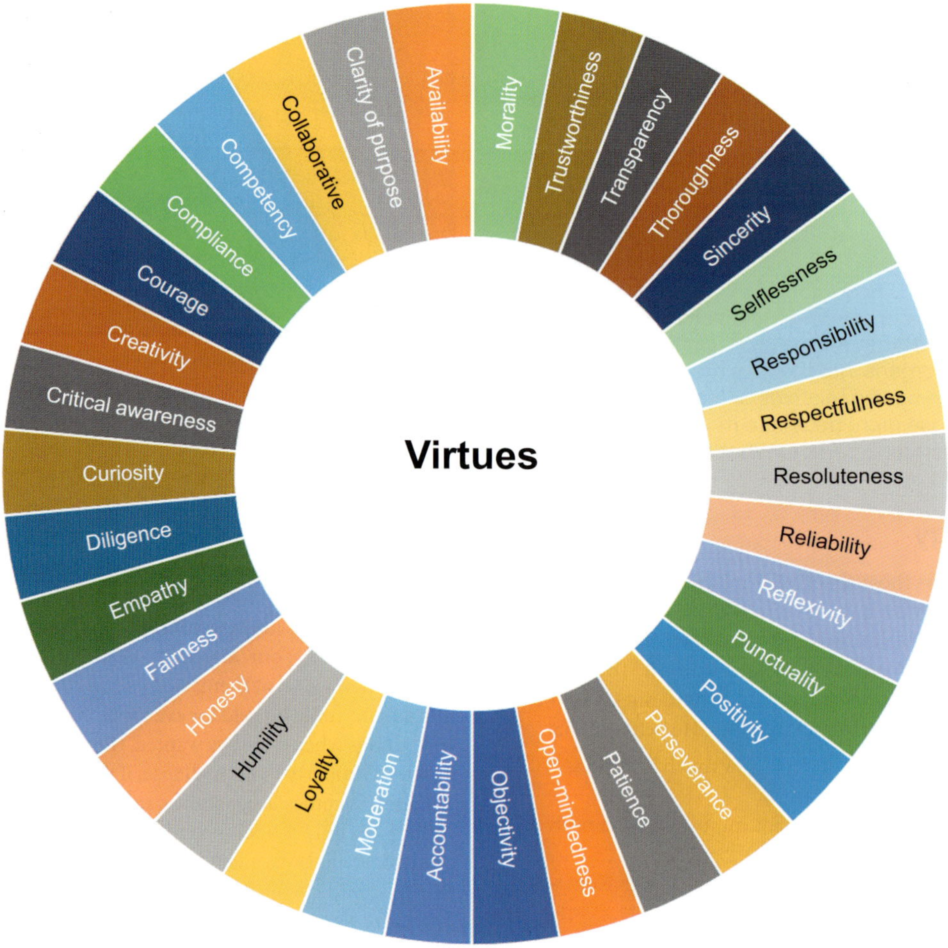

**Virtues**

Availability · Clarity of purpose · Collaborative · Competency · Compliance · Courage · Creativity · Critical awareness · Curiosity · Diligence · Empathy · Fairness · Honesty · Humility · Loyalty · Moderation · Accountability · Objectivity · Open-mindedness · Patience · Perseverance · Positivity · Punctuality · Reflexivity · Reliability · Resoluteness · Respectfulness · Respectfulness · Responsibility · Selflessness · Sincerity · Thoroughness · Transparency · Trustworthiness · Morality

**Fig. 1.11** A 'wheel of some virtues' to prompt discussion and debate. (Courtesy Neelam Wright.)

The disadvantages of Kantianism are:

- It depends on freedom of will and rationality: are we perfectly free and rational?
- It seems to be absolutist in nature: the imperative 'do not lie' is intractable—it means 'do not lie EVER', even if it prevents great harm from occurring.
- The moral rules can seem abstract and unable to deal with the complexities of real-life ethical dilemmas.
- Two duties (imperatives) may conflict, so what happens then?

- Not all people may be considered rational individuals, for example, children, people with learning difficulties or people with cognitive or intellectual impairments, and this appears to make them exempt from the duties rational individuals owe to each other.

Duties often go hand in hand with rights. When someone has a 'right', it usually implies someone else has a 'duty' to respect that right. This may entail a duty to do something or to refrain from doing something. Ronald Dworkin (1977) suggests that rights are special kinds of fact—moral facts—which carry more influence in moral disputes. This way of thinking sees moral rights as 'insistent normative demands' that take precedence over other types of moral argument. Rights can be positive or negative:

- A negative right: generally confers a freedom from interference, for example, the 'right to life' involves a freedom from being killed.
- A positive right: confers a duty on someone else to provide for the right holder, for example, the 'right to healthcare' imposes a duty on the government to provide health facilities and health professionals for citizens.

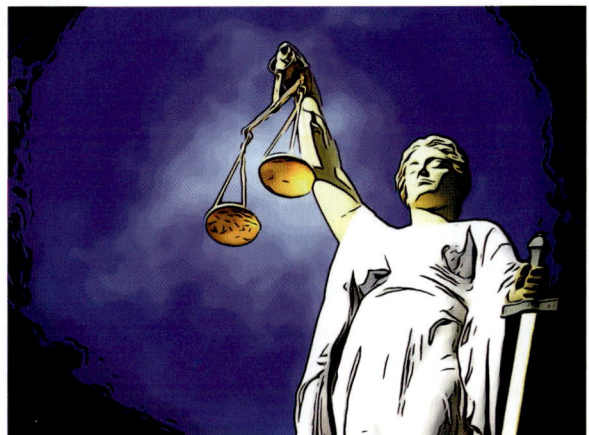

**Fig. 1.12** Lady Justice, a symbol of justice based on Justitia, is a Roman goddess—in Greek mythology named Dice or Dike—representing fair judgement and high moral standards. Her attributes indicate impartiality (blindfold or closed eyes), balanced assessment of the points brought forward by the disputing parties (scale) and the authority to convict and sentence (sword).

**CASE 1.3 THOUGHT EXPERIMENT: THE AXE MURDERER (AFTER IMMANUEL KANT)**

You are a committed deontologist and hold that it is impermissible to lie. A friend runs up to your door and begs you not to tell anyone where he has gone. He then runs off. Soon after, a person with an axe knocks on your door and asks where your friend went. As a deontologist you think that you should always tell the truth as it is a universalisable maxim; however, if you do, the axe murderer will kill your friend.

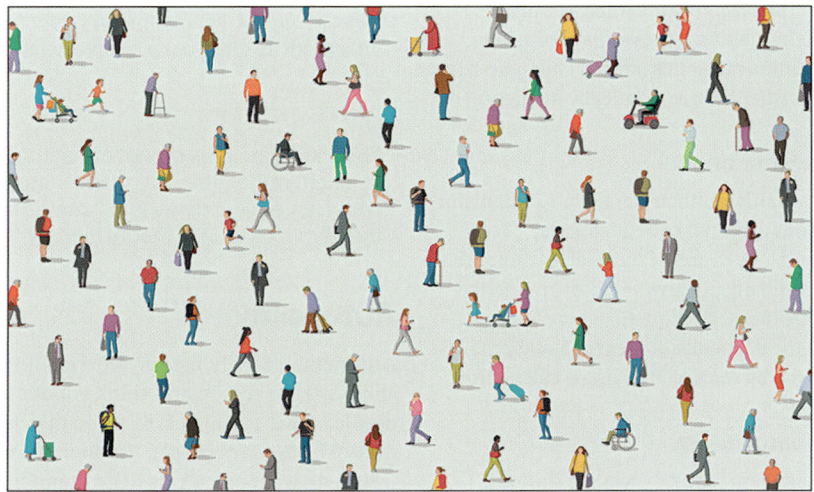

**Fig. 1.13** Increasing population diversity may increase conflict around values.

# Virtue ethics

Virtue ethics is one of the oldest schools of ethics, and in the western tradition it is derived from the works of the ancient Greeks, particularly Socrates, Plato and Aristotle. However, there are many other similar theories from other parts of the world. Virtue ethics focuses on the character and motivation of an individual rather than their actions or consequences. There are several parts to this theory, as outlined below.

1. It is teleological or goal driven. Aristotle claimed that just as the aim of medicine was health, so the aim of the good life was to achieve *eudaimonia* or flourishing.
2. Virtues are a golden mean between two extremes. Courage is a virtue; a deficiency of courage is cowardice, and an excess of courage is rashness.
3. People become virtuous by repeatedly doing virtuous actions, so that they become habits.
4. The amount of any virtue required and the correct action in any situation is known by developing *phronesis*, that is, prudence or practical wisdom.

Socrates (469–399 BCE) asked: 'How should one live, in order to achieve *eudaimonia* (happiness or flourishing)?' His answer was that the good life was the one lived in accordance with *arête* (virtue). Ancient virtues included wisdom, justice, courage, moderation and piety. According to virtue theory, it is the cultivation of virtue within one's character that is the function of morality. Philosophers such as Alasdair MacIntyre (born 1929) have advocated that the study of ethics should be directed towards how we ought to live our lives and advised which ethical characteristics we should try and develop. In a sense, virtue theory tries to concentrate on what it is that makes some people 'good' or 'virtuous' and how they are different from those who are not. The right thing to do in a given dilemma is that which a 'virtuous' person would do. Virtue theory emphasizes:

- The *interpretation* of certain facts of a dilemma, within a specific *context*. That is by looking at the values pertinent to those involved in a dilemma rather than abstract hypothesizing.
- *Reasoning by analogy* rather than reasoning by deduction or from principles.

The advantages of the virtue theory:

- It is more personal than either utilitarianism or Kantianism: it supports those actions done out of benevolence, friendship, honesty and love in and of themselves rather than because they are 'maximizing positive value' or are carried out in accordance with 'moral duty'.
- It is more adaptive to the particular context of a dilemma rather than being bound by rules or applying a 'calculation' to a dilemma.

The disadvantages of virtue theory:

- A list of virtues is insufficient to justify why we should promote them.
- It is unhelpful in *resolving* moral conflicts.
- There is no universally agreed-on list of virtues to promote.

Some writers, however, have attempted to come up with a set of medical virtues. Pellegrino and Thomasma (1993) proposed a list of virtues, including trust, compassion, prudence, justice, fortitude, temperance, integrity and self-effacement. The key virtue in a physician's character is phronesis, which is 'both a moral and an intellectual virtue that disposes one habitually to choose the right thing to do in a concrete moral situation'. Unlike deontology or utilitarianism, virtue ethics does not lend itself so much to thought experiments.

# THE FOUR PRINCIPLES

The four principles of biomedical ethics are what spring to mind for most medical students and doctors when asked about ethics. It is the most widely taught ethical framework in UK medical schools and probably the most commonly used ethical framework by doctors in English-speaking countries. It was first devised in the 1970s by two Americans, Tom Beauchamp and James Childress, who introduced the idea of the 'four principles' or 'principlism'. The four principles are:

- **Autonomy:** Respecting patient decisions. This includes facilitating and respecting the autonomy of people whose mental capacity may be limited or fluctuant.
- **Beneficence**: Doing good or providing benefit.
- **Nonmaleficence**: Avoiding doing harm or minimizing harm if it is unavoidable (e.g. during surgery).
- **Justice**: The principle of ensuring fairness and equity in the distribution of risks and benefits. This includes the idea of treating equals equally, being equitable by catering for varying needs or recognizing relevant inequalities.

When using the four principles, it is important to remember that no one principle is more important than the others and that the principles can conflict. For example, respecting a patient's autonomy can conflict with treating your patients equitably (one form of justice).

**HINTS AND TIPS**

The four principles do not constitute an 'ethical theory' as such, rather, they are guidelines: a framework around which an ethical discussion can be based, regardless of the favourite ethical theory held by the participants.

# Autonomy

Autonomy literally means 'self-rule'. In essence, it refers to an ability: (1) to reason and think about one's own choices, (2) to decide how to act and (3) to act on that decision, all without hindrance from other people. Autonomy is more than simply being free to do what one wants to do. It implies that rational thought and self-awareness are involved in a decision. While many animals are free to do what they want, they are not autonomous because they do not critically evaluate the benefits and risks to themselves, or others, involved in their decisions.

In respecting a person's autonomy, we recognize that they are entitled to make decisions that affect their own lives. Justification for this principle is most obviously found in Kantian theory: the idea that people should be treated not simply as means but as ends in themselves. However, support for autonomy can also be found in those versions of *rule utilitarianism* which hold that the best outcomes arise when autonomy is respected. Depending on age (i.e. children) or illness, people may be more or less autonomous. We may judge that they have the capacity to make all decisions, some decisions or no decisions, and this may fluctuate over time. The degree to which a person is autonomous is central to the concepts of consent and capacity in medical ethics and law. This is discussed further in Chapters 3 and 4.

## Beneficence and nonmaleficence

Beneficence is the principle of doing 'good'. In healthcare, this generally means improving the welfare of patients. Nonmaleficence means 'not harming patients'. It is associated with the Latin phrase *primum non nocere* or 'first do no harm', which is often attributed to Hippocrates. As 'doing good' and 'not doing harm' seem to fall on a continuum, there is often confusion about where nonmaleficence ends and beneficence begins. One way of making a distinction is to see nonmaleficence as a duty towards all people, whereas beneficence, as we cannot help everyone, is a duty we choose to discharge on specific people. Medical staff, by accepting a patient, have chosen to act beneficently towards that person.

Another way to think about it refers to our actions: beneficence is a positive action—doing something—for example, inserting a catheter to relieve urinary retention; nonmaleficence is a negative action—not doing something—for example, not doing cardiopulmonary resuscitation in a frail patient with metastatic cancer. The principles of beneficence and nonmaleficence are broadly similar to the utilitarian principle of maximizing benefit and minimizing harm. But in the case of beneficence and nonmaleficence, the consideration is usually about a particular person, whereas utilitarian considerations can be about an individual or a collective group of people.

## Justice

Aristotle famously said that justice is about treating equals equally and unequals unequally. The question of who is an equal has never been satisfactorily answered. In healthcare, the principle of justice generally refers to the allocation or distribution of finite resources, including expertise and time, among the population. There is no easy answer as to what constitutes fair distribution or which patients are equals. The following are possible answers:

1. *Equality*: Each person receives an equal share of the resources available.
2. *Need*: Each person receives resources appropriate to how much that person needs.
3. *Desert*: Each person receives resources according to how much they deserve them in terms of contribution, effort or merit.
4. *Desire*: Each person gets what they want. Desire forms the basis of a utilitarian outlook: utilitarianism is important as it forms the basis for cost-effective analysis and quality-adjusted life years.

Justice is considered further in Chapter 5, which deals with commissioning and resource allocation in healthcare.

## VALUES-BASED MEDICINE

Consideration for individual values, including those of the patient, can be challenging in the context of modern healthcare, where complex and conflicting values are often at play. This is particularly so when patient values seem to be at odds with evidence-based practice or widely shared ethical principles or when the values of a health professional may affect the care provided.

Values-based practice is a framework developed originally in the domain of mental health. It maintains that values are pervasive and powerful influences in healthcare decisions and research and that their impact is often underestimated. It suggests that our current approaches lead us to ignore some important manifestations of values at both the general level—in legal, policy and research contexts—and the individual level in clinical practice. All students and trainees are continually exposed to areas of ethical difficulty throughout their training. Fulford (2004) describes the 'squeaky wheel principle' of values-based medicine. This suggests that we tend to notice values only when they are diverse or in conflict and may overlook them in contexts where they are assumed to be shared. Learners may have difficulty doing this alone or when there is a fear of speaking up in a group setting. Respectful discussion with others is essential to bring out a proper range of responses to ethical problems or value conflicts and to challenge individual views.

## THE CORE CURRICULUM IN MEDICAL ETHICS AND LAW

The Institute of Medical Ethics and Law (2019) core curriculum outlines essential areas underpinning practice as a UK Foundation Doctor. It has been endorsed by the GMC, which means it will form a basis for the standards expected from medical school graduates and hence medical students.

In Years 1 and 2, medical students are expected to:

- Recognize and understand core ethical and legal topics.
- Apply common ethical arguments using constructed case scenarios.

- Be able to understand and discuss differing viewpoints.
- Be aware of GMC requirements around student fitness to practise.

In Years 3 and 4, medical students are expected to:

- Be familiar with GMC professional codes of conduct.
- Recognize ethical and legal issues and be able to apply common ethical arguments to actual clinical encounters in different specialties and public health interventions.
- Recognize and conform with professional and legal obligations in practice.
- Demonstrate the ability to reflect on ethical practice of self, peers and teachers.

In Year 5 (and 6 when relevant), medical students are expected to be able to:

- Integrate ethical analysis of actual clinical encounters with clinical knowledge and skills and legal obligations.
- Elaborate on common ethical arguments.
- Propose decisions and/or actions based on this synthesis.
- Display professional attitudes and behaviours consistent with Good Medical Practice.
- Be aware of their own values.

As a doctor progresses through their career, they should be able to demonstrate increasing competence in how to identify, acknowledge and deal with ethical, legal and professional issues. Teaching and learning should be relevant to the stage of training and the specialty.

The updated curriculum also specifies a core content of learning for medical ethics and law, found in the bracketed chapters:

- Context of medical practice (all chapters)
- Foundations of medical ethics and law (see Chapter 1)
- Professionalism: 'good medical practice' (see Chapter 2)
- Confidentiality (see Chapter 2)
- Medical research (see Chapter 2)
- Decision-making and capacity (see Chapter 3)
- Children and young people (see Chapter 3)
- Mental health (see Chapter 3)
- Genetics (see Chapter 3)
- Beginnings of life (see Chapter 4)
- Towards the end of life (see Chapter 4)
- Justice and public health (see Chapter 5)

## POTTED TIMELINE OF KEY DEVELOPMENTS IN MEDICINE

7th century BCE: Earliest surviving Sumerian/Assyrian medical texts found on clay tablets. Both Sumerian/Assyrian and Ancient Egyptian civilizations had sophisticated medical systems linked to religious practices.

377 BCE: Death of Hippocrates. Widely seen as the father of the modern medical tradition, Hippocratic medicine focused on clinical observation and reason.

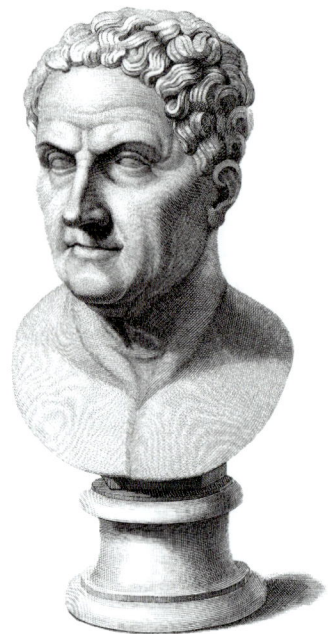

**Fig. 1.14** Claudius Galen (c.130–201 BCE) demonstrated that arteries contain blood, not air as had previously been thought. Artery means 'air containing' in Greek. After studies, he became a physician to the gladiators, where no doubt he witnessed spurting arteries. Later, he was based in Rome and became physician to Emperor Marcus Aurelius, writing approximately 500 publications. Galen remained the preeminent medical authority until the publication by Andreas Vesalius of *De Humani Corporis Fabrica* (*The Construction of the Human Body*) in 1543.

322 BCE: Death of Aristotle. As well as being a philosopher, Aristotle was an empiricist who wrote on many subjects, including biology, and used animal dissection to further the understanding of anatomy.

c.216: Death of Galen (Fig. 1.14). A Greek physician from Pergamon in Asia Minor, now Turkey, synthesized clinical medicine with scientific study. Following his death, the Graeco-Roman medical tradition began to ossify.

100–400: The earliest surviving works of Ayurvedic (Indian) medicine which describe, among other things, plastic surgical techniques and cataract operations.

832: The Bayt al-Hikma, or House of Wisdom, is founded in Baghdad. This was a centre for scholarship with Greek texts translated into Arabic and Syriac, including many medical works.

1037: Death of Ibn Sina (Avicenna), the Islamic philosopher-physician who wrote the Kitab al-Qanun or Canon of Medicine—a large medical encyclopaedia which proved influential in Islamic lands and across the West.

c.1100: The medical school at Salerno is founded. This led to many Ancient Greek works being translated into Latin

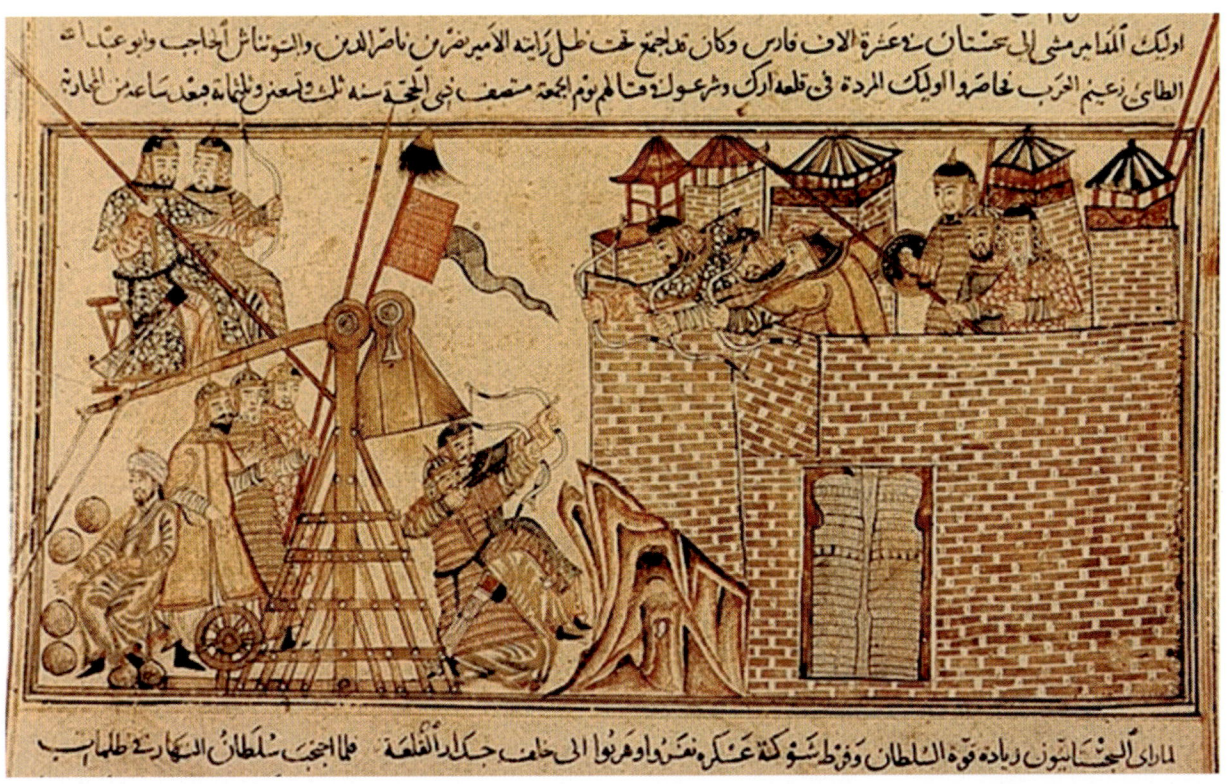

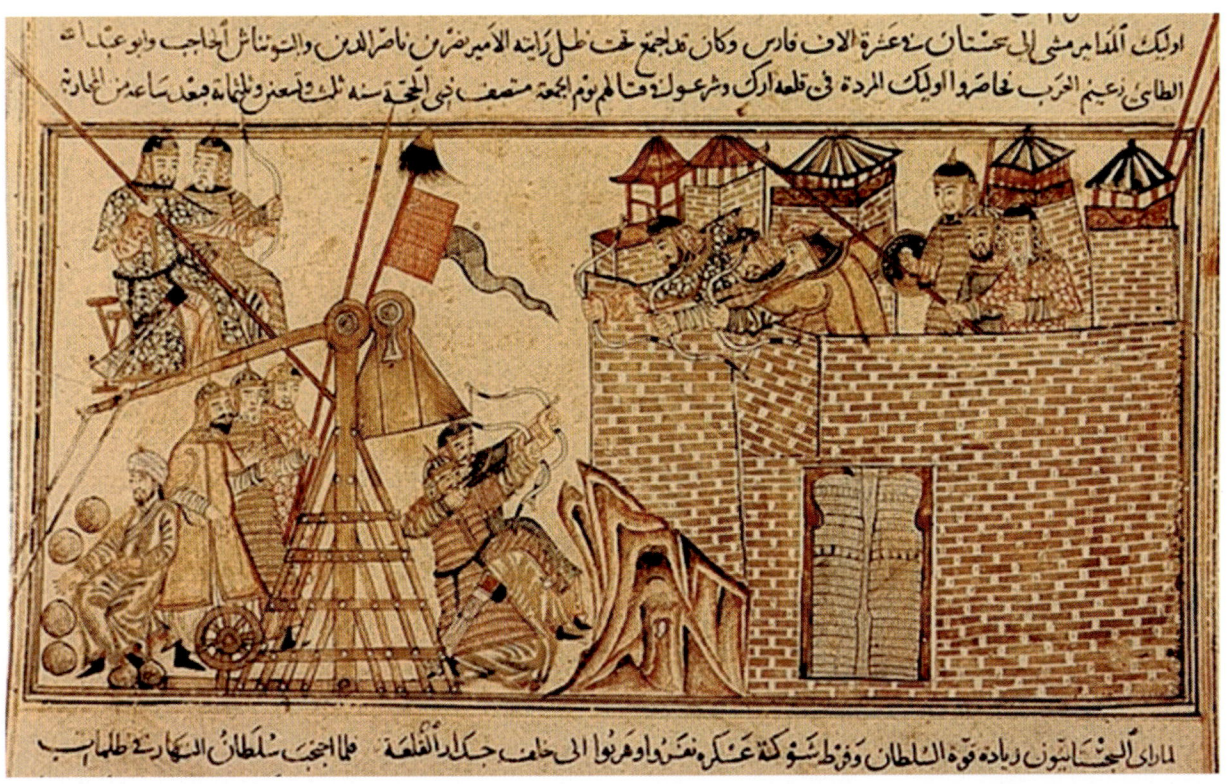

**Fig. 1.15** The invading Tatar army under Genghis Khan suffered an outbreak of the Bubonic plague. During his siege of the city Caffa (now called Theodosia) on the Black Sea coast, the Tartars came up with a plan to devastate their enemy by flinging plague-stricken corpses of their fallen soldiers over the city walls to purposely infect their enemy. The plan worked, and the inhabitants of Caffa were forced to surrender their city to the Mongol invaders. It is believed that some of the survivors of the initial attack left Caffa for Constantinople and other Mediterranean ports, contributing to the pandemic known as the Black Death.

and the introduction of Arabic and Jewish medical knowledge into Europe.

1347: Start of the Black Death (Fig. 1.15).

1492: Columbus lands on Hispaniola. The populations of the Americas had not been exposed to the diseases of the Old World before, and vast numbers died as a result.

1543: Vesalius publishes his work on anatomy, overturning many of the beliefs that had persisted since Galen.

1628: William Harvey demonstrates how the heart pumps blood around the body.

1704: The Rose Case in the UK House of Lords allows Apothecaries to prescribe medicines, creating the forerunners of General Practitioners.

1745: The Company of Surgeons in London separates from the Barber's company.

1798: Jenner publishes his work on smallpox vaccination (Fig. 1.16).

1858: Formation of the UK GMC to help distinguish qualified doctors from unqualified quacks.

1865: Ignaz Semmelweis dies. He recognized the importance of handwashing before patient contact after comparing mortality rates between midwifery students and medical students.

1865: Elizabeth Garrett Anderson qualifies as a doctor through the Society of Apothecaries, the first female in the United Kingdom to do so.

1867: Joseph Lister publishes on antiseptic procedures for the operating theatre, which leads to a significant decline in mortality.

1895: Roentgen discovers X-rays.

1903: Marie and Pierre Curie win the Nobel Prize for their work on radiation (Fig. 1.17).

1928: Alexander Flemming discovers penicillin (Fig. 1.18).

1939–1945: World War II. This led to medical innovations, including in the field of plastic surgery. The war also saw a programme of human experimentation and murder by both the Nazi and the Imperial Japanese regimes under the auspices of medical research.

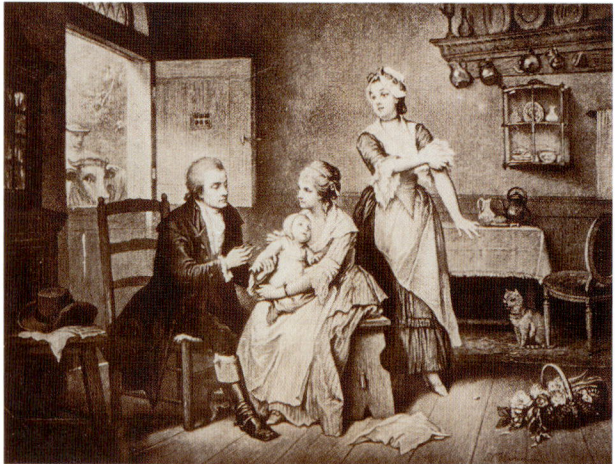

**Fig. 1.16** Edward Jenner vaccinating an infant.

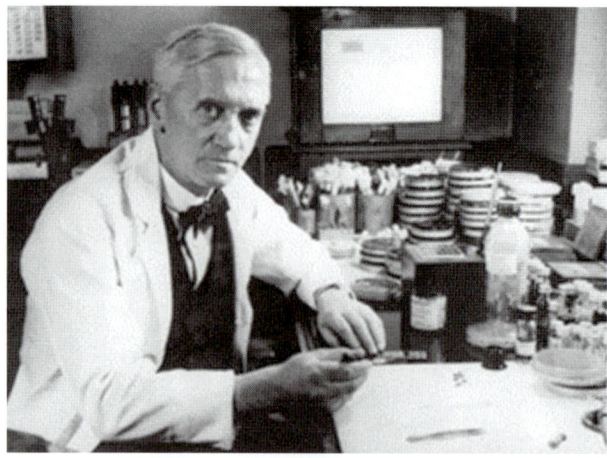

**Fig. 1.18** Alexander Fleming (1881–1955) in his laboratory. In 1945 he shared the Nobel Prize with Ernst Boris Chain and Howard Walter Florey for the discovery of penicillin and its curative effect in various infectious diseases.

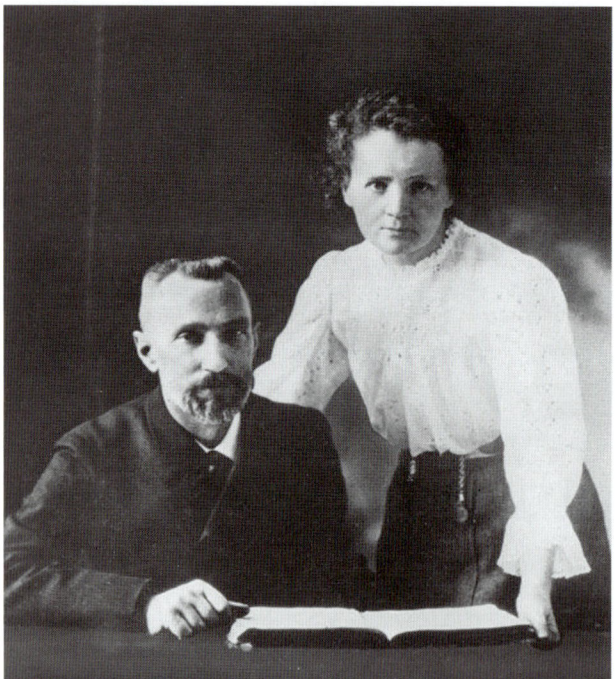

**Fig. 1.17** Pierre and Marie Curie in 1903.

1945: Nuremberg Trials for war crimes. Many of the doctors tried were released and returned to practising medicine.

1946: The NHS Act was passed, establishing a national health service free at the point of delivery for all. It was not universally welcomed by the UK medical establishment.

1960: The contraceptive pill became commercially available.

1967: Abortion Act passed.

1967: First heart transplant carried out by Christiaan Barnard in South Africa. The patient died 8 days later.

1972: Charnley hip invented. Although hip replacements had been around for some time, they had not been particularly effective until Charnley's design.

1972: End of the Tuskegee Experiment. Black patients with syphilis were left untreated so that researchers could better understand the progression of the disease.

1978: Birth of Louise Brown, the first child conceived by in vitro fertilization (IVF) (Fig. 1.19).

1981: Recognition of HIV as a public health crisis.

2003: Human genome fully mapped.

2020: COVID-19 pandemic.

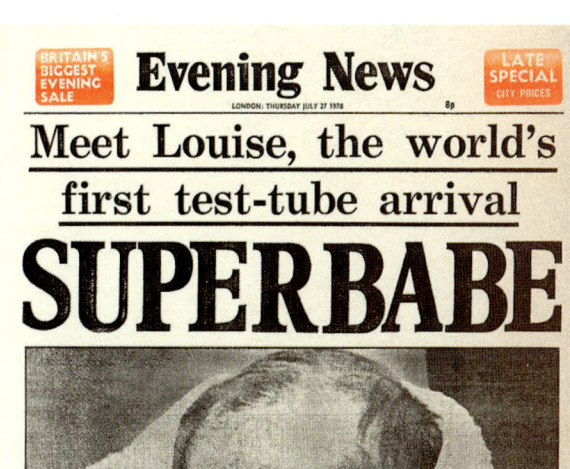

**Fig. 1.19** Newspaper front page (27 July 1978) announcing the birth of Louise J. Brown, the first IVF baby, born on 25 July 1978. (From *Evening News*.)

## References

*Abortion Act* 1967, c. 87. https://www.legislation.gov.uk/ukpga/1967/87/contents

*Adults with incapacity (Scotland) Act* 2000, asp 4. https://www.legislation.gov.uk/asp/2000/4/contents

*Barnett v. Chelsea and Kensington HMC* [1969] 1QB 428.

Beauchamp, T. L., & Childress, J. F. (2013). *Principles of biomedical ethics* (7th ed.). New York: Oxford University Press.

*Bolam v. Friern Hospital Management Committee* [1957] 1WLR 583.

*Bolitho v. City and Hackney Health Authority* [1997] UKHL 46.

Campbell, A. V., & Higgs, R. (1982). *In that case: Medical ethics in everyday practice*. London: Darton, Longman and Todd.

*Coronavirus Act* 2020, c. 7.https://www.legislation.gov.uk/ukpga/2020/7/contents/enacted

Dworkin, R. (1977). *Taking rights seriously*. London: Duckworth.

Fulford, K. (2004). Ten principles of values-based medicine In J. Radden (Ed.), *The philosophy of psychiatry: A companion* (pp. 205–234). New York: Oxford University Press.

Fulford, K., Dickenson, D., & Murray, T. (2002). *Healthcare ethics and human values: An introductory text with readings and case studies*. Oxford: Blackwell.

General Medical Council. (2023) *Good medical practice 2024*. GMC https://www.gmc-uk.org/-/media/documents/gmp-2024-final---english_pdf-102607294.pdf

*Health and Social Care Act* 2008, c. 14. https://www.legislation.gov.uk/ukpga/2008/14/contents

*Health and Social Care Act* 2012, c. 7. https://www.legislation.gov.uk/ukpga/2012/7/contents

*Human Fertilisation and Embryology Act* 2008, c. 22. https://www.legislation.gov.uk/ukpga/2008/22/contents

*Human Rights Act* 1998, c. 42. https://www.legislation.gov.uk/ukpga/1998/42/contents

Institute of Medical Ethics. (2019). *Core curriculum for undergraduate medical ethics and law*. Institute of Medical Ethics. https://ime-uk.org/wp-content/uploads/2020/10/IME_revised_ethics_and_law__curriculum_Learning_outcomes_2019.pdf

*Mental Capacity Act* 2005, c. 9. https://www.legislation.gov.uk/ukpga/2005/9/contents

*National Health Service Act* 2006, c. 41. https://www.legislation.gov.uk/ukpga/2006/41/contents

*National Health Service (Wales) Act* 2006, c. 42.https://www.legislation.gov.uk/ukpga/2006/42/contents

*National Health Service (Consequential Provisions) Act* 2006, c. 43. https://www.legislation.gov.uk/ukpga/2006/43/contents

Pellegrino, E., & Thomasma, D. (1993). *The virtues in medical practice*. New York: Oxford University Press.

*Pretty v. United Kingdom 2346/02* [2002] ECHR 427.

*Public Health (Control of Disease) Act* 1984, c. 22. https://www.legislation.gov.uk/ukpga/1984/22/contents

*R (on the application of Tracey) v. Cambridge University Hospital NHS Trust* (2014). EWCA Civ 822. https://www.judiciary.uk/wp-content/uploads/2014/06/tracey-approved.pdf

## Further Reading

*Health and Social Care Act* 2022, c. 31. https://www.legislation.gov.uk/ukpga/2022/31/contents/enacted

Hoeyer, K. (2006). 'Ethics wars': Reflections on the antagonism between bioethicists and social science observers of biomedicine. *Human Studies*, 29, 203–227. https://doi.org/10.1007/s10746-006-9022-9.

*Medical Act* 1983, c.54. https://www.legislation.gov.uk/ukpga/1983/54/contents

Porter, R. (1997). *The greatest benefit to mankind: A medical history of humanity from antiquity to the present*. London: HarperCollins Publishers, London.

Stirrat, G. M., et al. (2010). Medical ethics and law for doctors of tomorrow: The 1998 Consensus Statement updated. *Journal of Medical Ethics*, 36(1), 55–60. https://doi.org/10.1136/jme.2009.034660.

*The embassy of good science* [online]. https://embassy.science/wiki/Main_Page.

Medical professionalism as a concept has evolved significantly over time, reflecting changing societal expectations, advances in medical technology and the complexity of healthcare delivery. At the turn of the last century medical professionalism centred on moral obligations and ethical conduct, with emphasis on virtues like altruism, honesty and integrity. Discussions were often framed in the context of the Hippocratic Oath, which served as a moral compass for the doctor. Professionalism has expanded to include broader issues of patient care, health systems and the role of the doctor in society. Curricula of professional regulatory bodies reflect these trends and now often include patient safety, communication skills, interprofessional working, leadership, continuing education and—of course—ethics and law as core dimensions (Fig. 2.1).

## OATHS AND DECLARATIONS

- Are promises to uphold a publicly and professionally accepted set of values.
- Support trust in the profession and by extension social status of the profession.

*The Hippocratic Oath* (~425 BCE) is attributed to the Greek physician Hippocrates (Fig. 2.2). Hippocrates is associated with the value of scientific rationality in medical practice. The historic oath contains some enduring values: consideration of the patient's best interests, confidentiality, not doing 'whatever is deleterious and mischievous' and teaching medicine. It does not mention autonomy or justice. Some medical schools use adapted versions today.

Two modern declarations arose after World War II when the medical profession in Germany had become complicit in the activities of the Nazi party.

- *The Declaration of Geneva* (1948, most recently revised 2017) is a modern Hippocratic Oath. It requires doctors to make the health of their patients their 'first consideration', uphold patient autonomy, be nondiscriminatory and attend to their 'own health, well-being and abilities' in order to practise at a high standard (Anonymous, 2017).
- *The Declaration of Helsinki* (1964, revised 2013) deals with medical research involving human subjects. The rights and interests of an individual patient must take precedence over the broader interests of advancing knowledge for public or scientific gain (World Medical Association, 2013).

The International Code of Medical Ethics adds statements on conflicts of interest, teamwork, environmental sustainability, personal boundaries and reporting of concerns (Parsa-Parsi 2022).

## CONSCIENCE AND PERSONAL BELIEFS

Doctors may hold personal beliefs or values that conflict with those of their patients and colleagues. The General Medical Council (2023a) recognizes beliefs are important to people holding them and that doctors should be able to practice medicine in accordance with their beliefs, as long as they are acting legally and not:

- Treating patients unfairly.
- Denying patients appropriate medical services.
- Causing patients undue distress.

In both the *Abortion Act* 1967 and the *Human Fertilisation and Embryology Act* 1990 (amended 2008) there are conscientious objection clauses, and similar clauses are likely if physician-assisted suicide/euthanasia is ever legalized in the United Kingdom. For more, see Chapter 4. Doctors have a right to conscientiously object to other treatments or procedures including, but not limited to, providing contraceptive services (Fig. 2.3) or withdrawal of treatment in end-of-life patients. It might be helpful to find out how your medical school manages situations of potential conscientious objection in undergraduate assessments.

The General Medical Council (2013a and 2023a) guidelines state:

- You must not unfairly discriminate against patients by allowing your personal views to affect your professional relationship with patients or the treatment you provide.
- You must explain to patients if you have a conscientious objection to a particular procedure, that the patient has the right to see another doctor. You must ensure they have enough information to be able to do this, and if it is not practical for the patient to arrange to see another doctor you must help arrange it.
- You must not express to your patients your personal beliefs—including political, religious or moral beliefs—in ways that exploit their vulnerability or that are likely to cause them distress.

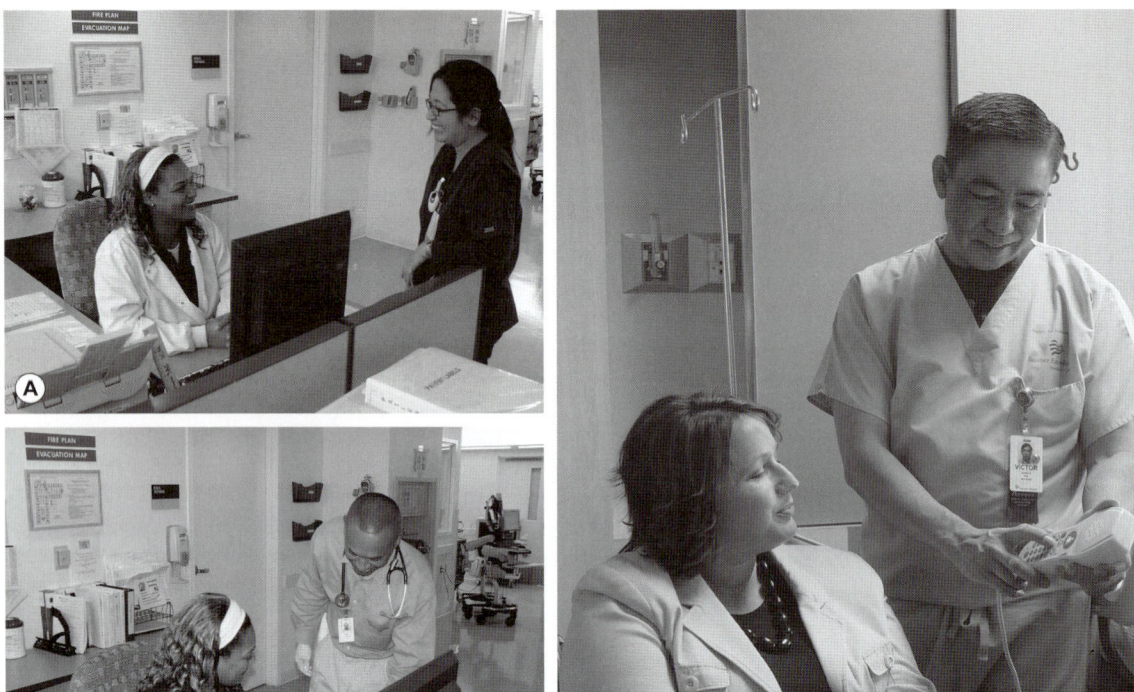

**Fig. 2.1** Emphasis on the practical aspects of professional conduct, including conflict resolution and resilience, reflect current conceptions of medical professionalism as upholding ethical principles while effectively navigating the complexities of modern clinical practice.

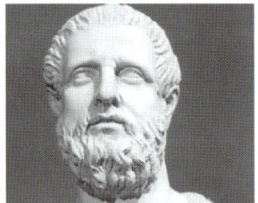

**Fig. 2.2** Hippocrates (460–370 BCE).

### CASE 2.1 PERSONAL BELIEFS AND A GENERAL MEDICAL COUNCIL FITNESS TO PRACTISE HEARING

B was a 19-year-old patient at Bethesda Medical Practice in 2022 and attended a general practitioner appointment with Dr S to discuss mental health symptoms. His mum waited outside. B left the consultation for a short time and re-entered to discuss the spiritual approach that had been offered. A complaint was made later on behalf of B by his mum. The tribunal hearing found the patient was known to be vulnerable on account of his mental health; that Dr S had discussed religious and/or spiritual beliefs, clasped hands and prayed with B without consent; and this had distressed the patient. The overall finding was of professional misconduct and a warning was placed on the GMC registration of Dr S.

Attempting to evangelize patients is considered to be an inappropriate use of medical influence over a potentially vulnerable patient. Personal boundaries and power imbalance in the doctor–patient relationship are considered further later.

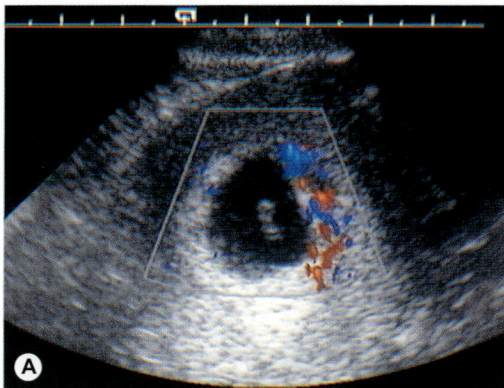

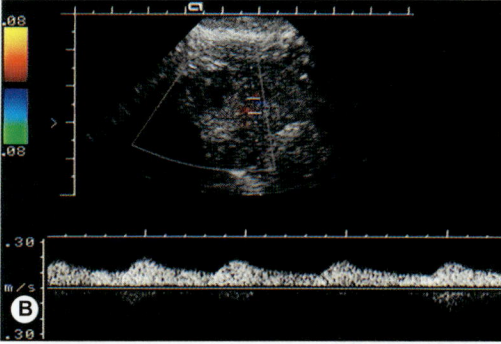

Fig. 2.3 Some doctors have a conscientious objection to termination of pregnancy: you are advised to consider your personal position. (A) Normal colour flow pattern in the trophoblast of a normal 7-week intrauterine pregnancy. This patient subsequently had a termination. (B) Vascular trophoblast in the adnexal region. Colour and spectral Doppler demonstrating low-resistance flow, implying active trophoblast and suggesting a need either for administration of methotrexate as medical treatment or surgery.

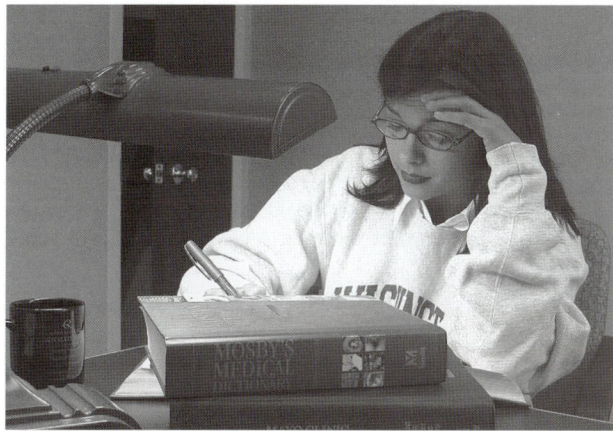

Fig. 2.4 Medicine is a demanding course of study in preparation for joining the profession. Examination stress on medical students can alter immunologic parameters.

## DUTIES FOR MEDICAL STUDENTS AND DOCTORS

Duty-based medical ethics theories are deontological and are discussed in Chapter 1 along with consequentialist and virtue ethics theories which are not strictly duty based but may generate duties. Professional bodies such as the UK General Medical Council (GMC) also set out duties for medical students and doctors. Although medical students are not fully qualified and have legal restrictions on their developing practice, they are bound by many of the same behavioural standards as doctors (Fig. 2.4). This is because medical students are, in the words of the GMC, 'tomorrow's doctors'. Patients may see students as knowledgeable because they recognize that students take histories, perform examinations and practise some clinical skills that qualified doctors also do. Students must be aware their behaviour outside the clinical environment, including their personal lives, may impact their fitness to practise. This derives from the Aristotelian idea that excellence and virtue are features of a whole person and stem from repeatedly doing virtuous acts, whether 'at work' or elsewhere. Medical education literature advocates that the development of a professional identity benefits from shared professional values becoming internalized, which translates into consistency in professional behaviours.

Therefore:

- Students have a duty to ensure patients know they are students and not doctors. Consider whether medical students should introduce themselves, or be introduced, as *medical students* or as *student doctors*? Is the title 'student doctor' likely to mislead a patient into thinking that the person seeing them is medically qualified?
- Students have a duty to behave professionally in clinical and educational settings and are subject to the same ethical duties as doctors such as maintaining confidentiality and only performing procedures in which they are competent.
- Consistency in professional identity is developed over time by attending the learning opportunities and clinical placements offered through medical school, as these offer ongoing insight into and modelling professional values and behaviours.
- Students have a duty to avoid behaving in an antisocial or criminal manner outside the clinical setting, for example taking recreational drugs, drink driving, disorderly behaviour in public.

*Remember*: students have a professional duty to make sure that patients know they are medical *students* and not doctors.

A medical student whose behaviour falls below an acceptable standard may not be allowed to graduate and/or register with the GMC.

## PROFESSIONAL REGULATION: 'DOCTORS', 'MEDICAL PROFESSIONALS' AND THE GENERAL MEDICAL COUNCIL

The UK GMC was established by law in 1858, and its overarching purpose of protecting the public is set out in the *Medical Act 1983*. The GMC was originally intended to help patients distinguish qualified doctors from unqualified people posing as 'doctors'. Today all practising UK doctors must register, whether they work for the National Health Service (NHS) and/or for other providers. Good Medical Practice is a core guidance document first published in 1995 (General Medical Council 2023a). The GMC is preparing to start regulating physician associates and anaesthesia associates as well as doctors; and with this in mind the core guidance now addresses 'medical professionals' rather than 'doctors'.

ETHICS

### THE DUTIES OF MEDICAL PROFESSIONALS REGISTERED WITH THE GENERAL MEDICAL COUNCIL (2023)

Patients must be able to trust medical professionals with their lives and health. To justify that trust you must make the care of patients your first concern and meet the standards expected of you in all four domains.

#### Knowledge, skills and development

- Provide a good standard of practice and care and work within your competence.
- Keep your knowledge and skills up to date.

#### Patients, partnership and communication

- Respect every patient's dignity and treat them as an individual.
- Listen to patients and work in partnership with them, supporting them to make informed decisions about their care.
- Protect patients' personal information from improper disclosure.

#### Colleagues, culture and safety

- Work with colleagues in ways that best serve the interests of patients, being willing to lead or follow as circumstances require.
- Be willing to share your knowledge, skills and experience with colleagues, whether informally or through teaching, training, mentoring or coaching.
- Treat people with respect and help to create a working and training environment that is compassionate, supportive and fair, where everyone feels safe to ask questions, talk about errors and raise concerns.
- Act promptly if you think that patient safety or dignity may be seriously compromised.
- Take care of your own health and well-being needs, recognizing and taking appropriate action if you may not be fit to work.

#### Trust and professionalism

- Act with honesty and integrity and be open if things go wrong.
- Protect and promote the health of patients and the public.
- Never unfairly discriminate against patients or colleagues.
- Never abuse patients' trust in you or the public's trust in your profession.

Governments can order a Public Enquiry when there are serious public concerns about any societal matter. Public Inquiries into paediatric heart surgery at the Bristol Royal Infirmary (1984–95) and General Practitioner Harold Shipman (2003, considering serial murders over more than 20 years) have led to changes in UK professional regulation. The GMC now regulates medical education and practice from the point of entry to medical school until retirement.

To be added to the GMC General Practitioner or Specialist Register, a doctor typically takes postgraduate training and examinations overseen by the relevant Royal College or Faculty. The training and examinations are separate from the GMC, although the GMC maintains the registers. Trade union membership is also separate from the GMC and is optional. The British Medical Association and The Hospital Consultants and Specialists Association are the two main trade unions for UK doctors.

Providing a good standard of patient care requires up-to-date knowledge and skills, and this positions continuing education and training relevant to your area of practice as essential to an ongoing medical career. This can be as a learner and/or teacher. As a colleague you have an ethical obligation to support those around you to maintain their competencies in roles that may include supervisor, teacher, mentor or appraiser.

## Key functions of the GMC:

- Maintain a register of doctors who are licensed to practise medicine in the United Kingdom.
- Set and monitor professional standards in discussion with patients, doctors, employers and educators.
  - This includes undergraduate and postgraduate medical education.
  - For fully qualified doctors this includes annual appraisal and 5-yearly revalidation.
- Addressing concerns about an individual doctor's fitness to practise; outcomes can range from recommending remedial training or supervised practice, to temporary or permanent removal from the medical register.
- Providing the Professional and Linguistic Assessment Board test: doctors from outside the European Union have to pass before they can practise in the United Kingdom.
- Providing an appropriate 'certificate of good standing' for a UK-registered doctor moving abroad to practise in a territory covered by a different medical regulator.

---

**CASE 2.2** *BAWA-GARBA V. GENERAL MEDICAL COUNCIL* (2018)

Dr Bawa-Garba was the most senior specialist paediatric trainee at work when 6-year-old Jack Adcock was admitted to Leicester Royal Infirmary in February 2011. Jack had vomiting and diarrhoea and died later that day of sepsis. His death was unexpected and subsequently investigated by the hospital, with the conclusion that multiple issues had contributed. Dr Bawa-Garba had worked a 13-hour shift without a break and had just returned from maternity leave to a new hospital without any induction. As well as medical staffing shortages, there were difficulties with the computer system used to review test results. In 2015 Dr Bawa-Garba and the nurse looking after Jack, Ms Amaro, were found guilty of gross negligence manslaughter and given 2-year suspended prison sentences by the courts. Ms Amaro was struck off by the Nursing and Midwifery Council in 2016. In 2017 following GMC processes Dr Bawa-

Garba's fitness to practice was found to be impaired by the Medical Practitioners Tribunal (MPT) and she was suspended from practice for 12 months.

The Medical Practitioners Tribunal (MPT) service is determined by the *Medical Act 1983* and runs hearings for doctors whose practice is called into question by the GMC. The MPT is independent of and accountable to the GMC and to Parliament. The GMC appealed the initial MPT outcome, saying the sanction against Dr Bawa-Garba was not sufficiently severe. In 2018 the High Court held in favour of the GMC and that Dr Bawa-Garba should be erased from the medical register to protect public confidence. Dr Bawa-Garba went to the Court of Appeal, where it was found that a criminal manslaughter conviction should not result in automatic erasure from the medical register and the case should be considered as a whole. Dr Bawa-Garba later completed training and joined the Specialist Register in Paediatrics in 2022.

The Dr Bawa-Garba Case: key points
- GMC fitness to practise proceedings can result in a fitness to practise hearing conducted by the independent Medical Practitioners Tribunal Service.
- Gross negligence manslaughter and culpable homicide criminal court cases are extremely rare in medicine. A criminal conviction for manslaughter does not lead to automatic erasure from the medical register.
- The GMC role mainly focuses on the individual doctor and upholding public confidence in the profession, not the system of care in which the doctor works.
- Since Dr Bawa-Garba's case the GMC has stated its priorities around supporting reflective practice, freedom to raise concerns, treating doctors fairly, improving doctor's well-being and induction for doctors returning to work or starting a new role.

There were concerns here about disproportionate individual professional scapegoating in the context of failures in the system of care.

## HEALTH PROFESSIONS AND TEAMWORK

There are many regulated health professions: doctors, nurses and midwives, pharmacists, dentists, opticians and the allied health professions (see Clinical Notes below). The emerging roles of physician associate and anaesthesia associate are expected to become GMC regulated, although they are not doctors. Nursing associates are regulated by the Nursing and Midwifery Council and bridge a gap between healthcare support workers and registered nurses. Social workers are usually employed by the Local Authority (the local council). Around 10% of the UK population provides informal care to a close family member or friend, and although not regulated, their contribution to 'the team' is often vital.

## CLINICAL NOTES

### ALLIED HEALTH PROFESSIONS REGULATED BY THE HEALTH AND CARE PROFESSIONS COUNCIL

- Arts therapist
- Biomedical scientist
- Chiropodist/podiatrist
- Clinical scientist
- Dietitian
- Hearing aid dispenser
- Occupational therapist
- Operating department practitioner
- Orthoptist
- Paramedic
- Physiotherapist
- Practitioner psychologist
- Prosthetist/orthotist
- Radiographer
- Speech and language therapist

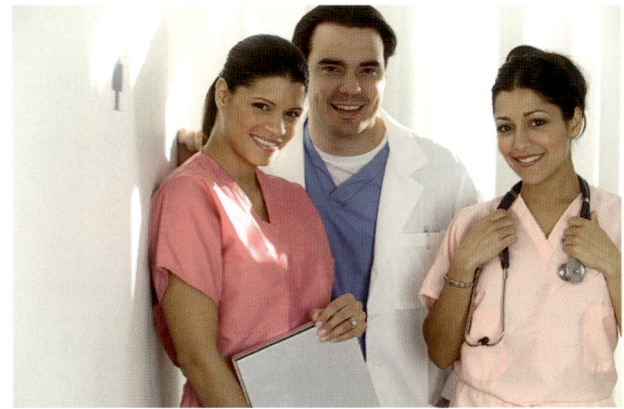

**Fig. 2.5** Is this teamwork?

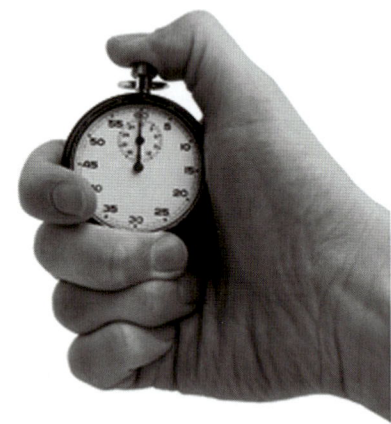

**Fig. 2.6** Clocking on and off and professionalism—what do you think, do they go together?

The GMC requires doctors to work with colleagues to best serve patients' interests (Fig. 2.5). Service pressures may be high for various local and/or wider reasons. Poor communication and conflict do sometimes occur both within and between professions. Boundaries between different roles are sometimes unclear or overlap. For example, some nurses can prescribe, and some operations or part-procedures are performed by surgical care practitioners (SCPs)—experienced nurses or operating department practitioners with additional specific training. The British Medical Association (2023) position is that doctors should not prescribe or request an investigation using ionizing radiation for a patient solely based on the recommendation of a physician associate, anaesthesia associate or SCP. Considered, clear and consistent communication and respect for everyone in the team give the best opportunity to optimally use the available skill mix. The role of a (senior) doctor is usually associated with holding the ultimate responsibility for clinical decisions.

The *Working Time Regulations 1998* required full compliance by 2009 and legally restricted working hours. Nonetheess over half of doctors with formal roles as trainers and nearly two-thirds of doctors in training were at moderate or high risk of burnout in 2022 to 2023 (General Medical Council, 2023b). Doctors frequently report being asked to work at high intensity and working beyond their rostered hours. Changing medical rota patterns have increased the pressure for advanced nurse practitioners and other professional roles like physician associates to develop (Fig. 2.6).

## CLINICAL NOTES

### WORKING TIME REGULATIONS 1998—BRIEF OVERVIEW

- Maximum average of 48 hours a week over a reference period (17–26 weeks).
- A weekly rest period of at least 24 hours.
- 11 hours of consecutive rest per day.
- Minimum 20-minute rest break for any shift over 6 hours.

## CLINICAL NOTES

### TEAMWORK IN PRINCIPLE AND IN PRACTICE

Excerpt from Leadership and Management for all Doctors (General Medical Council, 2012): 'You must tackle discrimination where it arises and encourage your colleagues to do the same. You must treat your colleagues fairly and with respect. You must not bully or harass them or unfairly discriminate against them. You should challenge the behaviour of colleagues who do not meet this standard'.

NHS Employers (2023) workforce statistics:

- 98% of staff experienced incivility in the workplace.
- 18.7% of staff overall experienced bullying or harassment, rising to 25% among staff with disabilities. Staff identifying as bisexual, homosexual and from Black and minority ethnic backgrounds were more likely to experience bullying or harassment. *To this we add that sometimes professionals face inappropriate behaviours from patients, family members and carers, which also needs to be challenged.*

In summary, healthcare today is provided by a team of varied clinical professionals who may also be separate from each other in time and/or space. There are usually essential supports provided by nonclinical administrative and managerial staff as well, although these roles have no dedicated professional regulator. While this offers opportunities for patient centred care, the culture of organizations—how people treat each other—plays a role in how an individual experiences their working environment. There can be downstream effects for better or worse, seen in higher or lower rates of absenteeism and rates of staff retention or turnover.

### CASE 2.3 ILLUSTRATIVE CASE: EFFECTIVE MULTIDISCIPLINARY TEAM WORKING

Peter is 65 years old and has been recently diagnosed with advanced pancreatic cancer. He is referred to the hospice outpatient clinic for symptom management. He loves his food and is struggling with appetite, so the chef and a dietician get involved. He also loves to exercise, and a physiotherapist supports him in using the exercise bike in the patient gym on-site. He used to work in the luxury travel business and really appreciates the aromatherapy and massage therapy on offer. The doctor makes a new prescription for analgesics. The hospice outpatient nurse liaises with the community nursing team (district nurses) when Peter is no longer able to attend the hospice as his condition changes, and he also asks to see the chaplain.

*Which of the professionals involved with the patient are subject to regulation? Does regulation go far enough, or does it go too far? Who else may be important in providing care to Peter?*

## DISCLOSURE OF MISTAKES AND MISCONDUCT

Mistakes happen in all workplaces; in healthcare the consequences can be particularly grave. The NHS is still striving for a widespread 'just culture' of fairness, openness and learning—where staff feel able to speak up when things go wrong rather than fearing blame.

If you make a mistake, a reasonable course of action is to:

- Inform your clinical supervisor and rectify the mistake where possible.
- With support from your supervisor, explain and apologize to the patient.

### COMMUNICATION

### DUTY OF CANDOUR

***Health and Social Care Act 2008 (Regulated Activities) Regulations 2014***

When things go wrong with care and treatment, a patient must be informed and given reasonable support and an apology. A legal duty rests with the healthcare organization in the United Kingdom, and doctor(s) are often party to communications consistent with professional guidance (General Medical Council and Nursing & Midwifery Council, 2015).

## Concerns about a colleague

If you believe the behaviour of a colleague brings into question their fitness to practise:

- Consider if patients are at risk: General Medical Council (2023a) guidance says 'You must be compassionate towards colleagues who have problems with their performance or health. But you must put patient safety first at all times'.

- If you feel able, you might choose to approach your colleague directly. You may be successful in encouraging your colleague to take time off work and seek timely professional assessment.
- If you are uncomfortable approaching your colleague directly, or if approaching them proves unsuccessful, then voice your concerns to an appropriate person from the employing organization, for example your colleague's educational supervisor, the education dean or the medical director.

Remember that you still have obligations of confidentiality towards your colleague and any patients involved. A colleague may subsequently seek a consultation with their own GP and may self-refer or agree to be referred to an Occupational Health service. An Occupational Health physician has the duty to prioritize patient safety in the organization they are working for, as well as consider the needs of their individual patient. There is also Practitioner Health, a confidential NHS primary care mental health and addiction service with expertise in treating health and care professionals.

## Whistle-blowing

The *Public Interest Disclosure Act* 1998 is sometimes called the 'Whistle-Blowing Act'. It aims to protect any worker who discloses concerns via the appropriate channels in the public interest. Employees who claim they have been dismissed or overlooked for promotion as a result of a disclosure can bring their case before an employment tribunal. The Act does not cover volunteers and self-employed individuals.

---

**CASE 2.4** *DAY V. HEALTH EDUCATION ENGLAND & OTHERS* (2017)

Dr Chris Day made a disclosure about understaffing in an Intensive Care Unit in 2014 within Lewisham and Greenwich NHS Trust linked to two patient deaths. He made disclosures to both the Trust and the Health Education England. Dr Day later lost his job and national training number and sought to bring a whistle-blowing claim against the employing Trust and the national training body Health Education England (HEE, now merged into NHS England). Dr Day's right to a whistle-blowing claim against HEE was initially rejected on the grounds that he was not directly employed by them. This was overturned in the Court of Appeal and clarifies the position for all doctors in training, as well as for agency workers and others in triangular relationships in healthcare and other sectors of employment. At the time of writing (2024) further aspects of this case are yet to be settled.

---

## INDEMNITY, NEGLIGENCE AND EXPERT WITNESSES

Doctors working in NHS general practice and hospitals are covered by a state-backed clinical negligence scheme, significantly reducing their personal risk. It is very strongly advised to take out additional personal medical indemnity annually because the state-backed scheme does not cover all eventualities.

Personal indemnity can provide other support and this can vary with the indemnifying company. For example, it may include support with GMC fitness to practise investigations, indemnity for report writing or private clinical work, representation at disciplinary investigations, preparation responses to patient complaints, assistance with criminal investigations arising from clinical practice (e.g. gross negligence manslaughter), representation at the coroner's court and indemnity for Good Samaritan acts.

*A claim for clinical negligence requires:*

- There was a duty of care.
- The duty of care was breached.
- The breach in the duty of care *caused* the harm (physical or psychological).

It is usually straightforward for a claimant/patient to prove a duty of care existed. A breach in duty of care is determined against 'a reasonable standard of care' or that of an 'ordinarily competent practitioner'—which generally speaking is not the same as *a gold standard of best practice*. Also, in a given clinical situation different doctors may justify taking different courses of action. So a breach in the duty of care is sometimes more difficult to prove. It can also be difficult to prove that it was the breach of duty of care that caused the harm, not other factors.

Expert witnesses may be consulted (Fig. 2.7). These are doctors with considerable clinical experience in the area of medical

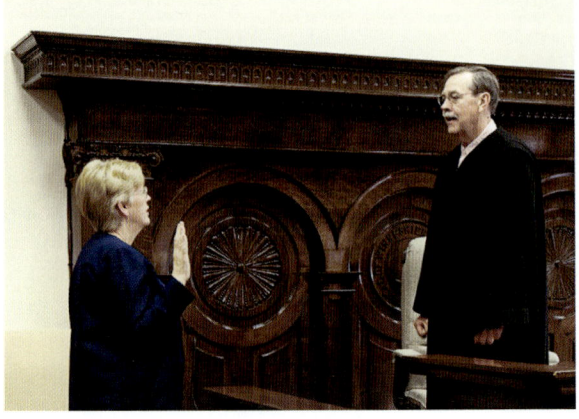

**Fig. 2.7** An expert witness taking the oath in court.

practice relevant to the individual patient case who generally have done extra training in how to act as an expert witness. The duty of an expert witness is to the court and requires them to be impartial; the expert witness is not there to favour either the claimant (patient) or defendant (doctor).

---

## ETHICS

### KEY POINTS

The Bolam and Bolitho tests are applied to medical negligence claims.

- Bolam test: Are the actions of the doctor endorsed by a responsible body of medical opinion from the relevant specialty at the material time of the case in question?
- Bolitho test: Does the responsible body of medical opinion have a logical basis in the opinion of the court, and has it considered the risks and benefits of competing options?

---

### CASE 2.5  *BOLAM V. FRIERN HOSPITAL MANAGEMENT COMMITTEE* (1957)

This involved an adult consenting to electroconvulsive (ECT) therapy which was then given without muscle relaxant and without restraining the patient; during ECT the patient had severe muscle spasms and fell off the bed, fracturing his pelvis. The doctor had followed usual practice for the times, including not informing the patient of small but serious risks associated with ECT, so the claim failed.

---

### CASE 2.6  *BOLITHO V. CITY AND HACKNEY HEALTH AUTHORITY* (1997)

This involved a child with breathing difficulties who died in hospital, where the senior doctor did not receive a call to attend because the on-call bleep being carried had a low battery. The doctor argued that even if they had attended, the child would not have been intubated. Expert witness opinion supported the reasonableness of not intubating in the particular circumstances, so the claim for negligence failed. The court found this to be logical. It was a breach of duty not to attend, but the breach did not cause the harm.

---

## INDUSTRIAL ACTION

- Industrial action, or a strike, is when a mass of employed workers collectively refuse to fulfil their contractual duties because of a dispute with their employer. Workers are not paid for times when they go on strike.
- The *Trade Union and Labour Relations (Consolidation) Act* 1992 provides statutory immunities. This means the trade union(s) and individual workers can lawfully organize and take part in a strike without risking certain retaliatory actions (e.g. being sued or fired). To qualify for statutory immunity and be a 'protected industrial action' certain conditions must be met, including:
  - Trade dispute: There must be a trade dispute and the action called relates to that.
  - Ballot and notice: Worker ballot and employer notice procedures are met.
- To receive trade union support and protection, a doctor needs to be a paid-up member of one of the trade unions with recognized authority to coordinate a strike. It is not essential to be a member of a trade union to take part in a strike.

---

## ETHICS

### MINIMUM SERVICE LEVELS LEGISLATION

A specialized agency of the United Nations called 'The International Labour Organisation' (2001) says minimum service levels are justifiable in some situations to protect essential services where there is a danger to life, personal safety or health of some or all of the population. This potentially means certain groups of workers have limits imposed on their right to strike.

The UK Government is considering amendments to the *Strikes (Minimum Service Levels) Act* 2023 specifically to protect hospital services. The context includes strikes by consultants and junior doctors, nurses and ambulance service staff and industrial action in non–health sector employees. Currently healthcare organizations rely on goodwill from the trade union(s) and individual members of staff to provide some cover during periods of industrial action. These agreements, called 'derogations', are not always made and could be associated with serious safety incidents for patients.

*What services and what level of cover do you think are appropriate to be mandated by minimum service levels legislation for doctors during periods of industrial action?*

## CONFIDENTIALITY

Confidence in confidentiality arrangements is key to a trusting and therapeutic relationship between patients and doctors. The right to confidentiality follows from a right to autonomy: self-determination includes deciding who knows what about oneself. Medical consultations include disclosure of sensitive information to inform care, not for any other reason. Clinical information 'belongs' to the person who disclosed it and ought not to be shared with third parties without specific consent or overriding good reason. If patients do not have confidence in confidentiality arrangements, they may not present for assessment or may under-report symptoms. The obligation of confidentiality persists after death. Sometimes the coroner/coroner's court will require information after a patient has died.

---

### HINTS AND TIPS

**FROM THE GENERAL MEDICAL COUNCIL (2021)**

'Patients have a right to expect that their personal information will be held in confidence by their doctors.'

---

### CASE 2.7 ILLUSTRATIVE CASES FOR CONFIDENTIALITY

Dr A saw Ms Z in clinic last week and blood tests were requested as she had been feeling tired all the time for 2 months. Dr A goes out at lunchtime to stretch their legs and buy a sandwich and happens to bump into Ms Z's mum, who asks what is happening with her daughter. Dr A responds in general terms, that patients can only be discussed inside the surgery and does not confirm that Ms Z is a patient. It is a breach of confidentiality for Dr A to even confirm that Ms Z, an adult patient, has been for a consultation. Dr A does not know what Miss Z wants her mum to know.

In the afternoon Dr A is back in the clinic and sees Mr T to review blood pressure medications. Mr T asks, 'While I'm here, doctor, can I pick up my wife's prescription?' Dr A first must be sure that Mr T's wife is happy for her prescription to be collected by her husband and/or that her husband knows its contents.

---

## Statutory basis of confidentiality and patient access to healthcare records

The UK 'common law duty of confidentiality' is developed over time as courts make decisions on particular cases and thereby set legal precedents. It means personal information shared in confidence must not be disclosed without a legal authority or overriding justification, or unless the patient consents to disclosure.

The *Data Protection Act* 2018 describes the statutory duty to maintain the confidentiality of medical records and other personal information stored. It applies to electronic and paper records. It is a UK law which compliments the *European Union General Data Protection Regulations* (*Regulation (EU) 2016/679*). There are eight principles of the *Data Protection Act* (DPA):

1. Information is processed fairly and lawfully.
2. Information is obtained for specified and lawful purposes.
3. Information is adequate, relevant and not excessive in relation to the purpose obtained for.
4. Information is accurate and kept up-to-date—including contact details for patients.
5. Information is not kept for longer than necessary.
6. Information is not used in ways contrary to the rights of the data subject (the patient).
7. Appropriate measures are taken to prevent unauthorized disclosure of information (Fig. 2.8).
8. Information is not transferred to areas that cannot provide the above assurances.

**The DPA gives a patient the right to:**

- Be informed about what information is being held and why.
- Access their personal data, that is have a copy of their medical record; a fee may be charged.
- Have inaccuracies corrected.
- Seek damages as a result of misleading information.

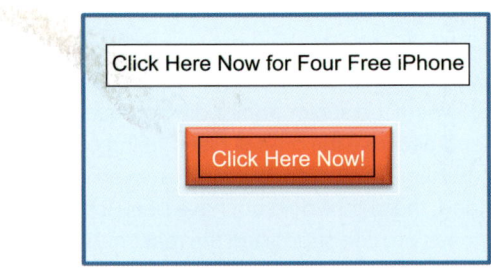

**Fig. 2.8** Many healthcare organizations rely to a large extent on computerized patient records and other electronic systems which must be kept secure. This requires ongoing organizational investment in cybersecurity measures and individual staff to be alert to 'phishing' attempts in various forms.

## When should confidential information be disclosed?

Sometimes confidentiality needs to be broken, and doctors frequently seek additional support or guidance before doing this—including from senior colleagues involved with the patient and perhaps from their medical indemnifier. It is important to remember that absolute guarantees of confidentiality cannot be given to patients, because they may reveal circumstances to you that you have an overriding duty to share—often in order to prevent other harms. Where safe to do so, you will generally still inform the patient of your intention to make a disclosure.

information outweighs the rights to privacy for the patient and the associated risk to public confidence through overriding normal confidentiality.
- Wounds that are not self-inflicted and are caused by gunshot or knife attack should usually be reported to the police.

## Other challenging scenarios

- If a patient is a victim of neglect, physical or sexual abuse and in your assessment is unable to give valid consent and you believe disclosure will prevent further harm, you must disclose information to the appropriate responsible person or statutory agency. This may involve domestic abuse situations like coercive control.
- Third-party interests
  - Where maintaining confidentiality creates a risk of serious harm or death.
  - Disclosure is required for the prevention or detection of a serious crime.
    - The *Counter-Terrorism and Security Act* 2015 contains the 'Prevent' duty and it is a crime *not* to disclose information related to potential acts of terrorism.
    - Police requests for medical information to help with investigations need to provide sufficient information to assist medical decision-making as to whether a disclosure is appropriate, and if so, how much information to disclose.
- Driving.
- *The Driver and Vehicle Licensing Agency (DVLA)* is responsible for deciding if a person is medically fit to hold a driving licence. If a patient has a condition that impairs their ability to drive, inform them of their legal duty to inform the DVLA. If the patient cannot understand this advice, for example in dementia, you should inform the DVLA. If a patient refuses to accept your diagnosis, advise them to seek a second opinion and not to drive pending further advice. If a patient continues to drive when they are unfit, make every effort to persuade them to stop. If they cannot be persuaded, then inform the DVLA. Inform the patient of your intention and write to confirm that a disclosure has been made.
  - A patient's motor insurance may not be deemed valid if they are medically unfit to drive and have an incident, so you must consider the possibility the patient may still be driving and inform the patient if you consider them medically unfit to drive.
- Medical Fitness to Drive Guidance is split into neurological, cardiovascular, diabetes mellitus, psychiatric, drug or alcohol misuse or dependence, visual, renal, respiratory and miscellaneous conditions (Driver and Vehicle Licensing Agency, 2024).

## CASE 2.8  ILLUSTRATIVE CASE: MR L IS HIV POSITIVE AND DEMANDS CONFIDENTIALITY

Mr L is HIV positive and demands you tell no one else of his diagnosis, including the wider healthcare team. Key points include confidentiality and preventing risk to third parties.

HIV/AIDS is different from many other infectious diseases: there is no cure, patients can live unaffected for long periods and still be infective, and there is some stigma associated (Fig. 2.9).

Factors favouring confidentiality and not disclosing include:

1. The right to privacy based on respect for autonomy.
2. Erosion of confidence in the medical consultation, leading to worse consequences (e.g. fewer people with HIV seeking treatment).

Factors favouring the breaking of confidentiality include:

1. Risk of inappropriate treatment for Mr L if other members of the healthcare team only have a partial medical history, including drug interactions with antiretrovirals.
2. Potential risk to Mr L's current sexual partner if sex is unprotected.
3. Potential risk to other healthcare professionals—for example some dental and surgical procedures can involve accidental contact with blood.

In practice, start by explaining to Mr L why you think it is necessary that the healthcare team knows about his HIV status. He can be informed that all healthcare staff and students have a duty of confidentiality. In particular, a general practitioner (GP) is not well placed to manage the patient's overall condition, including prescribing other medicines safely, unless also informed about HIV status.

If Mr L continues to refuse disclosure to his GP, his wishes usually ought to be respected. Rarely, if the patient is violent or severely mentally disturbed, disclosure to the GP without consent may be appropriate.

What about disclosing information to Mr L's current partner? If he has communicated an intention to engage in risky unprotected sex, there may be a duty to warn the partner if Mr L cannot be persuaded to do so.

1. The harm of breaking confidentiality is the loss of patient trust that follows. This may discourage future health-seeking behaviours. There may be further harms such as relationship strain and stigmatization if the diagnosis becomes more widely known.
2. The main benefit of disclosure is reducing the risk of serious harm to Mr L's current sexual partner. It seems reasonable that preventing HIV infection is a good enough reason to break confidentiality. A patient does not have an absolute right to confidentiality: as a doctor you always need to consider the risks to other relevant people. The GMC advises that information can be disclosed to protect a person from the risk of death or serious harm: however, information must only be disclosed to those at active risk.
3. When the courts are asked about breaking confidentiality, decisions generally weigh the public interest in maintaining confidentiality (confidentiality encourages patients to seek help) against either third-party or public interest in disclosure (protection of people at risk).

## PROFESSIONAL BOUNDARIES

It is the responsibility of the doctor to maintain appropriate professional boundaries and avoid conflict of interest situations. A conflict of interest can be actual or perceived by others. Both are important for the doctor to anticipate given the duty to maintain trust at an individual level and in the profession as a whole.

The doctor–patient dynamic often involves a power imbalance. The doctor has access to expertise and resources which the patient needs, and the patient has physical and/or mental and/or emotional vulnerabilities in varying degrees.

Common boundary considerations include:

- Inappropriate sexual behaviour.
- Doctors treating family, friends and themselves.
- Accepting gifts from patients and colleagues.
- Doctors as patients/concerns about a colleague.

### Inappropriate sexual behaviour

General Medical Council (2023c) guidance is not to pursue a sexual or improper emotional relationship with a patient or someone close to them (Fig. 2.10). Personal illness can render any self-assured person temporarily vulnerable to exploitation. Illness in a close family member or friend can be similarly destabilizing. The principle is for the doctor not to abuse the imbalance of power and to uphold trust.

Sexualized behaviour has been defined as acts, words or behaviour intended to arouse or gratify sexual impulses and desires. If a

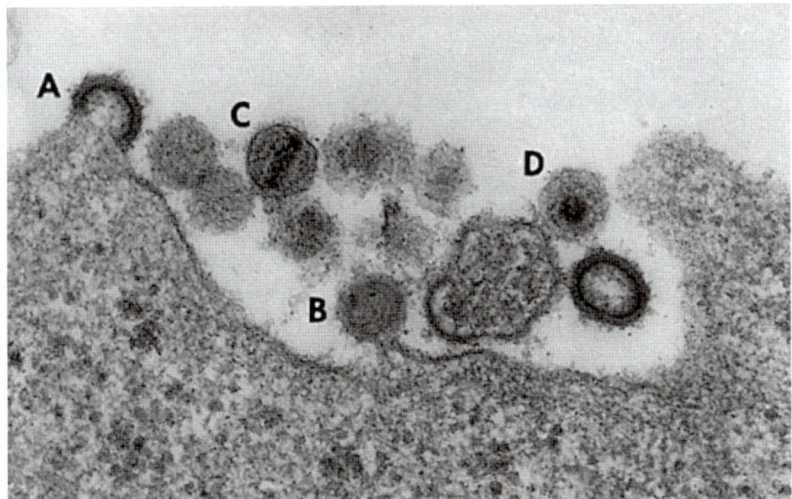

**Fig. 2.9** Transmission electron micrograph of HIV-1. Virions are shown at all stages of morphogenesis: early (A) and late (B) budding forms and cell-free mature virions (C and D) with condensed central cores.

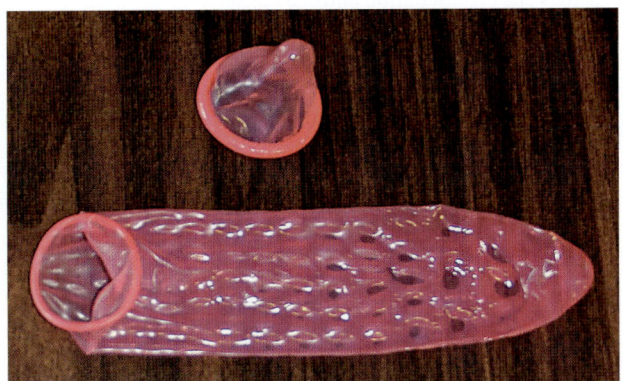

**Fig. 2.10** Male condoms.

**ETHICS**

**PRACTICE POINT**

If you are unsure whether you are—or could be seen to be—abusing your professional position, consider discussing the situation with an impartial colleague, indemnity organization, the British Medical Association or (confidentially) with a member of the GMC Standards and Ethics team.

## Chaperones

A chaperone helps to manage professional boundaries, typically for intimate examinations (General Medical Council 2023d). A chaperone needs to be appropriately trained. They witness the doctor's conduct with a patient when either the doctor or the patient requests it. For example, the patient may be particularly vulnerable and/or the doctor may require protection against the risk of allegations of indecent assault. The use of chaperones has been particularly encouraged since 2000 when GP Clifford Ayling was convicted of multiple counts of indecent assault.

## What is an intimate examination?

1. Examining the breasts, genitalia, rectum.
2. Any examination involving touching or being close to the patient *may* be considered intimate *by a patient or doctor,* for example fundoscopy in dimmed lighting, abdominal palpation, palpating for an apex beat.

patient or someone close to them displays sexualized behaviour, a doctor should try to re-establish a professional boundary. Where this is not possible, sometimes doctors have to end the professional relationship and ask a colleague to take over care.

Relationships with former patients may be inappropriate as well. Relevant factors include the length of time since the professional contact ended, the nature and duration of the previous professional contact, the nature of patient vulnerability at the time and whether they are still vulnerable, and whether there is ongoing involvement in care for other individuals close to the former patient. Pursuing a relationship with a former patient is more likely to be, or be seen to be, an abuse of position if you met the patient in a psychiatric or paediatric setting.

3. Cultural and religious factors influence whether an examination is considered intimate and whether a chaperone is needed.
4. Patients may consider themselves, or could be considered, vulnerable—regardless of whether the examining clinician considers them to be sexually attractive.

---

### CLINICAL NOTES

#### PRACTICE POINTS

- Avoid assumptions about when a patient, of the same or different sex to you, may or may not require a chaperone.
- If you as the doctor require a chaperone—explain to the patient and seek their consent.
- The patient may have objections to another person being present and has the right to decline a chaperone. If you as the clinician feel vulnerable, you can refuse to carry out the examination or procedure and arrange alternative care for the patient.
- Document the offer of and consent to a chaperone, and if relevant the full name and position of who filled that role; ideally the chaperone will also make an independent note in the medical record.
- A chaperone should have appropriate prior training.
- Give the patient privacy to undress and dress.
- Use curtains and appropriate drapes to maintain patient dignity during the examination.
- Explain what you are doing throughout; avoid irrelevant or personal comments.
- The chaperone stays present for the minimum appropriate period, not necessarily and not usually for the whole consultation.
- Record any concerns you or the patient have about the examination.

---

**When to be particularly cautious:**

- Vulnerable patients, for example with mental health symptoms.
- Patients who have made previous allegations of indecent assault.
- If the patient suggests explicitly or implicitly they find you sexually attractive.
- If you find the patient sexually attractive.

Remember that nonurgent examinations can be deferred if necessary.

## Intimate examinations under anaesthetic

Students may learn vaginal and rectal examination techniques in this setting. General Medical Council (2023e) guidance exists to protect patients from unethical practices:

- Obtain prior consent, usually in writing, for intimate examinations under anaesthetic (Fig. 2.11).
- Doctors supervising a student should ensure that valid consent has been obtained.
- Students are also under an obligation to make sure that consent is obtained.

## Doctors treating family, friends and themselves

GMC Good Medical Practice (2023a): 'You must, wherever possible, avoid providing medical care to yourself or anyone with whom you have a close personal relationship.' This is because your professional judgement can be affected by your close personal relationship. In an emergency, for example a cardiac arrest, you may start resuscitation and call for help.

You must also avoid providing clinical care to yourself. Self-prescribing, for example, may involve drugs of addiction or inaccurate diagnosis and lacks the rigour of independent assessment and may prevent treating doctors from understanding all the medicines being taken. Such behaviours can lead to fitness to practice proceedings (General Medical Council, 2023e).

---

### CASE 2.9 ILLUSTRATIVE CASE FOR PROFESSIONAL BOUNDARIES

*You arrive early for the morning clinic. Two colleagues are off sick and there is lots of paperwork. As you start reading the first letter, there is a knock on your door. The receptionist says one of the hospital consultants, whom you know is friends with the senior GP partner, has 'popped in on the off chance' of seeing a GP before work. Would you make special allowances for a colleague? Why might you and why might you not?*

Would you be more likely to see them before morning surgery if they:

- Are a relative?
- Are a personal friend?
- Used to be your boss?
- Used to be your school teacher?
- Are a local celebrity?
- Are a local politician?
- Are a local religious leader?
- None of the above?

---

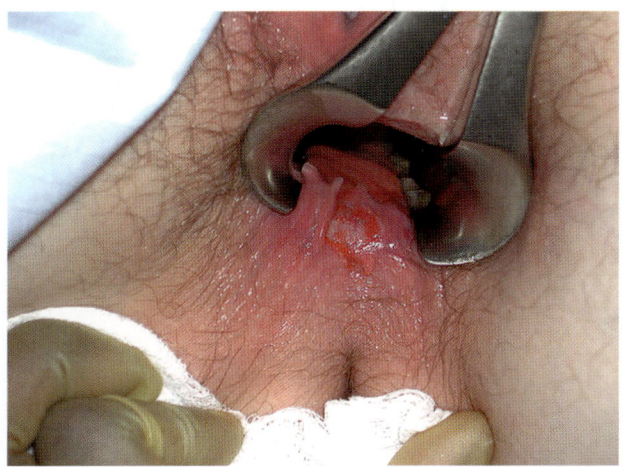

**Fig. 2.11** Anal fissure demonstrated at examination under anaesthetic. You must ensure appropriate patient consent has been obtained in advance for intimate examinations, including those under anaesthetic.

**CLINICAL NOTES**

**GIFT SCENARIOS**

Consider whether it would be appropriate for a doctor to accept any of the following:

- A box of chocolates from a patient, who then asks for a 2-week supply of sleeping tablets.
- A case containing six bottles of Champagne, from a grateful patient after his general practitioner (GP) spots a skin cancer in time for it to be removed with clear margins.
- Free educational meetings at a local private hospital, led by consultants at that hospital.
- A limited edition luxury car from a 90-year-old patient to their favourite geriatrician.
- A cheque for £300 towards a new piece of equipment for a GP health centre from a patient who has just been diagnosed with a terminal illness.
- An all-expenses-paid trip to a dermatology conference in the South of France, courtesy of a leading brand of topical steroids.

You must be prepared to explain and justify your decisions. If you see good reasons for making special allowances, consider where you will set your limits. Doctors can be put under pressure by those seeking to blur boundaries for their own interests. Friends and family members short on time, or medical colleagues doubtful about confidentiality or the impact of disclosures on their careers can seek informal consultations. Upholding clinical boundaries can protect doctors from pressures that might otherwise be coercive.

## Financial dealings and gifts

GMC Good Medical Practice (2023a): 'You must not ask for or accept—from patients, colleagues or others—any incentive payments, gifts or hospitality that may affect or be seen to affect the way you propose, provide or prescribe treatments, refer or commission services for patients.'

Problems can arise around:

- Gifts from patients.
- A patient telling a doctor they are a future beneficiary in their will.
- A doctor having a financial interest in a facility where they wish to refer their patient.
- Educational lunches sponsored by pharmaceutical companies (Fig. 2.12).

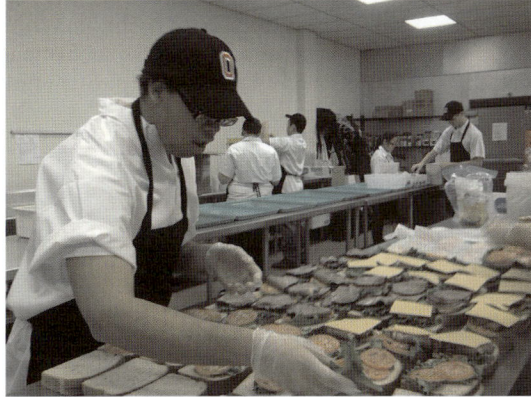

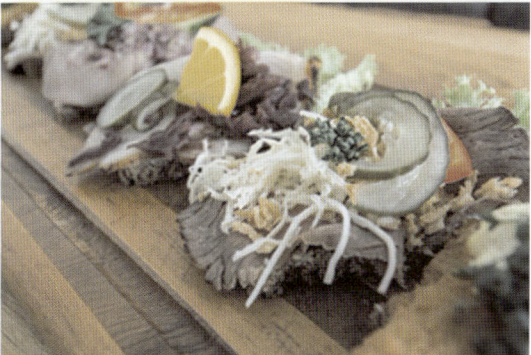

**Fig. 2.12** There is said to be no such thing as a free lunch.

A gift from a grateful patient may seem harmless, but professional bodies urge caution. Gifts or loans are sometimes offered by patients, consciously or unconsciously, as a means of establishing an improper sense of closeness.

Doctors need to be sensitive to potential issues where they are made beneficiaries of the will of a patient. They need to avoid involvement in assessing patient capacity to make legal and financial decisions and be sensitive to the possibility that their future financial interests might be seen to have an impact on clinical decision-making. If such conflicts of interest cannot be avoided, then they should be disclosed to those with a relevant interest.

You may accept *unsolicited* gifts from patients or their relatives if this does not affect and does not appear to affect your professional work, other patients' trust in you or the public trust in the profession. You should refuse gifts or bequests where they could be perceived as an abuse of trust. Many organizations have a policy position on gifts; a more relaxed approach may be taken to low-value personal gifts such as confectionery that can be shared among the team or flowers.

## SOCIAL MEDIA CONDUCT

The standards expected of doctors are the same, whatever the medium of communication. The principle is that you are still representing the profession, just online and electronically, and you still need to maintain public trust in the profession. The confidentiality of your personal communications with friends and family cannot be guaranteed. Take care not to share patient-identifiable information.

Some examples of social media platforms:

- Networking: Facebook, LinkedIn
- Content communities: YouTube
- Blogs: X (Twitter)
- Forums: doctors.net

### CLINICAL NOTES

#### GMC: DOCTOR'S USE OF SOCIAL MEDIA

- Review your privacy settings for all social media profiles; remember social media providers cannot guarantee your confidentiality.
- If a patient contacts you through your private profile, indicate that you cannot mix social and professional relationships, and if appropriate, direct them to your professional profile.
- Comments or posts about individuals or organizations online are subject to the same laws of copyright and defamation as written or verbal communications, whether made in a personal or professional capacity.

General Medical Council, 2023f.

### CASE 2.10 DOCTORS' PRIVATE WHATSAPP GROUP, MISCONDUCT AND GENERAL MEDICAL COUNCIL (GMC) WARNINGS

- Police investigations into a third party unexpectedly led to concerns about the conduct of doctors in a private WhatsApp group between 2014 and 2016.
- The GMC became involved, obtaining the full WhatsApp transcript by court order.
  - The thread contained messages that were offensive, racist, misogynistic, discriminatory and disrespectful to people with other protected characteristics and included one category A prohibited image and five extreme pornographic images.
- Concerns were referred to the Medical Practitioners Tribunal Service (MPTS) on the basis that no one had removed themselves from the group or used any channels to report concerns and were thereby bringing the profession into disrepute.
- The doctors appealed against the referral to MPTS mainly on the grounds of a right to respect for their personal correspondence, but this was not upheld.
- MPTS found evidence of misconduct but not ongoing impairment of fitness to practice, as the doctors showed remorse and insight and were considered unlikely to repeat the behaviours; GMC appealed against the MPTS decision and warnings were placed on the medical register for those involved.

## CLINICAL GOVERNANCE

'Clinical governance is a system through which NHS organizations are accountable for continuously improving the quality of their services and safeguarding high standards of care by creating an environment in which excellence in clinical care will flourish' (Scally & Donaldson, 1998). It involves monitoring systems and processes to provide assurance of patient safety and quality of care across the organization. This concept was introduced into the NHS in 1999.

Adherence to and involvement in developing protocols, audit, peer review, patient satisfaction and complaints systems, incident investigations, dissemination and incorporation of learning are all part of a culture of quality control. There can be a tension between institutionally controlled standardization of clinical decisions and the freedom to make clinical decisions in the interests of an individual patient.

# Evidence-based medicine (clinical effectiveness)

Evidence-based clinical practice developed in the 1980s, seeking to integrate the best research evidence with clinical experience and patient values. This followed earlier conversations in the 1970s about hierarchies of evidence.

# Clinical audit

Since the early 1990s participation in audits has been a requirement for UK doctors. It is a cycle of comparing actual practice with pre-agreed standards. A 'criterion and standard' in a clinical audit describes 'what should be done and in what proportion of cases' for a particular clinical situation. For example, 'was a mid-stream urine sample sent to the laboratory when empirical antibiotics were started for presumed urinary tract infection' is a criterion, and the standard might be set at 95% for a general adult inpatient population to allow for some clinical situations where it is not reasonably possible to obtain a mid-stream urine sample. Criteria and standards must be up to date, research based and adapted to the (local) service. In practice this means seeking agreement with clinical teams. This is important because the general purpose of audit goes beyond measuring current practice, to developing practical solutions to improve future care in that area. For audits to be useful, clinicians must be receptive to feedback and change their practice. Each organization will generally have an administrative and/or clinical audit lead.

Patients, public and the media can become interested in the outcomes of clinical audits. Some audits are conducted at a national level, such as MBRRACE-UK (Mothers and Babies: Reducing Risk through Audits and Confidential Enquiries across the United Kingdom). This combines the work of the national Confidential Enquiry into Maternal Deaths, which has run since 1952, and national surveillance of late foetal losses, stillbirths and infant deaths. As an example, data continue to show that mothers from Black, Asian and mixed ethnic backgrounds are at higher risk of maternal death than White mothers (MBRRACE-UK 2023).

- National Audit of Care at the End of Life (NACEL)
- National Audit of Dementia (NAD)
- National Audit of Metastatic Breast Cancer (NAoMe)
- National Audit of Primary Breast Cancer (NAoPri)
- National Bowel Cancer Audit (NBoCA)
- National Cancer Audit Collaborating Centre
- National Clinical Audit of Psychosis (NCAP)
- National Early Inflammatory Arthritis Audit (NEIAA)
- National Emergency Laparotomy Audit (NELA)
- National 'Epilepsy 12' Audit
- National Kidney Cancer Audit (NKCA)
- National Lung Cancer Audit (NLCA)
- National Maternity and Perinatal Audit (NMPA)
- National Neonatal Audit Programme (NNAP)
- National Non-Hodgkin Lymphoma Audit (NNHLA)
- National Obesity Audit
- National Oesophago-Gastric Cancer Audit (NOGCA)
- National Ovarian Cancer Audit (NOCA)
- National Paediatric Diabetes Audit (NPDA)
- National Pancreatic Cancer Audit (NPaCA)
- National Prostate Cancer Audit (NPCA)
- National Respiratory Audit Programme (NRAP)
- National Vascular Registry (NVR)
- Paediatric Intensive Care Audit Network (PICANet)
- Sentinel Stroke National Audit Programme (SSNAP)

There is also the National Confidential Enquiry into Patient Outcome and Deaths, a continuing national audit programme funded by the National Patient Safety Agency and Department of Health but independent of government and professional associations (Figs 2.11–2.12).

---

**CLINICAL NOTES**

**NHS NATIONAL CLINICAL AUDIT PROGRAMME (HEALTHCARE QUALITY IMPROVEMENT PARTNERSHIP 2024)**

- Falls and Fragility Fracture Audit (includes the Hip Fracture Database) (FFFAP)
- National Adult Diabetes Audit (NDA)
- National Audit of Cardiovascular Disease Prevention in Primary Care (CVDPrevent)

---

**ETHICS**

*FREEDOM OF INFORMATION ACT* 2000

The FOI Act gives the public a general right of access to almost all types of recorded information held by public authorities. FOI access requests can be made by anyone, including investigative journalists. Patient-specific information remains confidential, and there are other exceptions.

## Errors and significant event analysis

Significant event analysis differs from clinical audit. Significant event analysis reviews the details of an individual case or cases where there has been a significant occurrence; this may not necessarily mean a poor outcome for the patient. The aim is to learn lessons to inform changes in clinical practice or processes. Clinical incident reporting systems collect data on incidents with lower levels of concern. Most incidents that occur are multifactorial in origin: the so-called Swiss cheese model (Fig. 2.13). Factors are typically a combination of active failures, for example unsafe actions by staff, and latent conditions, for example excess time pressure or understaffing.

## NHS complaints procedures

Complaints procedures are a method of conflict resolution which patients and next of kin can pursue. They do not provide a route to financial compensation. Patients may take complaints to court as well as pursue NHS complaints processes.

Before a formal complaint is made, it may be possible to address the concerns directly. This may or may not involve the Patient Advice and Liaison Service, which is a department in most hospitals. Most complaints are managed locally, with those complained about responding either in writing or in person to the complainant. Hospital Trusts provide a lay conciliator to facilitate meetings. With honest and open communication the complainant and those complained about can often see each other's points of view, with explanations and apologies given as appropriate. Often there is satisfactory resolution at this level.

A complainant remaining dissatisfied with local processes can complain to the NHS Ombudsman. The Ombudsman is a civil servant independent of the NHS, responsible for reporting to Parliament. It is up to the Ombudsman whether or not to further investigate any complaints.

## MEDICAL RESEARCH

Research can ultimately improve the human condition and add new knowledge to the sum of human understanding. The potential to learn and to reduce future human suffering is secondary to the human rights of the individual research participant. Human rights abuses were committed in the name of medical research in the 20th century.

### CLINICAL NOTES

#### KEY POINTS

- Audit reviews actual clinical practice against the currently accepted standard of clinical practice.
- Research generates new knowledge.
- The human rights of research participants take precedence over the quest for new knowledge.
- Before starting medical research in the United Kingdom there must be Research Ethics Committee approval (Fig. 2.14).

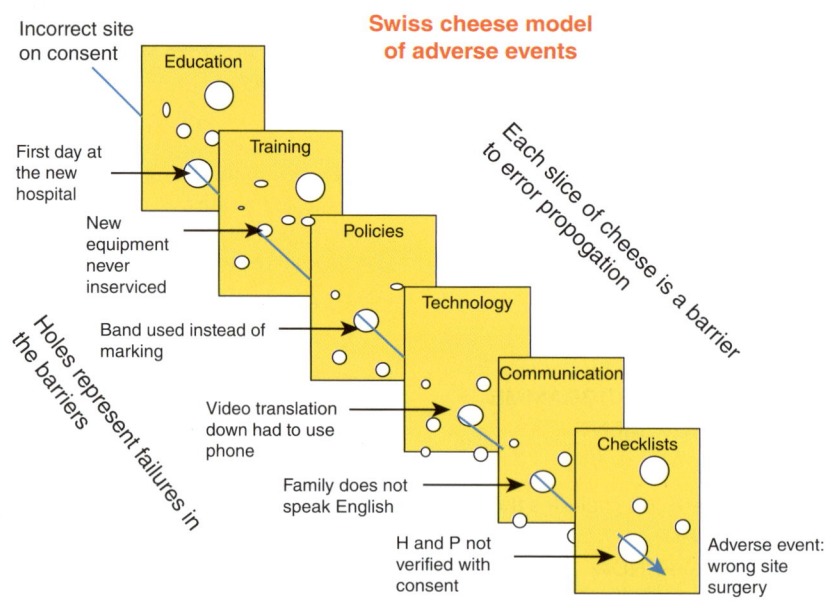

**Fig. 2.13** The Swiss cheese model of adverse events. H and P, *History and physical examination*. (From Stein, J. E., & Heiss, K. (2015). The Swiss cheese model of adverse event occurrence—Closing the holes. *Seminars in Pediatric Surgery, 24*(6), 278–282.)

### 1932–70

The US Public Health Service studied the progression of syphilis among ~400 Black males in Tuskegee. They were denied effective treatment (penicillin) even after it became available.

### 1940–45

Medical experiments were carried out in Nazi Germany under the direction of Dr Josef Mengele. Human subjects were treated like, or worse than, animals in medical research. Similar experiments were also carried out in territories occupied by Imperial Japan.

### 1949

The 'Nuremberg Code' arose from the case of *United States v. Brandt*. Brandt was Hitler's personal physician, although the case also heard 19 other doctors and three biomedical scientists.
1. *Absolute* need for *voluntary* consent.
2. Justification in terms of potential 'fruitful results'.
3. Proper design and previous animal experiments.
4. Avoidance of 'unnecessary physical and mental suffering and injury'.
5. Conducted by 'scientifically qualified persons'.
6. Stop the study if it becomes clear harm is resulting, or if the human subject wishes to.

### 1964

The Declaration of Helsinki (World Medical Association, 2013) facilitated research to potentially include the young and those lacking mental capacity. It is less restrictive than the Nuremberg Code.

### 1968

Nonstatutory research ethics committees were established in the United Kingdom to consider clinical trial proposals.

### 1984–90

UK guidelines by the Royal College of Physicians require research to be subject to ethical review before commencing.
- A patient expressing a strong preference for a particular treatment is probably ineligible to participate.
- Randomization of treatment without patient consent is unethical.

### 1999

International Conference on Harmonization Guidelines for Good Clinical Practice (Dixon, 1999) defines an international standard for research on human subjects. It aligns with the principles of the Declaration of Helsinki and aims for unified standards across Europe, Japan and the United States.

### 2004

The *Medications for Use (Clinical Trials) Regulations 2004* aim to standardize the regulation of medical research throughout the European Union.

### 2009

The Integrated Research Application System is a single online system for applying for approvals for health and social care research in the United Kingdom.

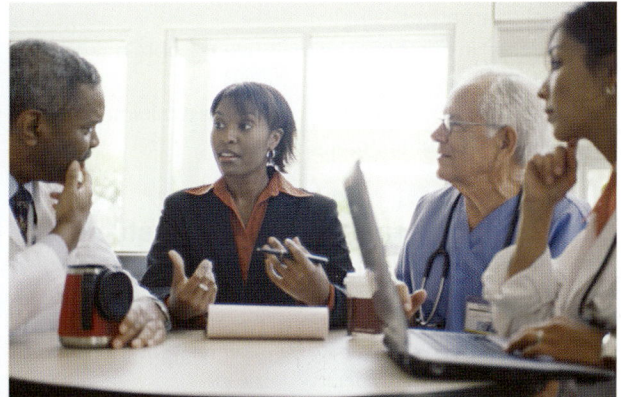

**Fig. 2.14** Multidisciplinary ethics committees review and approve or decline approvals for medical research.

## Ethical issues

1. *Equipoise*: It must be *unknown* whether the new treatment is more effective than current treatments. There will be reason to believe the new treatment could be more effective, perhaps from animal studies.
2. *Principle of least harm*: Study design allows only the minimal amount of potential harm to the individual. This usually means comparing a new treatment against the current treatment(s) rather than against a placebo. Potential benefits must outweigh the potential risks of treatment.
3. *Voluntary, informed consent*: Patients must understand potential risks and benefits and be informed that they can refuse from the outset or withdraw from the study at any time without affecting their ongoing healthcare. So there must be no coercion to participate and no abuse of power.

4. *Therapeutic misconception*: This occurs when research participants confuse the context of experimental research with their usual medical care. This can undermine the autonomy of patient choice to consent. Therapeutic misconception generally includes some degree of *therapeutic misestimation*—overestimating the benefits of taking part and/or underestimating the risks. It can help to state that research goals are based on research questions, not the participant's condition, and that benefits to the individual participant are not expected.

5. *Therapeutic versus nontherapeutic research*: Therapeutic research gives patients an experimental treatment and assesses effectiveness. Nontherapeutic research involves healthy individuals. Many people believe nontherapeutic research should involve lower levels of risk because there is less scope for benefit. This distinction was dropped from the 2000 Helsinki Revision, but remains important regarding children and other situations where a person is enrolled in a trial in their *best interests*.

# Research on subjects from vulnerable groups

A person lacking the ability to make autonomous choices is vulnerable (Fig. 2.15). This includes children and those with serious mental illness or incapacity. It also includes groups more vulnerable to exploitation such as prisoners.

## Research in children

Children cannot always give valid consent. Children aged over 16 are presumed to have the capacity to consent to medical treatment and, therefore, to consent to therapeutic research. Children under 16 *may* be sufficiently competent to consent. If a child is incompetent, research consent can be obtained from a person with parental responsibility. Research participation must be in the best interests of the child. It is usual to seek the child's assent to participate, even if they cannot give fully informed consent.

## Research in adults with mental incapacity

In the United Kingdom, a third party cannot consent to research participation on behalf of an adult, so entry for a trial is decided on the basis of the patient's best interests, and the responsibility is with the researcher. In practice, a 'consultee' is identified, often family or next of kin. This demonstrates a willingness to communicate and, where relevant, a desire to find out what the patient's wishes would have been if they were able to express them. However, the consultee cannot give consent.

Research on adults lacking capacity is covered by the *Mental Capacity Act* (MCA) 2005, *Clinical Trial Regulations* 2004, *Data Protection Act* 2018 and the *Human Tissue Act* 2004.

- The Research Ethics Committee must have grounds to believe the research cannot be carried out as effectively with people capable of giving consent.
- Research cannot do anything contrary to a valid advance decision by a participant.
- Research cannot proceed if the person appears to be unwilling or objects (does not assent).

## Animal research

Animal research is a debated area. It can be useful to consider:

1. Is the experiment well designed and will it produce significant results?
2. Could the experiment be done without animals?
3. Can animal suffering be reduced, for example if the experiment involves new surgical techniques, will the animals be given anaesthesia and agents for muscle paralysis?
4. With primate research, 'would we be happy doing this research to humans with a mental capacity that is equivalent to that of the animals being used?'

Further to the *Animal (Scientific Procedures) Act* 1986, a Select Committee reported (Parliament House of Lords, 2002):

- It is acceptable for humans to use animals in research and wrong to cause unnecessary or avoidable suffering.
- There is a continued need for animal experiments in applied research and in research aimed purely at extending knowledge.
- There is scope to pursue the three Rs of animal research.

**CLINICAL NOTES**

**THREE RS OF ANIMAL RESEARCH:**

**R**eplacement of conscious, living animals by nonsentient alternatives.

**R**eduction in number of animals used to obtain information.

**R**efinement of procedures to produce a minimal amount of suffering.

## Researching healthcare staff and students

Invitations to take part in research are a regular part of university life. Beyond the clinical setting, this can include sociological, psychological and educational research. These studies still must pass through a university (or other relevant) research ethics committee who considers:

1. What harms can be caused by research? For example distressing conversations in social research and duty to

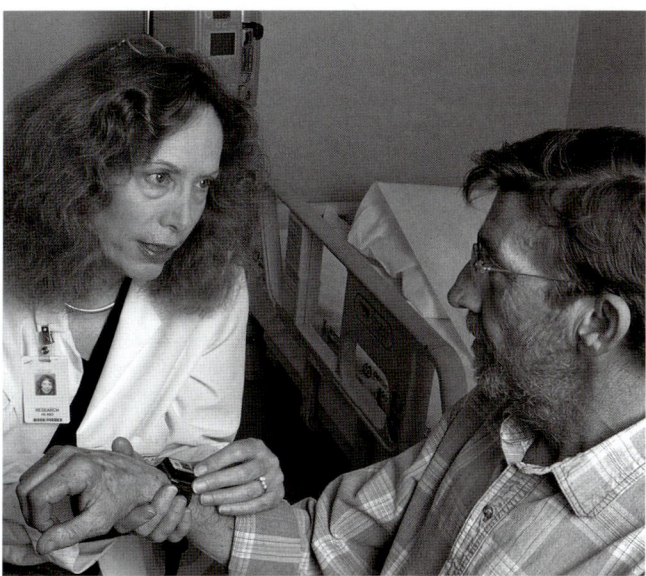

**Fig. 2.15** Research participants are selected based on factors such as age, sex, condition and location. They must then be informed about certain aspects of the proposed research in order to make a decision about participating. That decision, which is written and signed, is known as 'informed consent'.

report unethical or illegal conduct disclosed by participants.

2. Researcher safety. For example travelling alone to interview people in their own homes.

3. How will the personal information of participants be protected, for example data storage, data for publications?

## Publication ethics

Publication ethics is important for upholding trust in academic journals. Issues include:

1. Falsifying results, for example journals have statisticians who advise if results are 'too perfect'.

2. Authors and reviewers failing to disclose sources of major bias, for example being a shareholder in a company (financial), on the board of a charity or other campaigning organization linked to the area of interest (personal).

3. Gift authorship—where a named author did not contribute to the work.

4. Plagiarism—using someone else's work without acknowledgement and claiming credit.

5. Submitting the same work to multiple journals.

6. Research without Research Ethics Committee approval.

The Committee on Publication Ethics (COPE) (www.publicationethics.org) was established in 1997 by a group of medical journal editors in the United Kingdom. Now there are thousands of members worldwide across all academic fields.

---

**CASE 2.11  CASE STUDY ON NHS ORGAN RETENTION (THE 'ALDER HAY SCANDAL')**

The public enquiry into cardiac surgical deaths at Bristol Royal Infirmary led to disclosures that many NHS hospitals were keeping collections of human organs. Often this was 'for research purposes'. Postmortem organ removal, examination and retention had been a common medical practice for decades. This was frequently done without the knowledge of or informed consent from the patient in life or family after death and was criticized as a reflection of medical paternalism. Most of the attention became focused on Alder Hay Hospital in Liverpool and a collection of ~2000 sample pots from 850 infants accumulated during 1986 to 1996. Across the wider NHS over 100,000 body parts were being held. Informed consent was placed at the centre of reform, expressed in the *Human Tissue Act* 2004.

---

# References

*Abortion Act* 1967.

*Animals (Scientific Procedures) Act* 1986.

Anonymous. (2017). World Medical Association Declaration of Geneva. *African Health Sciences*, *17*(4), 1203. https://doi.org/10.4314/ahs.v17i4.30.

*Bawa-Garba v. General Medical Council* [2018] EWCA CIV 1879.

British Medical Association. (2023). *BMA junior doctors committee and GP registrar committee statement on MAPs*. BMA. https://www.bma.org.uk/news-and-opinion/bma-junior-doctors-committee-and-gp-registrar-committee-statement-on-maps#:~:text=It%20is%20the%20BMA's%20position,PA%2C%20AA%2C%20or%20SCP.

*Bolam v. Friern Hospital Management Committee* [1957] 1 WLR 583.

*Bolitho v. City and Hackney Health Authority* [1997] UKHL 46.

Children Act 1989.

*Counter-Terrorism and Security Act* 2015.

*Data Protection Act* 2018.

*Day v. Health Education England & Others* [2017] EWCA Civ 329.

Dixon, J. R. (1999). The International Conference on Harmonization Good Clinical Practice Guideline. *Quality Assurance*, *6*(2), 65–74. https://doi.org/10.1080/105294199277860.

Driver and Vehicle Licensing Agency. (2024). *Assessing fitness to drive – A guide for medical professionals*. Swansea: Crown. https://assets.publishing.service.gov.uk/media/65a51345867cd800135ae844/assessing-fitness-to-drive-january-2024.pdf.

*Freedom of Information Act* 2000.

General Medical Council. (2012). *Leadership and management for all doctors (updated 2023)*. GMC. https://www.gmc-uk.org/-/media/documents/Leadership_and_management_for_all_doctors___English_1015.pdf_48903400.pdf https://www.gmc-uk.org/-/media/documents/Leadership_and_management_for_all_doctors___English_1015.pdf_48903400.pdf.

General Medical Council. (2013a). *Personal beliefs and medical practice*. GMC. https://www.gmc-uk.org/-/media/documents/personal-beliefs-and-medical-practice-20200217_pdf-58833376.pdf.

General Medical Council. (2021). *Confidentiality: Good practice in handling patient information*. GMC. https://www.gmc-uk.org/-/media/documents/gmc-guidance-for-doctors---confidentiality-good-practice-in-handling-patient-information----70080105.pdf.

General Medical Council. (2023a). *Good medical practice 2024*. GMC. https://www.gmc-uk.org/-/media/documents/gmp-2024-final---english_pdf-102607294.pdf.

General Medical Council. (2023b). *National Training Survey 2023 results*. GMC. https://www.gmc-uk.org/-/media/documents/national-training-survey-2023-initial-findings-report_pdf-101939815.pdf.

General Medical Council. (2023c). *Professional standards. Maintaining personal and professional boundaries*. GMC. https://www.gmc-uk.org/-/media/gmc-site/ethical-guidance/mdg-2023/maintaining-personal-and-professional-boundaries-english.pdf.

General Medical Council. (2023d). *Professional Standards. Intimate examinations and chaperones*. GMC. https://www.gmc-uk.org/-/media/documents/intimate-examinations-and-chaperones_pdf-58835231.pdf.

General Medical Council. (2023e). *Guidance on assessing the seriousness of concerns relating to self-prescribing, or prescribing to those in close personal relationships with doctors*. GMC. https://www.gmc-uk.org/-/media/documents/dc6649-prescribing-concerns-58666780.pdf.

General Medical Council. (2023f). *Using social media as a medical professional*. GMC. https://www.gmc-uk.org/-/media/documents/using-social-media-as-a-medical-professional-final-version_pdf-105395775.pdf.

General Medical Council and Nursing & Midwifery Council. (2015). *Professional standards. Openness and honesty when things go wrong: The professional duty of candour (updated 2022)*. GMC. https://www.gmc-uk.org/-/media/documents/openness-and-honesty-when-things-go-wrong--the-professional-duty-of-cand____pdf-61540594.pdf.

Healthcare Quality Improvement Partnership. (2024). *The National Clinical Audit Programme*. https://www.hqip.org.uk/a-z-of-nca/

*Human Fertilisation and Embryology Act* 1990 (amended 2008).

*Human Tissue Act* 2004.

International Labour Organisation. (2001). Chapter V – Substantive provisions of labour legislation: The right to strike. In: *Labour Legislation guidelines*. https://www.ilo.org/static/english/dialogue/ifpdial/llg/noframes/ch5.htm

MBRRACE-UK. (2023). Maternal mortality 2019-2021. In: *Mothers and babies: Reducing risk through audits and confidential enquiries across the UK*. https://www.npeu.ox.ac.uk/mbrrace-uk/data-brief/maternal-mortality-2019-2021

Medications for Human Use (Clinical Trials) Regulations 2004.

*Mental Capacity Act* 2005.

NHS Employers. (2023). *Tackling bullying in the NHS infographic*. NHS Employers. https://www.nhsemployers.org/articles/tackling-bullying-nhs-infographic.

Parliament House of Lords. (2002). *Animals in scientific procedures – Report (HL 150-I)*. London: The Stationery Office Limited by Authority of The House of Lords.

Parsa-Parsi, R. W. (2022). The International Code of Medical Ethics of the World Medical Association. *Journal of the American Medical Association*, *328*(20), 2018–2021. https://doi.org/10.1001/jama.2022.19697.

Public Health (Infectious Diseases) Regulations 1988.

*Public Interest Disclosure Act* 1998.

Regulation (EU) 2016/679 (General Data Protection Regulation).

Scally, G., & Donaldson, L. J. (1998). The NHS's 50th anniversary. Clinical governance and the drive for quality improvement in the new NHS in England. *British Medical Journal*, *317*(7150), 61–65. doi: 10.1136/bmj.317.7150.61.

*Strikes (Minimum Service Levels) Act* 2023.

*Trade Union and Labour Relations (Consolidation) Act* 1992.

World Medical Association. (2013). World Medical Association Declaration of Helsinki: Ethical principles for medical research involving human subjects. *Journal of the American Medical Association*, *310*(20), 2191–2194. https://doi.org/10.1001/jama.2013.281053.

## Further Reading

Committee on Publication Ethics (COPE). http://www.publicationethics.org.

General Medical Council & Medical Schools Council. (2016). *Professional behaviour and fitness to practise: guidance for medical schools and their students*. General Medical Council and Medical

Schools Council. https://www.gmc-uk.org/-/media/documents/professional-behaviour-and-fitness-to-practise-20210811_pdf-66085925.pdf.

Hall, D. (2001). Reflecting on Redfern: What can we learn from the Alder Hey story? *Archives of Disease in Childhood*, *84*, 455–456. https://doi.org/10.1136/adc.84.6.455.

*Health and Social Care Act* 2008 (Regulated Activities).

Medical Practitioners Tribunal Service. (2023). *Record of determinations – Medical practitioners tribunal. Public record. Dates 21/08/2023–04/09/2023. GMC reference number 2890748*. https://www.mpts-uk.org/-/media/mpts-rod-files/dr-richard-scott-04-sep-23.pdf.

NHS England and NHS Improvement. (2021). *The matron's handbook. For aspiring and experienced matrons*. London: NHS England and NHS Improvement.

Williams, N. (2018). *Gross negligence manslaughter in healthcare. The report of a rapid policy review*. Crown. https://assets.publishing.service.gov.uk/media/5b2a3634ed915d2cc8317662/Williams_Report.pdf.

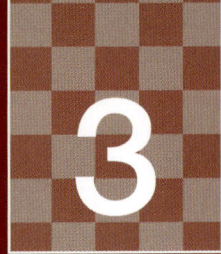
This chapter discusses wide-ranging issues with the common theme being the evolving social context of medical practice. First we consider traditional issues including consent and mental capacity, safeguarding and mental illness. We then turn to prominent and newer issues where medical practice interfaces with areas of significant social change; from the *Human Rights Act* 1998 and *Gender Recognition Act* 2004, we then consider cosmesis, iatrogenesis, genetics and new technologies.

## CONSENT

Consent is a core principle in medical law, following the ethical concept of autonomy. Patient consent to medical assessment and/or treatment protects the doctor against liability for trespass to the person (Fig. 3.1). Assessment or treatment provided without valid consent risks criminal prosecution for assault and battery. Assessment or treatment provided with inadequately informed consent risks litigation for damages. Adequate consent is needed in proportion to the level of intervention; it does not always need to be written:

- *Implied consent*: Patient behaviour suggests agreement. For example, the doctor advises the patient a blood test is needed and the patient holds out their arm to have this done.
- *Expressed verbal consent*: The patient explicitly agrees. For example, the doctor advises a rectal examination is required and offers a chaperone; the patient might agree for the examination and decline a chaperone (this should be documented, if you judge it is appropriate to proceed

on this basis). If you are unhappy to proceed without a chaperone you can delay the examination as long as the delay does not adversely impact on the patient (General Medical Council 2020a).
- *Written consent*: Needed for more invasive treatments including surgery (Fig. 3.2).

Following a discussion of risks, benefits and alternative approaches, in the context of factors that are significant to the patient; they sign a consent form to state that they have understood and agree. Be aware that a signed consent form is not conclusive proof of valid consent.

**ETHICS**

**THREE KEY ELEMENTS OF LEGALLY VALID CONSENT**

1. Voluntary: Consent or refusal must be given free of any pressures.
2. Fully informed: Consent or refusal must be based on adequate information.
3. Competence: The patient must be competent to consent to, or refuse, the treatment.

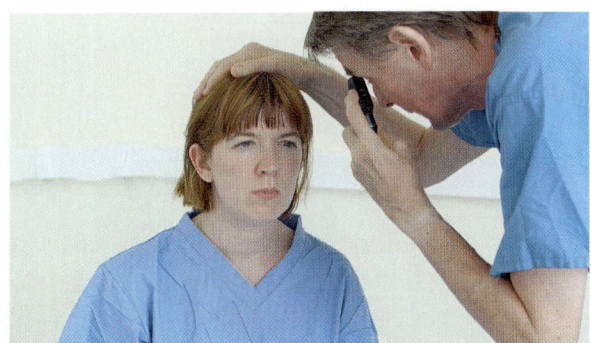

**Fig. 3.1** 'Intimate examinations'—sometimes a patient and doctor might have different ideas about what amounts to an intimate examination. For example, with an examination like fundoscopy in a darkened room or abdominal examination, use your judgement in the particular situation and consider sensitively enquiring about a chaperone.

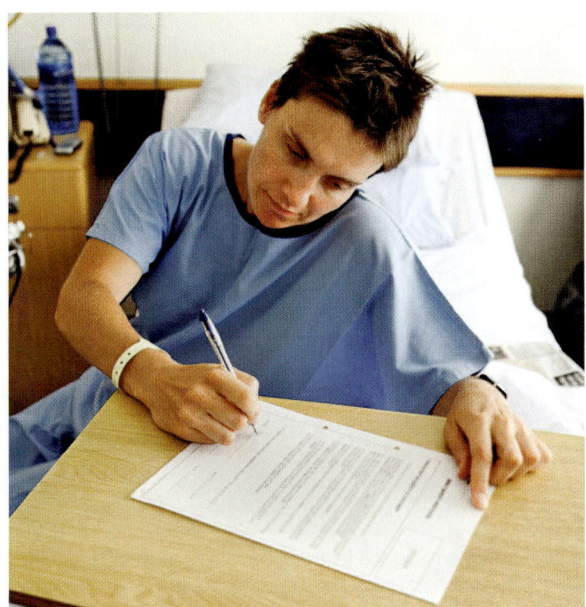

**Fig. 3.2** While important, a signed consent form is not conclusive proof of valid consent.

- The only justification for medical assessment and treatment in an adult patient without consent is by using the common law principle of best interest and only when they lack capacity to refuse. This may be in a medical emergency, for example cardiac arrest (Fig. 3.3).

## Voluntariness

Consent is invalid if the patient is subject to coercion or undue influence (Fig. 3.7).

---

### CASE 3.1 *RE T (ADULT: REFUSAL OF MEDICAL TREATMENT)* (1992)

T was 34 weeks' pregnant when she was injured in a car accident. Following conversations with her mother who was a Jehovah's Witness, T who was not herself a Jehovah's Witness subsequently refused a blood transfusion. T was later escalated to intensive care, was unconscious and a transfusion was seen as essential to save her life (Fig. 3.4).

Overriding T's earlier refusal, on hearing a range of family and health professional evidence the court held the normal right to self-determination had been compromised by the undue influence of the mother. It followed the duty of the doctors was to treat T according to their clinical judgement in her best interests and a blood transfusion could be given.

This case illustrates that while it is generally good practice to speak with the next of kin unless the patient asks you not to, family members have no automatic legal right to consent to or refuse treatment on behalf of a patient who is temporarily or permanently incapacitated.

Where doctors have doubts about the validity of an (advance) refusal of treatment for a serious condition, the courts can be involved swiftly for a declaration on the lawfulness of treatment.

---

## Sufficient information

Your duty is to provide enough information so the patient in front of you understands what will be done, why, and the benefits, risks and alternatives. Information considered important by the patient will differ depending on many factors including their clinical context, values, circumstances and life choices. The amount of information that is 'sufficient' is also a matter of judgement for each situation and requires you to explore the perspective of the particular patient. For example, a person blind in one eye may perceive the significance of risks of treatment on their seeing eye differently to a person with binocular vision. An opera singer might be especially interested in any potential side effects impacting their voice. The severe hypoxic complication in the Montgomery case, was a low frequency risk of <0.1% that was held significant considering the individual situation (Case 3.2). Generally speaking, the doctor is unable to decide independently what constitutes sufficient information for their patient.

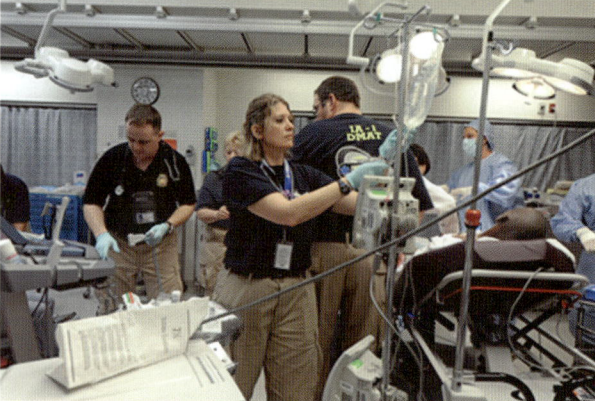

**Fig. 3.3** Treatment in good faith without the consent of an adult patient is typically done in an emergency situation under common law. In the absence of other information and when the patient is unable to give consent, it is assumed the patient in their own best interests would want their life to be saved if possible—for example.

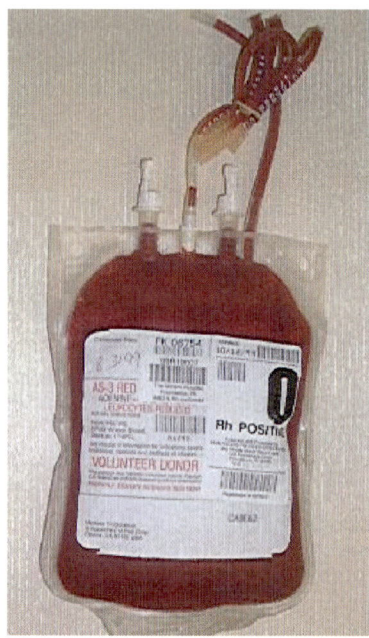

**Fig. 3.4** Blood ready to be transfused.

**CASE 3.2** *MONTGOMERY (APPELLANT) V. LANARKSHIRE HEALTH BOARD (RESPONDENT) (SCOTLAND) (2015)*

Nadine Montgomery was pregnant in 1999. She was known to have type 1 diabetes mellitus and small stature. She had asked if the size of her baby was a potential problem. She went on to deliver her son vaginally having not been counselled about the risks of shoulder dystocia (Fig. 3.5), which occurred. Delayed progression through labour led to her son Sam suffering a hypoxic brain injury and developing cerebral palsy. Nadine Montgomery said she would have requested the alternative of a caesarean section if she had known of the risks.

Finding in her favour, the Supreme Court overturned a previous decision by the House of Lords. Where previously *sufficient information* was a matter of medical opinion as per the Bolam and Bolitho cases (see Chapter 2), now the individual patient needs to be told what they want or need to know before they can give valid consent. The legal ruling reflects prevailing ethical currents supporting patient autonomy and shared decision-making and moves away from medical paternalism.

**The test of materiality:** In the individual case, is the court satisfied that a reasonable person in the patient's position would give significance to a given risk. If so, the doctor should discuss the material risks of treatment and reasonable alternative options (which may include no treatment).

To sue for negligence by means of *insufficient* consent the patient must prove:

- Information given was inadequate by accepted standards.
- With adequate information their consent would have been withheld at the time.

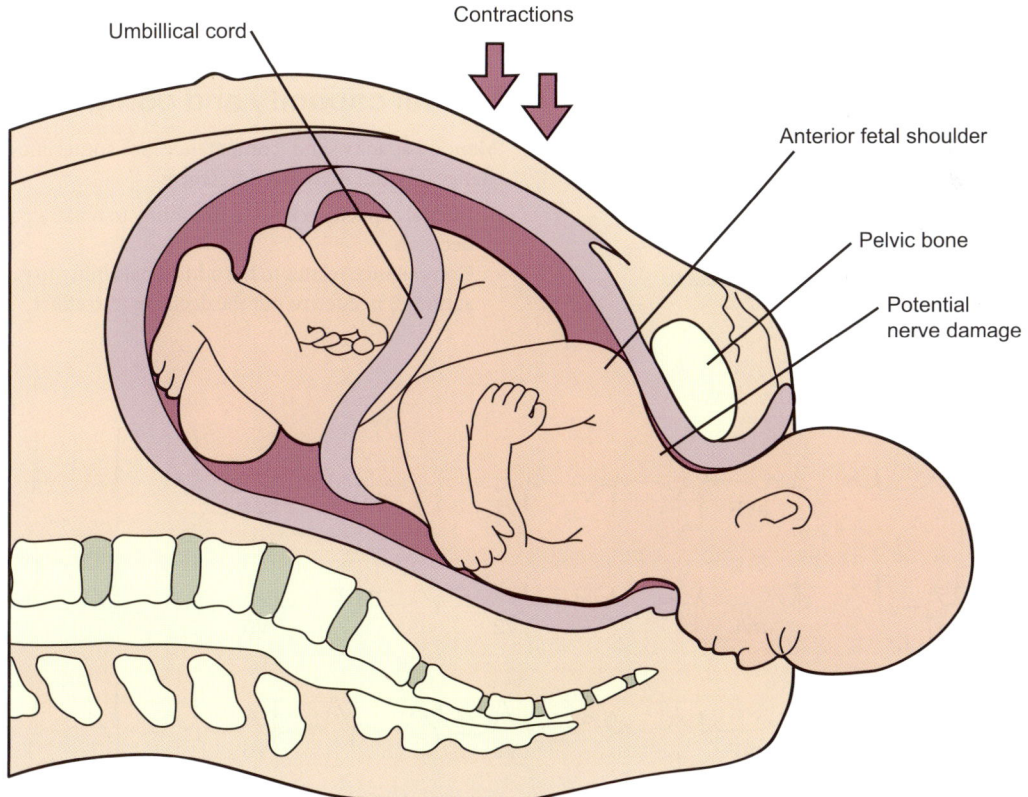

**Fig. 3.5** Shoulder dystocia causing Erb palsy.

- Harm resulted from the intervention for which informed consent was inadequate.

Insufficient consent was tested in the case of *McCulloch and others (Appellants) v. Forth Valley Health Board (Respondent) (Scotland)* (2023) (Case 3.3—where the claim failed) and in the case of *Birch v. University College London Hospital NHS Foundation Trust* (2008) (Case 3.4—where the claim succeeded).

### CASE 3.3 *MCCULLOCH AND OTHERS (APPELLANTS) V. FORTH VALLEY HEALTH BOARD (RESPONDENT) (SCOTLAND)* (2023)

Mr McCulloch died in 2012 from cardiac arrest. His cardiologist had concluded that the presentation was inconsistent with pericarditis (Fig. 3.6) and did not offer a nonsteroidal antiinflammatory drug (NSAID). A claim was brought alleging a breach in the duty of care by failing to inform the patient of NSAIDs as a possible treatment option.

Expert witnesses advised that some doctors would have prescribed NSAIDs in the clinical scenario, but a logical body of medical opinion would also support the decision not to. The Supreme Court held the 'professional practice test' (Bolam, Bolitho) is sufficient here. If in the doctor's opinion a treatment option is not a reasonable alternative, and this is supported by a reasonable body of medical opinion, the doctor did not act negligently.

*Reasonable treatment options to consider are defined by doctors (not patients or the court).*

### CASE 3.4 *BIRCH V. UNIVERSITY COLLEGE LONDON HOSPITAL NHS FOUNDATION TRUST* (2008)

Janet Birch was admitted with atypical symptoms of third cranial nerve palsy and had a background of type 1 diabetes mellitus. An MRI scan was recommended to exclude posterior communicating artery aneurysm or cavernous sinus pathology as differential diagnoses. There were no MRI slots available and she was transferred to a neurosurgical ward. Neurosurgeons opted to perform catheter angiography; a mildly invasive procedure with increased risks for the individual patient. The risks of catheter angiography were explained, and the procedure resulted in a stroke with significant disability.

While medical opinion supported the option of investigation with the catheter angiography in the circumstances of the case, it was found negligent not to have discussed the comparative risks of investigating with MRI instead.

*Reasonable investigative options must be discussed for consent to be sufficiently informed.*

## Mental capacity and competence

'Mental capacity' and 'competence' are sometimes used interchangeably, but there is a difference:

- Mental capacity relates to the ability to make a particular decision.
- Competence relates to the additional ability to perform the action(s) needed to put the decision into effect.

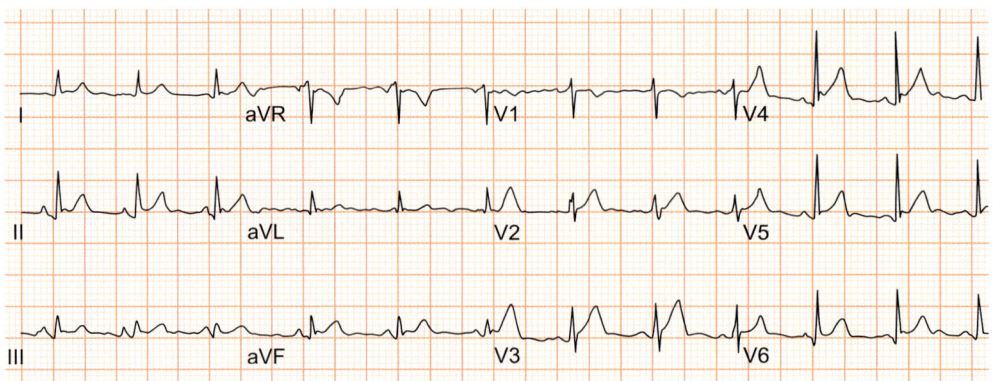

**Fig. 3.6** ECG in acute pericarditis showing PR segment depression (prominent in leads II and III) and ST elevation in multiple leads with concavity upwards.

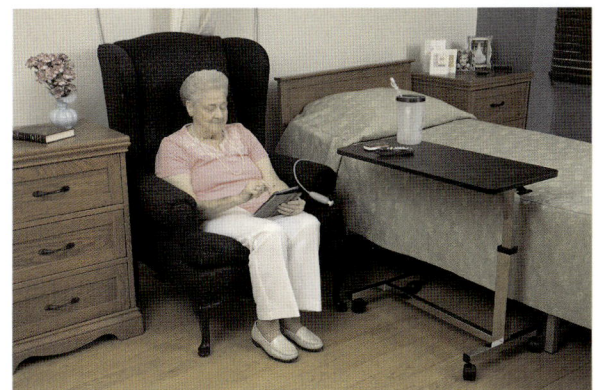

**Fig. 3.7** The liberty of vulnerable individuals often needs to be considered and should be safely maximized in long stay nursing and residential facilities.

- Hence a patient is 'competent to consent to (or refuse) treatment if they have the mental capacity to make that particular treatment decision'.

There are four elements to a capacity assessment. All must be met for the patient to be assessed as having capacity to make a particular decision:

1. Understand the relevant information.
2. Retain the relevant information long enough to make a decision.
3. Weigh the relevant information to make a choice.
4. Communicate that choice, using all practical means to aid communication.

This is included in the *Mental Capacity Act* 2005 and is sometimes called the 'Re C Test'.

---

**CASE 3.5** *THE 'RE C TEST' AND MENTAL CAPACITY — RE C (ADULT: REFUSAL OF MEDICAL TREATMENT) (1994)*

C was a patient with chronic paranoid schizophrenia who was detained in a secure psychiatric hospital in 1994. He developed gangrene of his foot and refused life-saving amputation.

C successfully brought a legal injunction to stop the proposed amputation without express written consent. It was found that while C had various delusional beliefs related to his schizophrenia that would have compromised his capacity to make other decisions; he was able to understand, retain, believe and weigh up the relevant information — and so make the

---

autonomous choice to refuse a potentially life-saving amputation.

The key difference between the 'Re C Test' and the test of capacity in the *Mental Capacity Act* 2005 is that patients are not required to *believe* that medical information is true in the MCA test.

This case also illustrates how a patient assessed as having capacity is allowed to make what some observers may consider an unwise decision.

**Key points about capacity:**

- Decision-specific: The patient may have the capacity to consent to or refuse a particular treatment, while not having the capacity to make other decisions.
- Mental illness: This does not necessarily diminish capacity to consent or refuse.
- Third-party influence: Capacity may be diminished by the undue influence of others—this sometimes needs to be considered in the setting of intimate partner violence, for example.
- Temporary disturbances: Capacity may also be temporarily diminished by exhaustion or pain.

## Further notes on the *Mental Capacity Act 2005*

- It applies to individuals aged 16 years and above—that is children aged 16 and 17 and adults—and intends to protect vulnerable people who cannot make their own decisions.
- A person aged below 16 years may be assessed as *competent* in certain circumstances, and the *Mental Capacity Act* does not apply to them.

### Five principles

- **Presumption of capacity:** All people aged 16 years and above are presumed to have the capacity to consent or refuse unless proved otherwise; people aged below 18 years are known as children in UK law and refusals of treatment by below 18 s can sometimes be overridden by a person with parental responsibility or by a court.
- **Support:** A person must be given all appropriate help to make their own decision before anyone concludes they are incapable.
- **Unwise decisions:** A person has the right to make what others may think is an unwise decision.
- **Best interests:** Decisions made on behalf of a person lacking capacity must be in their best interests.

- **Least restrictive:** Decisions and actions taken for a person lacking capacity should be least restrictive of their basic rights and future freedoms.

## Advance planning

- A Lasting Power of Attorney (LPA) can be nominated in anticipation of a (possible) future loss of capacity. There are two types: health and welfare, and property and financial affairs. The holder of an LPA only for property and financial affairs does not have any right to make health and welfare decisions.
- The person/patient creating the LPA can decide to restrict what decisions their attorney(s) can make.
- The *Court of Protection* can also make decisions on behalf of a person without capacity and may delegate to the *Office of the Public Guardian* the power to assign a 'court-appointed deputy'—often a relative or friend. If no one is available an *Independent Mental Capacity Advocate* can be appointed to make decisions in the best interests of the patient.
- 'ADRT'—Advance Decision to Refuse Treatment. These can only be made by a person aged 18 years or above. To be valid, the ADRT must be made at a time when the person still has capacity, and since making it the person must not have given any indication of having changed their mind or have behaved inconsistently with the decision. An advance decision to refuse life-prolonging treatment needs to be written, be clear about the specific circumstances to which it applies, be signed/dated by the patient and an independent witness and indicate an awareness that the treatment refusal amounts to a risk to life.

---

### Legal difference

The *Mental Capacity Act* 2005 does not apply in Scotland. Instead, the *Adults with Incapacity (Scotland) Act* 2000 is used. Where an individual is deemed to lack capacity, the following five principles are to be applied when making decisions on their behalf:

1. Benefit: The action must benefit the person with incapacity.
2. Least restrictive option.
3. Take into account the wishes of the person with incapacity.
4. Consultation with relevant others; this includes family and friends.
5. Encouraging the adult: as far as is practicable, the adult should be encouraged to manage their own affairs and to develop their ability to do so.

---

**HINTS AND TIPS**

**'I HAVE A LASTING POWER OF ATTORNEY'**

If someone close to the patient tells you they have a power of attorney, and you assess the patient lacks capacity for the clinical decision in question; you still need to be sure the attorney has been appointed for health and welfare decisions rather than property and financial affairs, and you need to know if the patient placed any restrictions on the decision-making scope of their attorney(s).

## Medical Treatment Without Capacity

Try to facilitate direct participation of the patient where possible. This can include arranging consultations at a time of day when the patient is most likely to be able to participate in decision-making due to fluctuating capacity or facilitating alternative modes of communication, such as through pictures when verbal communication is not possible. In an emergency to save life or prevent serious deterioration in health, you are protected by the 'doctrine of necessity' in providing medical treatment to a patient lacking capacity. When there is time it is best practice to consult those close to the patient as to what the patient would likely want, and what would be in their best interests.

## Deprivation of Liberty Safeguards and Liberty Protection Safeguards

DOLS were introduced in 2009 and replaced by LPS following the *Mental Capacity (Amendment) Act* 2019. The broad aim is to ensure a patient under constantly high levels of supervision or 'control' is not unreasonably denied their liberty, for example people in care homes or hospitals who lack the mental capacity to consent to their care arrangements. Consider:

- Restraint or sedation used to admit a person to an institution where the person resists.
- Staff exercising complete control over the care and movement of a person.
- A decision taken by the institution that the person will not be released into the care of others or permitted to live elsewhere.
- Where a request by carers for a person to be discharged to their care is refused.
- If a person is unable to maintain social contacts because of restrictions placed on their access to other people.

A written authorization is provided to support ongoing treatment or care for an initial period of 1 year at most; reauthorizations may be for longer periods (up to 3 years). DOLS were authorized by local authorities (councils); LPS will instead be authorized by NHS hospitals for their patients, by local health boards for community patients and by local authorities (councils) for everyone else including care home or hospice patients.

- DOLS applied from age 18 years, LPS will apply from age 16 years.
- DOLS was institution-specific, LPS will be person-specific and may involve multiple locations including the person's own home.
- LPS strengthen the duty to consult those caring for and close to the patient.

---

**ETHICS**

### WHAT IS A DEPRIVATION OF LIBERTY? (UK SUPREME COURT IN 2014)

Deprivation of liberty is linked to Article 5 of the European Convention on Human Rights

- The person is unable to make a decision about the care they receive or where they live and is unable to consent to the arrangements in place for their care because of a 'Mental Disorder'.
- The person is under 'continuous supervision and control'.
- The person is 'not free to leave'.
  Follows from the case: *P (by his litigation friend the Official Solicitor) (FC) (Appellant) v. Cheshire West and Chester Council and another (Respondents)* (2014).

---

# Potentially vulnerable people

## Cognitive impairment in adults

Adults may have lasting cognitive impairment for various reasons. Learning disability affects approximately 1.5 million people in the United Kingdom (2%–2.5% of the population). Approximately 1 million adults in the United Kingdom are affected by dementia, which increases in prevalence with age to 1 in 11 people aged above 65 years. Just because a person has a diagnosed learning disability, or dementia, or even if they are very old or appear frail—it does not necessarily mean they lack capacity to make or to participate in making, a particular decision about their life. Where a person has previously had a greater cognitive capacity, they may have previously expressed wishes or consistently behaved in ways which can help inform a decision that needs to be made now.

---

**HINTS AND TIPS**

### KEY POINT

Remember some people with learning disability and dementia syndromes are undiagnosed, and the severity and impact of these conditions can vary from mild to profound. You need to assess each person individually and in relation to the particular decision that is required at the time.

---

**CASE 3.6** *H.L. V. THE UNITED KINGDOM* (2004) EUROPEAN COURT OF HUMAN RIGHTS

*'THE BOURNEWOOD CASE'—A COMPLIANT BUT INCAPACITATED PATIENT*

In 1997 HL was a 48-year-old autistic male with profound learning disabilities. In the 32 years prior to 1994 he had lived at Bournewood psychiatric hospital and since 1994 had lived with Mr and Mrs E in their home under a resettlement scheme. One day he became agitated at a day centre and risked a serious injury to himself. He was taken to Accident and Emergency, given sedation and readmitted to Bournewood. If HL had tried to leave, he would have been detained under the *Mental Health Act* 1983. While he never tried to leave, he remained an informal patient and none of the protections under the *Mental Health Act* could be applied.

Although HL was released after several months, Mr and Mrs E took the case to court for unlawful detention. The House of Lords found the admission of HL without his capacity to consent or refuse was lawful and could be supported by the doctrine of necessity in his best interests; but it was noted this left a *compliant but incapacitated patient* without any legal safeguards against an extended admission. The European Court of Human Rights, considering Article 5, later found that HL had been unlawfully deprived of his liberty: it was unlawful because there was no readily accessible procedure to obtain an independent review. This led to the Deprivation of Liberty Safeguards (DOLS) being introduced in 2009.

DOLS and its replacement, the Liberty Protection Safeguards, intend to provide legal protection for vulnerable people deprived of their liberty who are not detained under the *Mental Health Act* 1983. This is a mechanism to prevent arbitrary decisions which deprive a person of their liberty and to give rights to challenge deprivation of liberty authorizations. It can be seen among the currents flowing away from medical paternalism.

## Children

Children in UK law are people aged below 18 years. Children aged 16 years and above are presumed to have the mental capacity to *consent to* treatment, following the *Family Law Reform Act* 1969. Treatment refusals by children are more complex.

## CASE 3.7 *GILLICK V. WEST NORFOLK AND WISBECH AREA HEALTH AUTHORITY* (1986)

The case arose after a Department of Health and Social Security circular advocating the preservation of confidentiality when the patient was requesting contraception, even if the patient was aged below 16 years. Mrs Gillick had 10 children, a number of whom were girls below the age of 16. She went to court to challenge the Health Authority's ability to give contraceptive advice to her children without her knowledge or consent (Fig. 3.8). The case was settled in the House of Lords, which decided against Mrs Gillick:

- The parental responsibility to 'control a child' exists to benefit the child not the parent; the best interests of the child have priority; children in the United Kingdom are not the property of their parents.
- The parental right yields to the child's right when the child reaches sufficient understanding and intelligence.
- Sufficient understanding and intelligence may be reached before the age of 16 years.
- The doctor must assess if the child understands the medical, social and moral aspects of the proposed treatment.

In the Gillick case, Lord Fraser produced guidelines for clinicians providing contraceptive advice or treatment to children below the age of 16. The clinician must be satisfied:

- The young person understands the medical advice.
- The young person cannot be persuaded to inform their parents.
- The young person is likely to begin or continue having sexual intercourse even without contraception.
- Unless the young person receives contraception, their physical or mental health or both are likely to suffer.
- The young person's best interests require them to receive contraceptive advice or treatment with or without parental consent.

In summary:

- Gillick competence: Children below 16 years demonstrating sufficient maturity can *consent to* medical advice and treatment, and they have a right to confidentiality.
- Fraser guidelines relate specifically to contraceptive treatment and advice for children below 16 years.

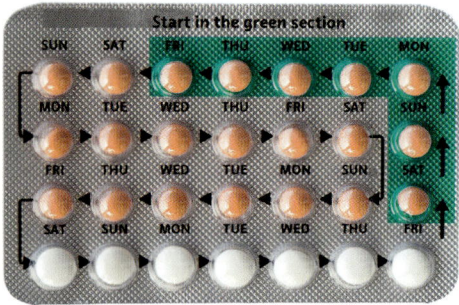

**Fig. 3.8** A 4-week pack of the combined hormonal contraceptive pill, with seven pills highlighted in green to indicate the start section for pill intake. The arrows and days printed on the pack indicate the sequence for the consumption of pills. This particular issue comes with seven white pills which are not hormonally active, intended to effect a withdrawal bleed.

Following the Gillick case, and considering the legal age of consent for sexual intercourse in the United Kingdom is 16 years: the *Sexual Offences Act* 2003 states that a doctor who provides contraceptive and sexual health advice or treatment to a Gillick-competent below 16 years will not be considered an accessory to a sexual offence. Note however that a child aged below 13 years is unable to legally consent to any form of sexual activity, so any such case requires safeguarding actions and is a case of statutory rape.

### Legal divergence

In Scotland, the Fraser guidelines do not apply. Instead, the *Age of Legal Capacity (Scotland) Act* 1991 is used, which applies similar criteria.

### Children and the refusal of treatment

The duty of a doctor includes offering treatment in the best interests of a patient. This may help to explain why a child may be assessed as competent to *consent to* treatment relatively more readily than being assessed as competent *to refuse* a recommended treatment, especially where the consequences of refusal are potentially serious. Courts have tended to conclude that a child (below 18) making an 'unwise decision' is not competent and for the parent(s) or the court to overrule a treatment refusal.

### ETHICS

#### KEY POINT

**0–18 years: guidance for all doctors (**General Medical Council, 2020b)
   *You should seek legal advice if you think treatment is in the best interests of a competent young person who refuses.*

**CASE 3.8** *NHS TRUST V. X (IN THE MATTER OF X (A CHILD) (NO 2)) (2021)*

X was a 15-year-old girl with sickle cell disease and along with her mother was a Jehovah's Witness. During the summer and autumn of 2020, she required repeated hospital admissions and life-saving blood transfusions for sickle cell crises. Urgent applications were made to the court for authorization to provide treatment—these were granted. A rolling-authorization was also sought to provide for similar situations up to the age of 18 years—these were refused on the grounds that any future situations would need to be considered in their actual context.

- A child does not have an absolute right to refuse medical treatment; whether they are below 16 and Gillick-competent or aged 16 to 17 years with capacity; the court can overrule a refusal of treatment and particularly where there is a risk of death or serious permanent harm from refusal.
- Court powers under the *Children Act* 1989 (updated in 2004) allow orders in the 'best interests' of an under 18, the starting position for which is held to be seeking the survival of a child to adulthood.

## Parental responsibility

A person with parental responsibility can consent to medical assessment and treatment on behalf of a child. Parental responsibility defines who can consent to *nonurgent* medical assessment and treatment if the child is incompetent. More than one person may have parental responsibility, but a doctor requires consent from only one.

---

**CLINICAL NOTES**

**PARENTAL RESPONSIBILITY (FROM GMC 0–18 YEARS: GUIDANCE FOR ALL DOCTORS)**

- Mothers and married fathers have parental responsibility automatically; this remains even in the event of later divorce.
- Unmarried fathers are named on the birth certificate.
- Married step-parents and registered civil partners can acquire parental responsibility through a Parental Responsibility Agreement with the mother or by getting a Parental Responsibility Order from the court.
- Parents lose parental responsibility if a child is adopted; parental responsibility passes to the adoptive parents.
- Parental responsibility can be restricted by court order.
- Local authorities have parental responsibility while a child is subject to a care order.
- People without parental responsibility, but who have care of a child, may do what is reasonable to safeguard or promote the child's welfare, for example step-parents, grandparents and childminders. You can rely on their consent if they are authorized by the parents. Ensure their decisions align with those of the parents, particularly for contentious or important decisions.
- Seek legal advice when in doubt about who has parental responsibility.

## SAFEGUARDING

Safeguarding relates to the duty to identify and keep a person free from abuse. There are many types of abuse, which can occur together in any combination. Any type of abuse can be just as impactful. UK Care and Statutory Support Guidance identifies ten types of abuse (Department of Health and Social Care, 2023; Social Care Institute for Excellence, 2015):

- Coercive control
- Discriminatory abuse
- Domestic violence or abuse
- Financial or material abuse
- Modern slavery
- Neglect or acts of omission
- Organizational or institutional abuse
- Psychological or emotional abuse
- Physical abuse
- Self-neglect
- Sexual abuse

Sometimes a person may be vulnerable to abuse and realize; other times a person may be vulnerable and not realize. Children and adults with cognitive impairment are particularly vulnerable, but abuse can affect anyone. The Office for National Statistics (2023) estimates that in a 1-year period the prevalence of domestic abuse is around 10% of the adult population (6% of females and 3% of males, based on incidents actually reported into the Crime Survey for England and Wales, which are likely to underestimate the true prevalence). The lifetime prevalence is one in four females, and one in six males. For comparison, the UK adult population prevalence of chronic kidney disease is around 6%, and type 2 diabetes mellitus around 9%. Beyond physical injuries; abuse can present as medically unexplained symptoms, persistent physical symptoms and mental health symptoms (Husain & Chalder 2021).

As a doctor, you may be the first person the patient has trusted with information about previous or ongoing abuse. You have a duty to act to try to prevent avoidable harm, and when possible it is best to do so with the patient's knowledge and consent. You may decide to speak to:

- Senior members of the clinical team.
- Organizational safeguarding lead (e.g. hospital/GP surgery)—usually a clinical colleague.
- Your local Adult's Social Work on-call team (from age 18, sometimes from age 16).
- Your local Children's Social Work on-call team (provision may vary at age 16 and 17).

A Social Worker is usually employed by the Local Authority ('the council'); has access to more information and will be familiar with liaising with the Police, Schools and any other relevant parties. A Social Worker is often better placed than a clinician to investigate and understand the totality of the risks in a given safeguarding situation and respond proportionately. Hospital admission is sometimes used for adults or children, providing a safe space for full assessment.

- You may meet and treat people who are vulnerable to being drawn into terrorism. Radicalization is comparable to other types of exploitation, and safeguarding principles should be applied to such situations. The *Counter-Terrorism and Security Act* 2015 creates a 'prevent duty' on NHS employers, including training staff appropriately in recognizing radicalization.

## Adult abuse, including abuse of older adults

Risk factors may relate to the victim, the carer or be shared by both.

- *The victim*: Dependency; communication difficulties, cognitive impairment, behavioural problems.
- *The carer*: Drug or alcohol misuse; lifestyle adversely affected by caring role; divided loyalties (e.g. older relative and young child); physical or mental health problems; role reversal (e.g. ageing child and aged parent) and isolation (real or perceived).
- *Shared*: Poor housing and poor long-term relationship.

  Warning signs may include:

- Unexplained injuries or recurrent accidents.
- Bruises or burns in unusual areas or shaped like an object.
- Odd patient behaviour (e.g. anxious, frightened or withdrawn).
- Difficulty gaining access to the patient.
- Refusal of necessary support services by the patient or carer.

**Adult abuse, including abuse of older adults**, can be ethically challenging. A person with mental capacity has the right to choose to remain in a vulnerable setting and to decline your offer to involve social services. If you suspect patient autonomy is compromised by reduced capacity or coercion, you may decide to involve social services.

## Child abuse

The 1989 United Nations Convention on the Rights of the Child obliges nations to ensure resources and services are available to serve the needs and interests of children. Children have a right to dignity, respect and the opportunity to participate in decision-making.

## *The Children Act* 1989 (amended 2004)

- Defines a child as a person below 18 years old.
- Identifies the welfare of the child as of *paramount importance* in court decisions.
- Defines how to make decisions where those with parental responsibility disagree.
- Provides ways to protect a child from harm in the event of those with parental responsibility being unable; this includes Emergency Protection Orders.
- Safety of a child is more important than other considerations, such as confidentiality.

## *Female Genital Mutilation Act* 2003

Female Genital Mutilation is illegal in the United Kingdom, and it is also illegal to take a child out of the United Kingdom for the purposes of FGM. It is a specific example of violence against females and girls with physical and emotional aspects: the female genital organs are physically injured or changed without medical reason. In females below 18 years this includes any genital piercing or tattoo. FGM can be severely painful with short and long-term consequences: mental health problems, uro-gynaecological symptoms and difficulties in childbirth with risks to the child and mother including death. Cultural practices vary from neonatal, to childhood or adolescence, to just before marriage or first pregnancy. Approximately 65,000 UK girls below 14 years are at risk, and the communities most at risk include Somalian, Kenyan, Sudanese, Eritrean, Egyptian, Nigerian and Sierra Leonean. FGM is also practiced in Turkey, Kurdistan, Yemen, Afghanistan, Pakistan (South), Thailand, Malaysia and Indonesia. In everyday speech 'female genital mutilation' is unlikely to be the phrasing used; instead be alert to references to 'cutting', 'female circumcision', 'initiation', 'Sunna', 'infibulation' or going to a 'coming of age ceremony'.

**CLINICAL NOTES**

**FEMALE GENITAL MUTILATION AND HEALTH PROFESSIONAL DUTIES**

- *You must report to the police any case of FGM that you discover in the course of your work when the patient is aged below 18 years at the time you become aware—this means either a history direct from the patient or an examination of the patient. This is a legal*

*(Continued)*

# MENTAL HEALTH

The definitions and contours of mental illness have changed over time. In 1851 'drapetomania' was described as an illness affecting slaves with the tendency to run away from their masters. The *Suicide Act* 1961 decriminalized suicide in England and Wales, meaning the survivor of a suicide attempt would no longer be prosecuted. Homosexuality was categorized as a mental disorder in the *Diagnostic and Statistical Manual of Mental Disorders* until 1973. As discussed elsewhere, terms like gender dysphoria and gender incongruence have entered the psychiatry lexicon, which continues to be in a state of flux. A fundamental difference with other areas of medical practice is that understandings of the biological basis for psychiatric conditions are relatively underdeveloped. Genomic medicine and functional imaging are helping to advance the debate about the nature of mental illness—a debate going back at least to Plato and Hippocrates (Malla, Joober & Garcia, 2015; Liston et al., 2022).

Mental illness (Fig. 3.9) potentially carries more ethical issues than physical illness. Some political regimes in the 20th century misused psychiatry to suppress dissenters (van Voren, 2016). Mental illness can be used to mitigate behaviours that might be considered antisocial, immoral or criminal. While aiming to help the patient; psychiatrists also inform court decisions on who is punished and who is treated, who is told to work and who receives benefits. For this reason psychiatrists are sometimes portrayed as 'double agents'. Patient confidentiality can cause tensions: in the case of Egdell (1989) an independent psychiatrist was challenged by a detained patient who sought application for release or transfer to lower-security accommodation. Dr Egdell learned the unfavourable assessment about the dangerousness of the patient was not being shared and broke confidentiality: this was supported by the courts because the disclosure was held to be in the public interest.

## The *Mental Health Act* 1983 (amended 2007)

- 'Mental disorder' means any disorder or disability of the mind.
- Enables detention for assessment and treatment of high-risk patients with mental illness.
- Includes independent review mechanisms to ensure these powers are not abused.
- Most patients with mental illness have capacity and agree to treatment voluntarily—do not use the MHA unless it is needed.

There are over 100 'sections' in the *Mental Health Act*. In particular:

- Section 2 is compulsory admission for assessment not exceeding 28 days.
  - Two registered doctors and an approved social worker or relative must agree.
  - Patients can access an independent mental health tribunal to consider early discharge from the section.
- Section 3 is compulsory admission for treatment, initially not exceeding 6 months.

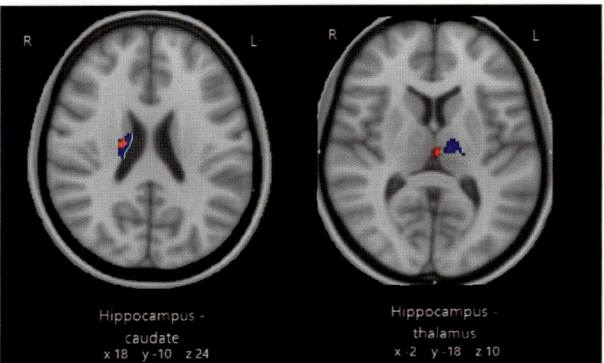

**Fig. 3.9** Altered hippocampal functioning is proposed to play a critical role in the development of schizophrenia-spectrum disorders.

- Two registered doctors and an approved social worker or relative must agree.
- Extendable the first time by 6 months, then for up to 3 years at a time.
- Patients can access an independent mental health tribunal to consider early discharge from the section.
- Section 5(2) allows a doctor to detain a person in hospital for up to 72 hours, until an assessment that decides if further detention under the *Mental Health Act* is needed.
- Section 5(4) allows a nurse to detain a patient in hospital for up to 6 hours, until they are reviewed by a doctor.
- Section 17 has provisions for a patient to be granted conditional leave to spend some time in the community as part of rehabilitation and treatment.
- Section 135 allows police to enter a person's home and take them to (or maintain them in) a place of safety for a mental health assessment to be done.
- Section 136 allows police to remove a person from a public place, when they seem to be suffering from a mental disorder, to a place of safety for a mental health assessment.
- Dependence on alcohol or drugs is not considered to be a disorder or disability of the mind (i.e. a mental disorder) under the MHA.
- The Second Opinion Assessment Doctor system is an important part of the *Mental Health Act* provisions—they have to be consulted in particular situations and at particular time points to check whether treatment is clinically appropriate and patient views and rights have been considered.

At the time of writing a draft Mental Health Bill is in English parliament and there may be updates to these laws. There have been concerns about rising rates of detention overall and over-representation of people from Black, Asian and minority ethnic groups in the detained population (Parliament, 2023). Reforms may raise the threshold for detention, shorten the review interval for those detained and expand access to advocacy services, aim to reduce the use of the MHA for people with learning disabilities and autistic people and improve the experience of patients.

---

**CLINICAL NOTES**

**TO USE THE *MENTAL HEALTH ACT* OR *MENTAL CAPACITY ACT*?**

- The *Mental Health Act 1983* (2007) primarily is for compulsory assessment and treatment of people who because of mental illness may be a danger to themselves or others; there is no age restriction.
  - An Advance Decision to Refuse Treatment can be overridden if the patient is correctly detained under the MHA *and* the medication is to treat mental disorder.

---

- If the patient has a power of attorney for health and welfare the attorney role becomes constrained in certain areas, in particular the MHA overrides the ability of the attorney to determine consent to certain mental health treatments and where the patient lives.
- The *Mental Capacity Act* 2005 primarily is to ensure the best interests and maximize the liberty of people without cognitive capacity aged above 16.
- In practice occasionally, either the MHA or MCA might be a justifiable option.
  - Risk-based proportionate restraint of the patient in either case is a significant ethical consideration.
  - Concerns continue about overreliance on the use of force, which sometimes needs to be used against a vulnerable patient to maintain patient or third-party safety.

## *Human Rights Act* 1998 (European Convention for Human Rights)

The *Human Rights Act* 1998 is UK legislation. The principles mirror the European Convention for Human Rights—an international treaty originally ratified in 1951 in the aftermath of World War II agreed by member states of *The Council of Europe* (a human rights organization, which is not the same as the European Union). It describes personal rights and freedoms, known as 'articles'—and applies to how the state treats an individual person. 'The state' means public authorities, including state-funded healthcare systems like the NHS. Individual rights sometimes have to be weighed against issues of individual responsibility and/or the public interest.

---

**CLINICAL NOTES**

**RIGHTS AND FREEDOMS MOST LIKELY TO HAVE RELEVANCE IN STATE-PROVIDED MEDICAL CONTEXTS**

- Article 2: Right to life
- Article 3: Freedom from torture and inhuman or degrading treatment
- Article 4: Freedom from slavery and forced labour
- Article 5: Right to liberty and security
- Article 8: Right to respect for private and family life
- Article 9: Freedom of thought, conscience and religion
- Article 10: Freedom of expression
- Article 12: Right to marry and start a family
- Article 14: Protection from discrimination in respect of these rights and freedoms

While 'the convention rights and freedoms' are all matters for the state and its organizations to uphold; professional codes of practice for individual medical practitioners share similarities with several 'articles' or otherwise complement them.

Regarding:

- Article 2: See Chapter 4.
- Article 3: Could be invoked where standards of healthcare in an organization give rise to serious concerns.
- Article 4: You sometimes need to be alert to identify a patient in a situation of modern slavery and follow safeguarding procedures.
- Article 5: May be invoked if the *Mental Health Act* is used incorrectly to detain a person.
- Article 8: Note the case in Chapter 2 about the Doctors' private WhatsApp group, which was shared in fitness to practice proceedings to help maintain the duty of the medical regulator to uphold public confidence in the profession. Article 8 is about an individual right to freedom from state interference in personal life, which can be limited in certain situations.
- Article 9: See Chapter 2.
- Article 10: May be relevant if there were attempts to suppress the raising of concerns (whistleblowing) about a public-funded healthcare organization.
- Article 12: Does not require the state to provide assisted conception services, but once they are provided it must be done without unjustified discrimination.
- Article 14: Has been raised in relation to concerns about equality of access to NHS assisted conception services for same-sex couples, for example.

---

**CASE 3.9  HUMAN RIGHTS ABUSES IN INSTITUTIONAL CARE SETTINGS**

Veilstone Care Home provided privately run, NHS-funded beds for adults with a learning disability. Ben was approximately aged 20 in 2010–11 and developed posttraumatic stress disorder related to episodes of excessive restraint, denial of family contact and the repeated use of a 'quiet room' as punishment. The High Court declared in 2023 that Ben's rights under Article 3 (torture and inhuman or degrading treatment) and Article 8 (the right to family and private life) were breached, and also that his Mum's rights were breached under Article 8 as her visits were prevented (Leigh Day, 2023).

Legal confirmation of human rights abuses is in addition to the criminal convictions of several former staff members at Veilstone some years before. Ben had previously been a resident at Winterbourne View near Bristol, where physical and psychological abuse of residents came to light via an undercover television documentary and individual staff members received criminal convictions.

Whorlton Hall Hospital in County Durham was also the subject of undercover television reporting in 2019 that showed patients being mocked and abused by staff. It also provided privately run, NHS-funded beds for people with a learning disability and autistic people with complex needs. Individual staff members received criminal convictions in 2023.

While the Veilstone case has legal significance for a judgement which confirmed human rights breaches on the part of the state; the broader ethical concern is the effective safeguarding of vulnerable people against all types of abuse—including physical and emotional seclusion, disproportionate restraint and threats. This particularly applies to people with a learning disability and autistic people and those detained under the *Mental Health Act* where there is a higher risk of care being provided within a 'closed culture' (Department of Health 2012a, 2012b).

Approximately 2000 people with a learning disability and/or autistic people are in 'inpatient' facilities in the United Kingdom, with a policy aim to reduce this and provide more community-based care.

## *Gender Recognition Act* 2004

Written by Ovid, the Metamorphoses in Greek Mythology cover various transformative themes and suggest that people both desiring and living in a changed gender have long existed. Medicalization of transgender individuals has long been a controversial topic and risks adding to social stigmatization and marginalization. The first gender-reassignment surgeries occurred decades before a diagnostic category was added to the *Diagnostic and Statistical Manual of Mental Disorders* (DSM) in 1980 and the *International Classification of Diseases* (ICD) in 1990. DSM is the standard classification of mental disorders by the American Psychiatric Association. ICD is a wide-ranging diagnostic system by the World Health Organization. The 2022 Text Revision of DSM (*DSM-V-TR*) uses the term Gender Dysphoria, with an emphasis on clinically significant distress and/or social functioning. ICD-11 (2022) uses the term Gender Incongruence, where it is no longer categorized with 'Mental and behavioural disorders' and instead is found under 'Conditions related to sexual health'. Terminology and classifications are debated and subject to further change.

The *Gender Recognition Act* 2004 created, for the first time in UK history, a legal way for a person to change gender. A process can be followed to obtain a Gender Recognition Certificate, which in turn can be used to instruct the Registrar of Births to issue a new birth certificate with the appropriate gender as the sex category. Sex category in current usage is based on anatomical, biological and/or genetic aspects of a person; while gender identity in current usage refers to the internal perception a person has of being a male, female or another gender identity. The *Gender Recognition Act* allows the gender identity of a person to come to occupy the sex category field on the UK birth certificate.

### CASE 3.10 *CHRISTINE GOODWIN V. UNITED KINGDOM* (2002) (EUROPEAN COURT OF HUMAN RIGHTS)

The 1937 birth certificate recorded a male sex category. She tended to dress as a female from an early age and did so outside work until 1984, after which she lived fully as a female. In 1990 the NHS provided gender reassignment surgery (also known as gender confirmation or affirmation surgery). Postoperatively, state records continued to identify her as a male. She tried to pursue a case of sexual harassment at work at an industrial tribunal and claimed it failed because she was legally a male. She was unable to access the state pension at the retirement age for females (at the time, earlier than for males), had to pay higher car insurance and was unable to marry a male.

The European Court of Human Rights held that a serious interference with private life arises when state actions conflict with an important aspect of personal identity. As the court held that a person has the right to establish the details of their personal identity, Article 8 was breached—the right to respect for private and family life. Article 12 the right to marry was also breached.

In forming a judgement, the court referenced social change since the human rights convention was first written, and medical developments including *the acceptance of the condition of gender identity disorder by the medical professions and health authorities* and technical treatment possibilities. The case led the way to the *Gender Recognition Act* 2004.

There have been considerations to update the *Gender Recognition Act* to make the path to a Gender Recognition Certificate faster and less medicalized. Currently England and Wales plan to continue requiring a psychiatrist report and do not propose to allow self-identification to suffice; while Scotland is considering moves towards self-identification. The *Equality Act* 2010 protects people from discrimination in the workplace and wider society and recognizes gender reassignment as a protected characteristic: this does not require a certificate to be produced. This means transgender patients may have some identification documents that differ from their birth certificate.

Medical training and expertise in this area of clinical practice are limited. NHS adult patient waiting times for first assessment by a specialist gender identity clinician are currently measured in years. Referrals to services have rapidly increased without proportionate additional clinical capacity. General Practitioners are sometimes asked to prescribe hormones before and after specialist involvement. Consider that:

- The patient may be motivated to buy unregulated hormones online or elsewhere without a prescription—check with your patient.
- Long waiting times without treatment may worsen distress and increase the risk of self-harm—check with your patient.

### CASE 3.11 *BELL AND ANOTHER V. THE TAVISTOCK AND PORTMAN NHS FOUNDATION TRUST AND OTHERS* (2021)

Keira Bell had transitioned to male as a teenager via hormonal treatment and double mastectomy and she later expressed regret. She came to see her previous gender dysphoria diagnosis as a symptom of other life challenges rather than a primary challenge itself and detransitioned to the extent she could. A case was brought about the prescribing of puberty-suppressing hormones to children and adolescents. There were concerns about the practice being 'experimental' with far-reaching and incompletely understood effects making it impossible to obtain informed consent. The court affirmed the usual test of Gillick competence applies similar to the original case about contraceptives; saying the clinical matters are routinely for clinicians, patients and their carers.

At the same time as the court process and in the context of widespread public interest, NHS England and NHS Improvement commissioned an independent review by Dr Hilary Cass into gender identity services for children and young people. The terms of reference note that services had moved in recent years from purely psychosocial therapies to also include hormone prescriptions, and increased rates of referrals were disproportionately for people born female. In 2011–12

*(Continued)*

**CASE 3.11 — Contd.**

there were ~250 UK children referred, and >5000 in 2021–22. Besides safety and long-term outcomes, there were concerns about access to limited state service provision. Final outcomes of The Cass Review (2022) are awaited: as there are significant gaps in the clinical evidence base, it seems likely that puberty-suppressing hormones will not be available as a routine state-funded NHS service and will only be available in the context of ethically approved research. There are ambitions to create a national network of childrens services based on the principles of research, ongoing education and training and clinical governance. This is likely to be a long process.

## CLINICAL NOTES

### CLINICAL PRACTICE

- Make efforts to identify, record, update and use the appropriate name and pronouns for all patients—this does not require evidence of a gender recognition certificate or new birth certificate.
- If you are unsure about the pronouns of the patient in front of you, consider sharing yours and/or asking the patient to confirm theirs. If you make an error with pronouns, then apologize and carry on.
- Transgender or gender nonconformity without distress is a normal human variation; the clinical assessment your patient needs may be *about something else entirely;* remember to take a medication history as usual and consider relevant anatomy.
- Gender identity and sexual orientation are separate constructs: if you need to obtain a sexual history from the patient then avoid assumptions based on gender identity.
- Disorders of sex development, for example XXY/Klinefelter syndrome, 45XO/Turner syndrome, androgen insensitivity syndrome, are distinct from gender identity matters but may coexist.
- Inequalities in health outcomes and experiences of healthcare for transgender people are an ongoing concern.
- In NHS-inpatient areas, transgender patients should generally be accommodated according to how they identify and this does not depend on a Gender Recognition Certificate; unless the medical condition requiring treatment is sex specific (e.g. a transgender

admitted for hysterectomy will usually need a gynaecology ward to access appropriate care); for nonbinary individuals and if in doubt, sensitively enquire with the patient and discuss practical options (NHS England and NHS Improvement, 2019). Notably this policy is called *delivering same-sex accommodation* and not 'same-gender accommodation'. The distinction may be important for other patients requesting same-sex facilities as a proportionate means of achieving a legitimate aim (e.g. privacy, dignity) (Equality and Human Rights Commission, 2022). Ultimately the rights and needs of all have to be balanced.
- Scientific and clinical knowledge, the ethical and legal landscape and service provision will likely see further important developments in the coming years.

Key ethical considerations typically revolve around whether biological sex or identified gender should have primacy in a given situation. A patient registered with a General Practitioner in England can self-identify the relevant gender and subsequently have a new NHS number allocated to them. A Gender Recognition Certificate is not required for this change and they are not required to have undergone any medical assessment or treatment. The General Practice is expected to print out any old medical records relating to the previous gender, redact the previous name and any gender specific terms (typically using a black marker) and scan the pages into the new patient record. Under current processes, transgender women registered as female will subsequently be invited for breast and cervical screening and will not be invited for abdominal aortic aneurysm (AAA) screening unless they request it, while transgender women registered as male will be invited for AAA screening and will not be invited for breast screening unless they request it. Similarly transgender men registered as female are invited for breast and cervical but not AAA screening, and transgender men registered as male are invited for AAA screening and will not be invited for breast or cervical screening but can request these. So in summary: default invitations to NHS screening programmes are determined by the gender in which the patient is registered with their General Practice and not their anatomical sex, and there will not be a truly continuous electronic record if the NHS number is changed (NHS England 2023; NHS Primary Care Support England 2023). What are the benefits of this, and what risks are posed to patient care in England?

## COSMESIS

The intersection of cosmesis with clinical practice is an evolving area. It includes surgical and nonsurgical cosmetic procedures

(General Medical Council, 2016). Generally speaking in the state-funded NHS, procedures purely for cosmetic reasons are not available. Following physical illnesses cosmetic procedures are offered: a common example is reconstructive breast surgery for patients affected by breast cancer. Recent years have seen growth in cosmetic procedures for nonmedical aesthetic purposes performed by registered medical, nursing and allied health practitioners as well as by unregistered practitioners.

- The British Association of Aesthetic Plastic Surgeons conducts an annual audit of cosmetic activity by registered doctors. In 2022 there was >100% increase in procedures to >31,000 compared to the year before—affected to some extent by reduced activity during COVID-19 lockdowns the year before. Nonetheless these are the highest annual activity figures recorded since the audit began in 2004. Females underwent 93% of these procedures (British Association of Aesthetic Cosmetic Surgeons, 2023).
- Far more nonsurgical cosmetic procedures are carried out—including approximately 900,000 botox injections annually in the United Kingdom (Department of Health & Social Care & Caulfield, 2023).

Physical and psychological *well-being* are commonly cited motivations for cosmetic procedures. It can be questioned to what extent these procedures benefit *health* and to what extent they represent commoditization of the human body. While the beauty and cosmetics industries are likely as old as humankind, increasing demand for cosmetic procedures has been associated with the emergence of social media technologies and 'reality' television shows. Most UK cosmetic practice occurs in the private sector and practitioners are not necessarily medically qualified or regulated:

- Nonsurgical cosmetic procedures include botox, laser hair removal, dermal fillers, chemical peels (Figs 3.10–3.12).
- The UK nonsurgical cosmetic industry was estimated at £3.6 billion pounds in 2019.
- High-street and do-it-yourself cosmetic procedures are or have been associated with concerns including the risk of putting profits before 'patient' care, inadequate consent for procedures including fostering unrealistic expectations and access for children or vulnerable adults.

In 2023 the UK Government ran a consultation around unregulated cosmetic procedures (Department of Health & Social Care & Caulfield, 2023). There is expected to be a new licensing scheme for practitioners and cosmetic businesses in England—to give assurance around qualifications, training, indemnity and hygienic premises. *SaveFace* holds an existing UK government approved register for providers of medical aesthetic treatments who are also a registered doctor, dentist, nurse or prescribing pharmacist.

*The Botulinum Toxin and Cosmetic Fillers (Children) Act* 2021 now makes it illegal for children below 18 years old to be provided with these injectable treatments for cosmetic reasons. The onus is on the provider to check the potential client's age. It is also illegal to assist in the making of an appointment for an underage person. The age restriction is set at 18 to match other age restrictions in England on comparable body modifications which carry health

---

**CASE 3.12 'ABC V. ST GEORGE'S HEALTHCARE NHS TRUST & OTHERS' (2020)**

A case where the father of ABC, during detention under the *Mental Health Act* after being found guilty of the manslaughter of her mother by reason of diminished responsibility, was found to carry the Huntington disease gene. This follows an autosomal dominant inheritance. A professional decision was made to preserve the confidentiality of the father, consistent with his wishes and not inform ABC of her risk. ABC was known to be pregnant at the time, and a doctor accidentally breached confidentiality after her baby was born—informing of the genetic status of her father. Having given birth in early 2010, ABC underwent genetic testing in 2013 and tested positive. She brought a case saying she would have opted for termination of pregnancy had she known in time, and that the doctors had a duty of care which included informing her of the genetic risk.

ABC had been the patient of a psychiatric team providing family therapy on account of the circumstances involving her father, so the psychiatrists owed her a duty of care. That duty amounted to weighing up whether the risks—to her father and to public trust in the health professions generally—of breaking confidentiality and providing information against her father's wishes were justifiable in the particular circumstances. The court found that, when balancing the interests of the patient and the at-risk relative (ABC), nondisclosure was supported by a responsible body of medical opinion ('the Bolam test'). So nondisclosure of genetic information to an at-risk relative was defensible and did not amount to a breach in the duty of care here. The fact was also considered that ABC had not subsequently informed her sister about the genetic risk—her sister by late 2010 was also pregnant: so doubts were raised as to whether ABC would in fact have undergone testing and termination of pregnancy had she been given the information in time.

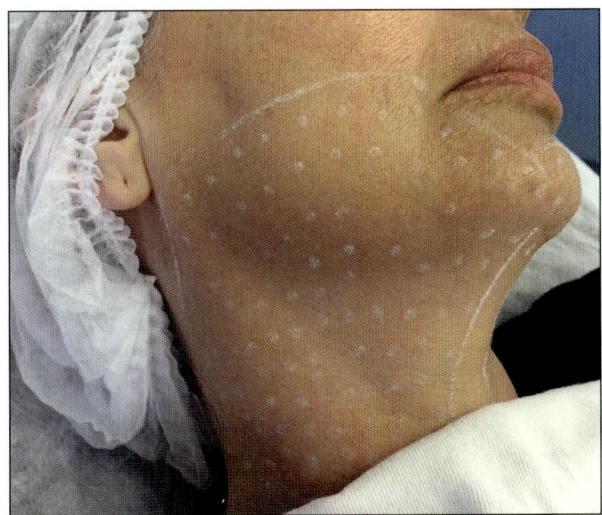

**Fig. 3.10** Representative injection points for the microbotox technique.

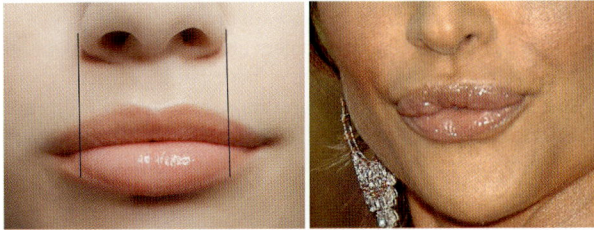

**Fig. 3.11** Filling the lips all the way to the oral commissure or overfilling the commissures in general can produce an unaesthetic 'duck-type' lip. Keeping the filler between imaginary lines dropped from the lateral alae are good indicators of where to stop the augmentation in the upper lip. (Courtesy Dr Joe Niamtu.)

risks (tattooing, sunbeds and teeth whitening) (Department of Health & Social Care, 2021). A parent or guardian above 18 years old cannot consent on behalf of the child. At the time of writing a child is not considered to have the capacity to consent to one of these procedures. Prior to the legislation it is estimated that 41,000 botox procedures for cosmetic reasons were performed on UK children in 2020. These treatments can be given *for medical reasons* to those below 18 years old, when approved by a registered doctor.

### CASE 3.13  SEMAGLUTIDE FOR COSMETIC WEIGHT LOSS

This has come to popular attention since 2022 through social media and celebrity influence. Currently semaglutide is only licensed in the United Kingdom for type 2 diabetes mellitus; in the United States it is also licensed for people with a body mass index (BMI) 27 kg/m² or more with at least one associated long-term condition (e.g. hypertension, type 2 diabetes mellitus, hypercholesterolaemia) or in patients with BMI >30 kg/m². Around 70% of Americans and nearly two-thirds of British people can be diagnosed as either obese or overweight. Cosmetic weight loss, however, is an unlicensed use for this drug. *How would you assess and advise a patient with no past medical history and a healthy BMI who is asking for this medication to help achieve a desired weight loss?*

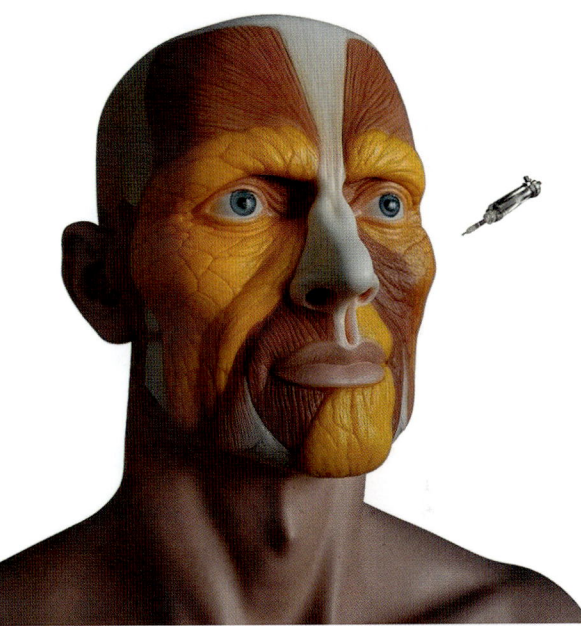

**Fig. 3.12** Medical illustration of potential facial fat loss and potential corresponding dermal filler injection sites to address this issue in Ozempic users. Ozempic is a drug that causes rapid weight loss, which can lead to a loss of fat in the temporal, cheek, tear trough, jawline, marionette and nasolabial fold regions, resulting in an aged and wrinkled appearance commonly known as 'Ozempic face'. The areas of potential fat loss and filler injection sites are highlighted in yellow.

What do you think about using a professional medical or other clinical qualification and regulated status to contribute to running a cosmetic business?

### IATROGENESIS

Iatrogenic illness is caused by medical intervention, investigation or treatment. This does not necessarily mean clinical practice has been substandard, unethical or illegal. For example consider a patient experiencing a complication from an operation who was appropriately consented for the risk of that complication, which is known to have an occurrence rate in the normal competent performance of that operation.

It has been argued that greater availability of health services fosters increasing dependence on doctors and health services in general—so called *social, cultural and structural iatrogenesis* (Illich, 1978). Historically people dealt with minor conditions themselves, whereas now patients frequently attend health services for reassurance and advice. UK family doctors aiming to reduce the pressure for appointments by taking on extra doctors or extending their clinics have found consultation rates rise and consultations take longer (Armstrong, 2003). The gradual increase in dependence on health services can be considered a form of sickness. Societal approaches to healthcare may make people feel less healthy through:

- Unrealistic health goals: For example the World Health Organization definition of health as a state of *complete physical, mental and social well-being* may convince people they could be healthier, have more well-being or are 'by definition' unhealthy.
- Implying that good health equates to consumption of healthcare services. Screening is one way in which 'healthy people'—and those with otherwise subclinical conditions—can become 'people at risk'.

---

**CASE 3.14** *CLOSTRIDIUM DIFFICILE* INFECTION, ANTIBIOTIC AND PROTON-PUMP INHIBITOR PRESCRIBING

Increasing rates of *C. difficile* infection have been linked to ageing populations, increased antibiotic use and acid suppression therapy in particular proton-pump inhibitors (PPIs) (Tawam et al., 2021; Patil & Blankenship, 2013). It has proven challenging to demonstrate a clear causal link between PPIs and *C. diff*, even though the association is accepted and plausible mechanisms exist.

At what point can we say a harmful outcome like *C. diff* infection is iatrogenic?

- Did the antibiotics prescribed empirically for an older adult in the community prevent a hospital admission or death due to pneumonia and sepsis? Or were the antibiotics unnecessary either because the infection was viral or because the person would have recovered normally in keeping with the natural history of the infection if they were given enough time to improve?
- Did the PPI prescription for the patient taking aspirin to reduce the risks of a further heart attack actually save an emergency ambulance, hospital admission or death from an atherosclerotic plaque event—by allowing them to tolerate aspirin safely for a prolonged period of time? Or was the PPI unnecessary because the individual patient was not going to have another atherosclerotic event or perhaps could have tolerated long-term aspirin without gastric upset?

---

## CLINICAL GENETICS

DNA was identified in the 1860s by Friedrich Miescher. James Watson and Francis Crick identified the double helix structure in 1953. Complete mapping—The Human Genome Project—began in 1990 and reached significant milestones in 2003 and 2022 (National Human Genome Research Institute, 2022). Several advances are now part of clinical practice, particularly for monogenic conditions. Any hopes about clinical genetics as a panacea for clinical practice and disease have not been realized. Many conditions are polygenically and epigenetically (behaviourally and environmentally) influenced. There have been concerns about genetic test results affecting applications for jobs and insurance coverage. Some people purchase direct-to-consumer genetic tests and may not have anyone to speak to about the results.

---

**COMMUNICATION**

**COMMUNICATION WITH PATIENTS**

- Genetic testing does not provide information about all possible conditions.
- Genetic tests are not all 100% accurate or predictive of future events.
- Some genetic test results need to be disclosed to insurers, but this is uncommon; in circumstances with a strong family history, it may be beneficial to share a negative result.

---

Clinical genetics practice invokes important and sometimes conflicting ethical considerations:

- A person may not want to know their genetic status; however if other family members are tested, the results may create a situation where the status of the original person can eventually be inferred without direct testing (Fig. 3.13).
- Reproductive choices may be impacted by knowledge of genetic status (see Chapter 4).
- Other people may be impacted by a given genetic status: when does the right to confidentiality and the principle of

autonomy for one person, who may be or become a parent (for example), become outweighed by the duty to provide justice or prevent harm to third parties, such as the other (potential) parent or existing children or an unborn child?

- Life insurance can be affected by knowledge of genetic status. While a family history cannot be changed, decisions on being tested need to be considered carefully. Predictive genetic test results must be disclosed for life insurance cover >£500,000 per person for Huntington disease in the United Kingdom (Association of British Insurers, 2023; HM Government & Association of British Insurers, 2018).

## CLINICAL NOTES

### KEY POINTS

- Genetic responsibility to self and others may lead us to consider the difference between the dominant legal discourse of *autonomy as individualistic* and the alternative ethical paradigm of *autonomy as relational* (Dove et al., 2017).
- The doctor's 'duty' to warn at-risk relatives can become an ethical quandary when confidentiality is wanted by a particular person (Grill & Rosén, 2021).

## ETHICS

### DEBATE BOX

- Does an individual have a responsibility to acquire genetic knowledge about themselves?
- Does an individual have a responsibility to share genetic results with relevant family?
- How does a health professional best consult with the carrier of a genetic mutation who does not wish to share information with relevant family?
- Does the health professional have a responsibility to share genetic results with relevant family?

## Applications of clinical genetics

Applications range from tests that may help before conception and all through the lifespan:

- Carrier testing
- Preimplantation testing or PIGD (preimplantation genetic diagnosis)
- Prenatal screening and tests
- Newborn screening and tests
- Predictive and presymptomatic testing

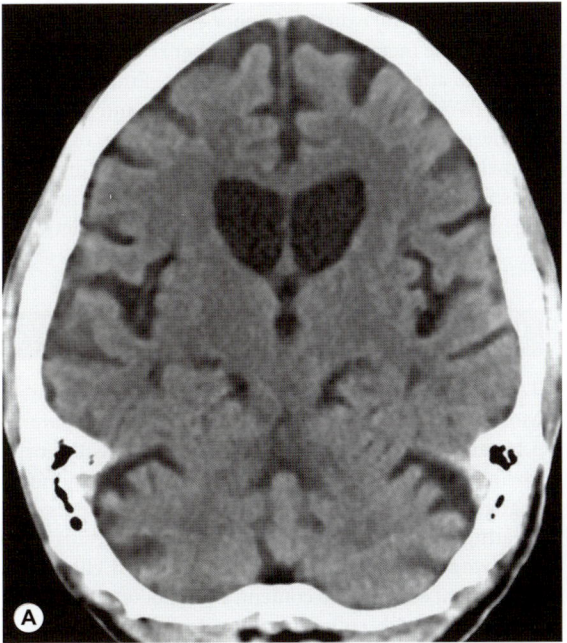
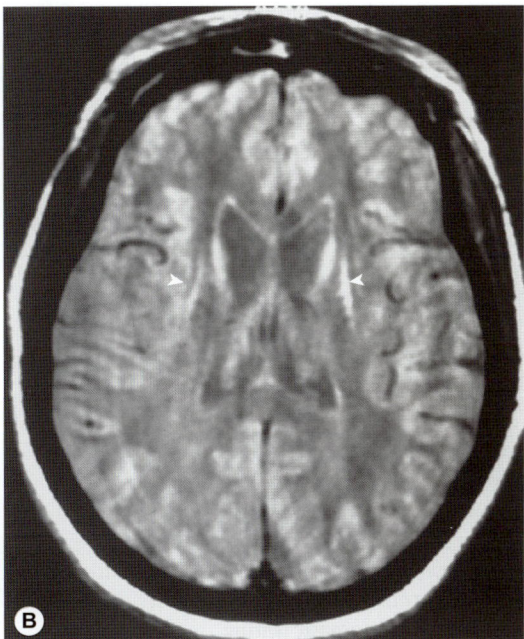

**Fig. 3.13** Huntington disease: (A) axial unenhanced computed tomography demonstrates caudate atrophy with ballooning of the frontal horns of the lateral ventricles; (B) proton density–weighted image in a different patient shows high signal intensity in the caudate nuclei bilaterally and in the putamina (*arrowheads*). This, again, shows frontal horn dilatation following atrophy of the adjacent caudate nuclei.

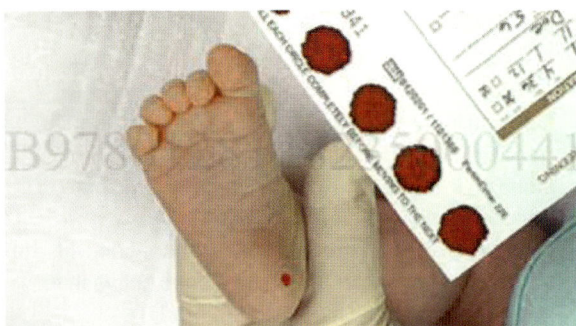

**Fig. 3.14** Site of heel prick and collection of blood sample on paper for newborn screening.

**Carrier testing** is usually done if one parent has a family history of autosomal recessive disease. If one parent is a carrier, the other parent may choose to be tested so they know in advance the risk of passing the condition to their children.

**Preimplantation testing (or preimplantation genetic diagnosis, PIGD)** detects genetic mutations in embryos made using assisted reproductive techniques like in-vitro fertilization.

**Prenatal screening** is routinely offered in the United Kingdom for Down syndrome, Edwards syndrome and Patau syndrome between 10 and 14 weeks of gestation via ultrasound and blood tests. If screening suggests a high risk then diagnostic testing with amniocentesis or chorionic villus sampling is offered. Strictly speaking these are not genetically inherited conditions, they are usually sporadically occurring chromosomal trisomies as a result of nondisjunction.

**Newborn screening**

The heel-prick blood spot in the United Kingdom looks for several autosomal recessive conditions (Fig. 3.14):

- Sickle cell.
- Cystic fibrosis.
- Inherited metabolic diseases:
  - Phenylketonuria
  - MCADD—medium-chain acyl-CoA dehydrogenase deficiency
  - Maple syrup urine disease
  - Isovaleric acidaemia
  - Glutaric aciduria type 1
  - Homocystinuria
- Congenital hypothyroidism is mostly sporadic but occasionally autosomal recessive.
- Severe combined immunodeficiency is mostly autosomal recessive and not currently tested in all areas.

**Predictive and presymptomatic testing**

BRCA1 and BRCA2 are the most common genes in hereditary breast and ovarian cancer, carried by around 1 in 400 people and follow autosomal dominant inheritance. Public awareness of these

conditions may have grown in recent years (Petrova, Cruz & Sáncheza, 2022; Basu et al., 2021).

- A 5% to 10% of bowel cancers are also thought to be genetic with the most common being Lynch syndrome (hereditary nonpolyposis colorectal cancer) which is also autosomal dominant.
- Huntington disease (Fig. 3.13) is considered in the case of *ABC v. St George's Healthcare NHS Trust & Others* (2020) (Case 3.12). Other conditions can also be tested for when relevant; for example, rare forms of familial motor neurone disease.

**HINTS AND TIPS**

**IN CLINICAL PRACTICE:**

- Take an appropriate family history.
- Take a social history which considers significant relationships the patient has.

## Pharmacogenomics

Individuals vary in their response to medicines and some of this is genetically influenced. For example (Dean & Kane, 2012), multi-ethnic population studies in the United States have estimated that around 5% of people metabolize codeine poorly, and such patients will experience poor efficacy. In contrast, 'ultrarapid' codeine metabolism with a higher risk of side effects is estimated to affect 28% of North Africans, Ethiopians and Arabs; 10% of Whites; 3% of African Americans and 1% of Hispanics, Chinese and Japanese. This gives a glimpse of how genetics knowledge, and possibly testing, may move us further along the journey of providing personalized clinical medicine (Royal College of Physicians & British Pharmacological Society 2022).

## HEALTH AND TECHNOLOGY

Technological developments continue to change the way we live. Most NHS General Practices became highly computerized (Fig. 3.15) and relatively paper-light in the 2000s, with hospitals following in the 2010s. Computers in the consultation room have changed the dynamic between doctors and patients, commonly creating a triadic relationship (Pearce et al., 2011). This can improve access to patient specific information, clinical guidelines and patient educational content, allow documentation and communication with colleagues; but it can equally interfere with patient communication, lead to inadvertent breaches of confidentiality and sometimes loss of confidence in the doctor's knowledge.

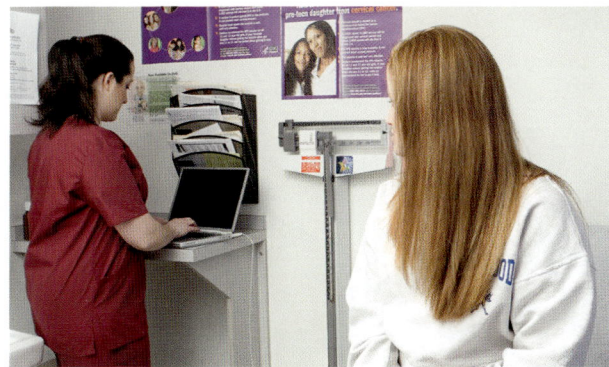

**Fig. 3.15** A consultation with the computer.

Electronic prescribing is now common; bringing automated prompts, reminders and warnings for the prescriber to consider. There are still an estimated 237 million medication errors annually in England, with 66 million errors being clinically significant. Many electronic referral and communication channels now exist between and within primary and secondary care. There are relatively newly used direct communication channels with patients, including text messaging and email. Such channels may increase the rate of activity and may have an impact on expectations about the speed of service provision. This may benefit some clinical situations and in other situations may diminish consideration for the use of time as a tool in the diagnostic and therapeutic process. The risk is a more investigational and interventional internal culture of and external expectation of medical practice which does not improve morbidity or mortality for patients.

Secure data storage and transfer is a concern with increased reliance on technology. For example, the websites of twenty NHS Trusts were found by investigational journalists to have been sharing browsing data with Meta (Facebook) for years (Das, 2023). Information shared varied from the unique IP (internet protocol) address of the person, their search words, to links clicked and viewed. There are concerns these data could be used for targeted advertising or linking personal identity to health conditions. *The British Medical Journal* reported in 2022 that hundreds of organizations including pharmaceutical companies, clinical commissioning groups and universities have breached patient data sharing agreements in recent years (Oxford, 2022).

Image transfer is now possible and for some conditions can reduce the need for the patient to travel for an appointment. Images of intimate body parts are not appropriate for such transfer, and the patient may have different boundaries to yours as to what they may feel comfortable to send electronically. Video consultation has become widely available as an option in recent years, accelerated by the COVID-19 pandemic. The overall proportion of remote consultations in NHS General Practice was 20% prepandemic, and in 2023 it was around 40%.

Some patients have equipment for remote monitoring at home—for example, blood pressure machines, pulse oximeters and thermometers. These can be useful in guiding the need for in-person assessment and the urgency. Patients without the means or access to home equipment potentially face a new type of disadvantage. 'Virtual wards' exist in some areas, where remote monitoring can be used to help appropriate patients stay at home for treatments and reduce hospital bed occupancy. Technological advancements over time in the medical and surgical specialities have created possibilities like implantable loop recorders, defibrillators and pacemakers in cardiology; continuous positive airway pressure machines in respiratory medicine; capsule endoscopy in gastroenterology; minimal access surgery in many specialities and various types of dialysis for renal and intensive care medicine—just to name a few.

The internet is now a vast and continually growing source of medical information of varying degrees of quality and relevance. Patients may consult it to their benefit or to their detriment. Professionals can help patients to identify reliable information sources (Figs 3.1–3.9).

## Artificial intelligence

Like most labour market sectors, AI is expected to replace or supplement humans to some extent in healthcare (Figs 3.17–3.19). Research is starting to offer evidence that interaction with robots is acceptable to patients and where it may be effective, but this is not universally agreed on (Chai et al., 2021; Chen et al., 2020). The degree and speed with which this impacts different medical specialities remains to be seen. Online chatbots will raise questions about fees for patients or

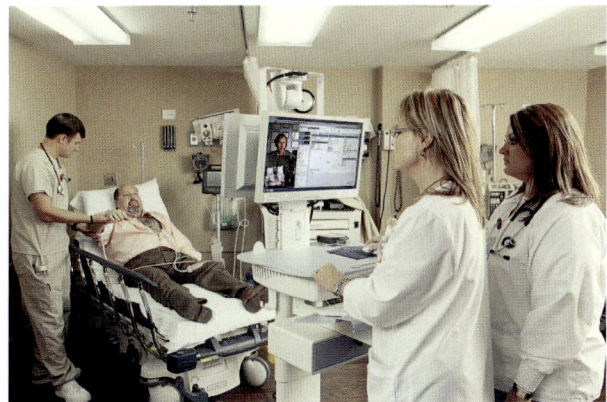

**Fig. 3.16** Patient undergoing a telemedicine consult with a large portable device displaying both patient and provider images, electronic medical record and auxiliary connections for a stethoscope and a continuous-wave Doppler.

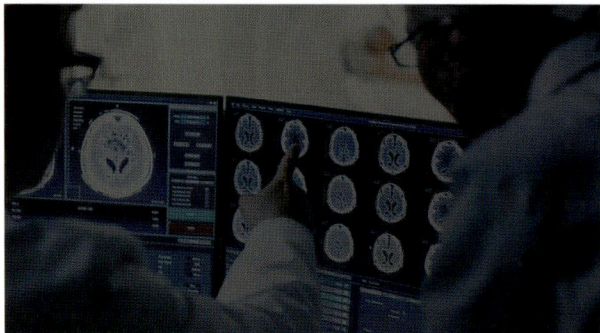

**Fig. 3.17** An artificial intelligence–based doctor assistance system.

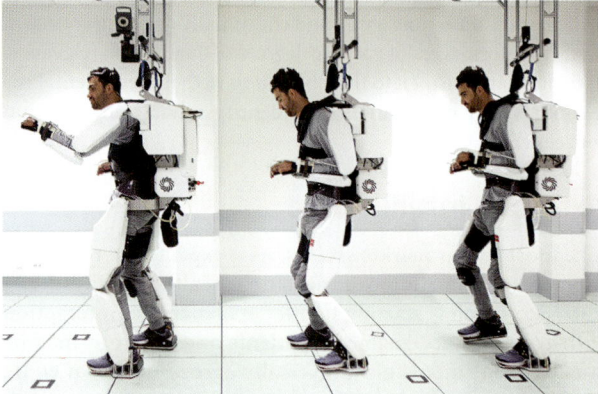

**Fig. 3.18** Brain–computer interface-controlled exoskeleton. An individual with quadriplegia moves with the assistance of robotic arms and legs controlled by decoding motor cortex activity in real time. The brain signals are recorded with two 64-electrode electrocorticography implants. (From Benabid et al. *The Lancet Neurology*, 2019, *18*(12) , 1112–1122.)

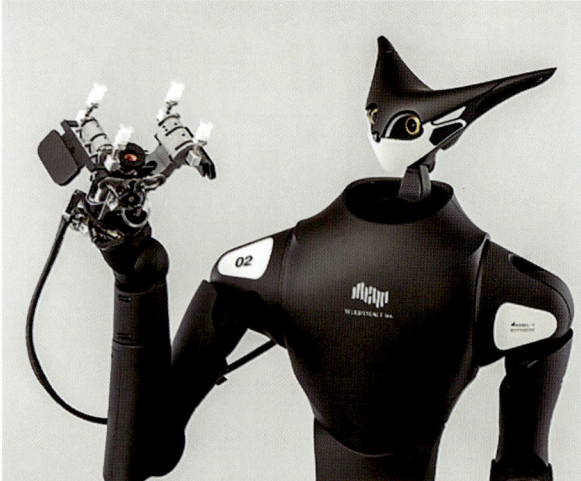

**Fig. 3.19** The Doctor will see you next?

insurers and data protection where accountability sits if a patient is harmed and how this intersects with medical education and training and professional regulation. Depending on the source material used by LLM (large language model) chatbots in their 'machine learning', they may perpetuate the collective unconscious biases of the original authors. Chatbots may be susceptible to 'learning' and potentiating the medical misinformation that can be relatively easily posted online. Chatbots are not currently suitable for diagnosing serious conditions or treating patients. They may be able to help in nonclinical health administration—for example booking or rearranging appointments. Technological developments have impacted on the need for different medical specialists before; for example, the development of coronary stenting from the 1990s onward led to a reduced need for cardiac surgeons (Figs 3.10–3.19).

## References

'*ABC v. St George's Healthcare NHS Trust & Others*' (2020) EWHC 455 (QB).

*Adults with Incapacity (Scotland) Act* 2000.

*Age of Legal Capacity (Scotland) Act* 1991.

Armstrong, D. (2003). Evaluating healthcare *In: An outline of sociology as applied to medicine* (5th ed., pp. 125–137). Hodder Arnold.

Association of British Insurers. (2023). *Consumer guide: Code on genetic testing and insurance.* Association of British Insurer.

Basu, N., et al. (2021). The Angelina Jolie effect: Contralateral risk-reducing mastectomy trends in patients at increased risk of breast cancer. *Scientific Reports*, *11*, 2847. https://doi.org/10.1038/s41598-021-82654-x. doi.

'*Bell and another v. The Tavistock and Portman NHS Foundation Trust and others*' (2021) EWCA Civ 1363.

'*Birch v. University College London Hospital NHS Foundation Trust*' (2008) EWHC 2237 (QB). https://www.bailii.org/ew/cases/EWHC/QB/2008/2237.html.

British Association of Aesthetic Cosmetic Surgeons. (2023). *Cosmetic surgery boom. BAAPS national audit reveals 102% rise in procedures during 2022.* The Royal College of Surgeons of England. https://baaps.org.uk/media/press_releases/1872/cosmetic_surgery_boom

*Botulinum Toxin and Cosmetic Fillers (Children) Act* 2021.

Chai, P., et al. (2021). Assessment of the acceptability and feasibility of using mobile robotic systems for patient evaluation. *JAMA Network Open*, *4*(3), e210667. https://doi.org/10.1001/jamanetworkopen.2021.0667.

Chen, K., et al. (2020). Effects of a humanoid companion robot on dementia symptoms and caregiver distress for residents in long-term care. *The Journal of Post-Acute and Long-Term Care Medicine*, *21*(11), 1724–1728. https://doi.org/10.1016/j.jamda.2020.05.036.

*Children Act* 1989 (amended 2004).

'*Christine Goodwin v. The United Kingdom*' (28957/95) (2002) ECHR (GC).

*Counter-Terrorism and Security Act* 2015.

Das, S. (May 27, 2023). NHS data breach: Trusts shared patient details with Facebook without consent. *The Guardian*. https://www.theguardian.com/society/2023/may/27/nhs-data-breach-trusts-shared-patient-details-with-facebook-meta-without-consent.

Dean, L., & Kane, M. (2012). Codeine therapy and CYP2D6 genotype. *Medical Genetics Summaries*. https://www.ncbi.nlm.nih.gov/books/NBK100662/.

Department of Health. (2012a). *DH winterbourne view review. Concordat: Programme of Action*. Department of Health.

Department of Health. (2012b). *Transforming care: A national response to Winterbourne View Hospital. Department of Health Review: Final Report*. Department of Health.

Department of Health & Social Care. (2021). *Botulinum toxin and cosmetic fillers for under 18s: Guidance for businesses*. Department of Health & Social Care.

Department of Health and Social Care. (2023). *Care and support statutory guidance: Using the Care Act guidance*. Department of Health and Social Care.

Department of Health & Social Care & Caulfield (2023). *Consultation launched into unregulated cosmetic procedures*. https://www.gov.uk/government/news/consultation-launched-into-unregulated-cosmetic-procedures.

Dove, E. S., et al. (2017). Beyond individualism: Is there a place for relational autonomy in clinical practice and research? *Clinical Ethics*, *12*(3), 150–165. https://doi.org/10.1177/1477750917704156.

Egdell, W. v. (1989). EWCA Civ 13.

*Equality Act* 2010.

Equality and Human Rights Commission. (2022). *Separate and single-sex service providers: A guide on the Equality Act sex and gender reassignment exceptions*. Equality and Human Rights Commissionhttps://www.equalityhumanrights.com/sites/default/files/guidance-separate-and-single-sex-service-providers-equality-act-sex-and-gender-reassignment-exceptions.pdf

*Family Law Reform Act* 1969.

*Female Genital Mutilation Act* 2003.

General Medical Council. (2016). *Guidance for doctors who offer cosmetic interventions*. GMC.

General Medical Council. (2020a). *Intimate examinations and chaperones*. Manchester: GMC.

General Medical Council. (2020b). *0–18 years: Guidance for all doctors*. Manchester: GMC.

*Gender Recognition Act* 2004.

*Gillick v. West Norfolk & Wisbech Area Health Authority* (1986) AC 112.

Grill, K., & Rosén, A. (2021). Healthcare professionals' responsibility for informing relatives at risk of hereditary disease. *Journal of Medical Ethics*, *47*, e12. https://doi.org/10.1136/medethics-2020-106236.

'*H.L. v. The United Kingdom*' *(45508/99)*' [2004] ECHR 720. https://hudoc.echr.coe.int/fre#{%22itemid%22:[%22002-4166%22]}.

HM Government & Association of British Insurers. (2018). *Code on genetic testing and insurance*.

*Human Rights Act* 1998.

Husain, M., & Chalder, T. (2021). Medically unexplained symptoms: assessment and management. *Clinical Medicine Journal*, *21*(1), 13–18. https://doi.org/10.7861/clinmed.2020-0947.

Illich, I. (1978). *Limits to medicine*. Caldar Boyars. (subsequently published and reprinted by Penguin Books).

Leigh Day. (2023). *Ben's case – Legal briefing 01.11.23 (Rubens, C., Millar, A. and Hyam, J)*. https://www.leighday.co.uk/media/5kifwpqv/cat-veilstone-legal-briefing.pdf

Liston, C., et al. (2022). Understanding the biological basis of psychiatric disease: What's next? *Cell*, *185*(1), 1–3. https://doi.org/10.1016/j.cell.2021.12.010.

Malla, A., Joober, R., & Garcia, A. (2015). "Mental illness is like any other medical illness": A critical examination of the statement and its impact on patient care and society. *Journal of Psychiatry and Neuroscience*, *40*(3), 147–150. https://doi.org/10.1503/jpn.150099.

'*McCulloch and others (Appellants) v. Forth Valley Health Board (Respondent) (Scotland)*' (2023) UKSC 26. https://www.supremecourt.uk/cases/uksc-2021-0149.html.

*Mental Capacity Act* 2005.

*Mental Capacity (Amendment) Act* 2019.

*Mental Health Act* 1983 (amended 2007).

'*Montgomery (Appellant) v. Lanarkshire Health Board (Respondent) (Scotland)*' (2015) UKSC 11. https://www.supremecourt.uk/cases/uksc-2013-0136.html.

National Human Genome Research Institute. (2022). *Fact sheet – Human genome project*. https://www.genome.gov/about-genomics/educational-resources/fact-sheets/human-genome-project.

NHS England. (2023). *Promotional material – NHS population screening: Information for trans and non-binary people*. United Kingdom https://www.gov.uk/government/publications/nhs-population-screening-information-for-transgender-people/nhs-population-screening-information-for-trans-people.

NHS England and NHS Improvement. (2019). *Delivering same-sex accommodation*. NHS England and NHS Improvement.

NHS Primary Care Support England. (2023). *Process for registering a patient gender re-assignment*. United Kingdom https://pcse.england.nhs.uk/sites/default/files/2023-08/process-for-registering-a-patient-gender-re-assignmentv10.pdf.

'*NHS Trust v. X (In the matter of X (A Child) (No 2)*' [2021] EWHC 65 (Fam). https://www.bailii.org/ew/cases/EWHC/Fam/2021/65.html.

Office for National Statistics. (2023). *Domestic abuse victim characteristics, England and Wales: Year ending March 2023*. Office for National Statistics.

Oxford, E. (2022). Hundreds of patient data breaches are left unpunished. *British Medical Journal*, *2022*(377), o1126. https://doi.org/10.1136/bmj.o1126.

'*P (by his litigation friend the Official Solicitor) (FC) (Appellant) v. Cheshire West and Chester Council and another (Respondents)*' (2014) UKSC 19.

Parliament. House of Commons & House of Lords Joint Committee on the Draft Mental Health Bill. (2023). *Draft Mental Health Bill 2022 report of session 2022–23 (HC 696 & HL Paper 128)*. London: By the authority of the House of Commons & the House of Lords.

Patil, R., & Blankenship, L. (2013). Proton pump inhibitors and *Clostridium difficile* infection: Are we propagating an already rapidly growing healthcare problem? *Gastroenterology Research*, *6*(5), 171–173. https://doi.org/10.4021/gr575w.

Pearce, C., et al. (2011). The patient and the computer in the primary care consultation. *Journal of the American Medical Informatics Association*, 18(2), 138–142. https://doi.org/10.1136/jamia.2010.006486.

Petrova, D., Cruz, M., & Sáncheza, M. (2022). BRCA1/2 testing for genetic susceptibility to cancer after 25 years: A scoping review and a primer on ethical implications. *Breast*, 61, 66–76. https://doi.org/10.1016/j.breast.2021.12.005.

'Re C (Adult: Refusal of Medical Treatment)' (1994) 1 All ER 819.

'Re T (Adult: Refusal of Medical Treatment)' (1992) EWCA Civ 18. https://www.bailii.org/ew/cases/EWCA/Civ/1992/18.html.

Royal College of Physicians & British Pharmacological Society. (2022). *Personalised prescribing. Using pharmacogenomics to improve patient outcomes*. Royal College of Physicians & British Pharmacological Society.

*Sexual Offences Act* 2003.

Social Care Institute for Excellence. (2015). *At a glance 69: Safeguarding adults: Types and indicators of abuse*. SCIE.

*Suicide Act* 1961.

Tawam, D., et al. (2021). The positive association between proton pump inhibitors and *Clostridium difficile* infection. *Innovations in Pharmacy*, 12(1), 10. https://doi.org/10.24926/iip.v12i1.3439.24926/iip.v12i1.3439.

The Cass Review. (2022). *Independent review of gender identity services for children and young people: Interim report February 2022*. Commissioned by NHS England and NHS Improvement.

van Voren, R. (2016). Ending political abuse of psychiatry: where we are at and what needs to be done. *BJPsych Bulletin*, 40(1), 30–33. https://doi.org/10.1192/pb.bp.114.049494.

## Further Reading

*Access to Medical Reports Act* 1988.

*Autism Act* 2009.

Coleman, E., et al. (2022). Standards of care for the health of transgender and gender diverse people, version 8. *International Journal of Transgender Health*, 23(suppl 1), 1–259. https://doi.org/10.1080/26895269.2022.2100644.

Department of Health. (2015). *Mental Health Act 1983: Code of practice. Presented to Parliament pursuant to section 118 of the Mental Health Act 1983*. The Stationery Office.

Garg, G., Elshimy, G., & Marwaha, R. (2023) Gender dysphoria. In: *StatPearls*. StatPearls Publishing.https://www.ncbi.nlm.nih.gov/books/NBK532313/

General Medical Council. (2024a). *Remote consultations*. https://www.gmc-uk.org/professional-standards/ethical-hub/remote-consultations.

General Medical Council. (2024b). *Trans healthcare*. https://www.gmc-uk.org/professional-standards/ethical-hub/trans-healthcare.

Li, Z., & Filobbos, G. (2020). What is the UK public searching for? A correlation analysis of Google trends search terms and cosmetic surgery in the UK. *Aesthetic Plastic Surgery*, 44(6), 2312–2318. https://doi.org/10.1007/s00266-020-01918-5.

Mencap. www.mencap.org.uk.

*Mental Health Act* 2007 Explanatory Notes (2007). Department of Health and the Ministry of Justice.

*Mental Health Units (Use of Force) Act* 2018.

Parker, M. (2012). *Ethical problems and genetics practice*. Cambridge University Press. https://doi.org/10.1017/CBO9781139107792.

Parliament. House of Commons. (2016). *Women and Equalities Committee. Transgender equality. First report of session 2015–16. Report, together with formal minutes relating to the report (HC390)*. By authority of the House of Commons.

Turnpenny, P. D., et al. (2021). *Emery's elements of medical genetics and genomics* (16th ed.). Elsevier.

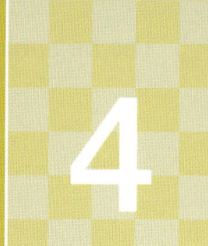

Many passionately debated issues in medical ethics and law involve the beginnings and ends of life. This chapter explores such issues including contraception, sterilization, abortion, in vitro fertilization (IVF) and surrogacy, as well as end-of-life decisions, euthanasia, the definition of death and organ transplantation. The first section of the chapter deals with the beginnings of life, and the second with the end.

## BEGINNING OF LIFE

In a normal pregnancy, the egg is fertilized by a sperm; develops into a zygote, morula, blastocyst; implants into the uterine lining at 8 to 10 days and then develops into an embryonic disc, before becoming an embryo (Fig. 4.1). The foetal heart begins to beat at 6 weeks, and by 8 weeks all major organs have started to form. A normal pregnancy is delivered at around 40 weeks' gestation but the limit of viability currently lies around 23 weeks (Mactier et al., 2020). Questions about the permissibility of abortion and assisted reproduction reach to the heart of the ethical and philosophical debates over when life begins, what the foetus is, how far we should be able to experiment on and alter the foetus and how far the autonomy of a pregnant female or person extends over the foetus.

## Key legislation covered in this section includes:

*Abortion Act* 1967 (amended 1990)
- *Human Fertilisation and Embryology Act* 1990 (amended 2008)
- *Offences Against the Person Act* 1861
- *Infant Life (Preservation) Act* 1929
- *Surrogacy Arrangements Act* 1985

    Key cases discussed include:
- *Paton v. British Pregnancy Advisory Service Trustees* (1979)
- *Re F (in Utero)* (1988)

*Janaway v. Salford Health Authority* (1989)
Key ethical issues discussed include conscientious objection, status of the foetus/embryo, rights of the pregnant person and of the foetus.

## THE FOETUS AND THE EMBRYO

A person's beliefs about the status of the embryo and foetus may become a common thread of argument that runs through a number of the issues in reproductive ethics, such as abortion, IVF, cloning and genetic screening. Gillon (2001) says this question is not so much ethical—to do with right and wrong, but epistemological—based on what you believe, in this case about the status of the foetus. According to the law in England and Wales and adapted from Herring (2010):

- A foetus is not a legal person.
- A foetus is not simply part of the mother either.
- It is not possible to bring legal proceedings in the name of the foetus.
- A foetus has interests that are protected by the law.
- A foetus is not directly protected by the European Convention on Human Rights.

### CASE 4.1 *PATON V. BRITISH PREGNANCY ADVISORY SERVICE TRUSTEES* (1979)

Mrs Paton became pregnant and became concerned about the pregnancy. She saw two doctors, both of whom agreed the pregnancy was a risk to her physical or mental health and that she was able to have an abortion under the conditions set out in the *Abortion Act* 1967. Her husband Mr Paton had not been consulted by Mrs Paton about the termination and sought a court injunction to stop the termination without his approval. The judge ruled that the partner had no ability to influence the choice of a female to access a termination, and that the foetus has no legal rights in law.

### CASE 4.2 *RE F (IN UTERO)* (1988)

F was a female with a history of mental disturbance and drug abuse. She became pregnant for a second time, and her first child had been taken into care. Fearing for the welfare of the unborn child, the local health authority applied to the Courts to make the unborn child a ward of the Court. The judge ruled that the court's jurisdiction did not extend over an unborn child, and that it would involve restrictions on a pregnant female's liberty that was not permitted under current legislation.

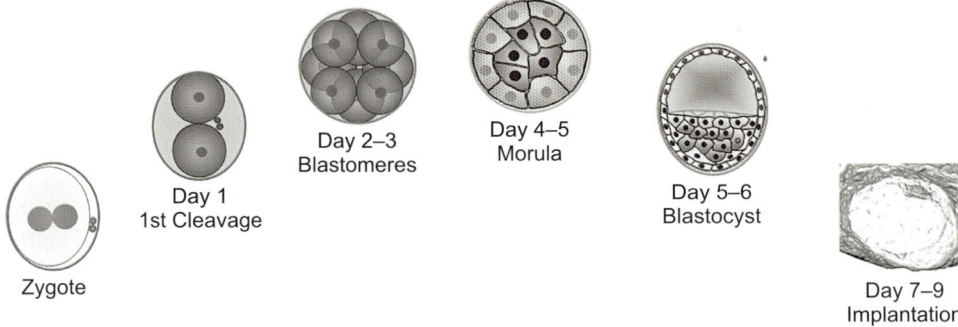

**Fig. 4.1** Early human development. The zygote is formed at fertilization with completion of the second meiotic division of the ovum. Soon after, the zygote undergoes the first cleavage. Blastomeres divide about once per 24 hours, compacting to form the morula at the 16- to 32-cell stage. Cells begin to differentiate and fluid begins to collect at one end of the morula as it becomes the blastocyst. Implantation occurs early in the second week. Legally, contraceptive treatments act prior to implantation.

The legal status of the foetus is thus relatively clear. However, the human embryo does not become a foetus until about the sixth week of pregnancy. Furthermore, how do we determine the *moral* status of the embryo and the foetus as it develops and progresses towards birth? A number of views and objections are presented later.

## The embryo/foetus is morally valuable because it is a human organism

This view holds that the embryo/foetus is valuable because it is *human* and as such deserves moral recognition. Therefore just as it is morally wrong to kill an adult or a child, it is equally wrong to kill a foetus or an embryo. All of these are seamless, continuous stages that can be traced back to conception and are all united in their membership of the human species. But:

- Is killing a zygote or primitive embryo really as morally bad as killing a child?
- Why do most jurisdictions that permit abortion only permit it in the early stages of pregnancy and heavily curtail or prohibit late term termination?

### CASE 4.3 THOUGHT EXPERIMENTS ABOUT THE EMBRYO AND THE FOETUS

1. You are working in a laboratory and there is a fire. You can either save a 5-year-old child or an embryo in a test tube. Would you be morally justified in saving the embryo over the child? If not, why?
2. You are working on the gynaecology ward. Two patients come in requesting an abortion, both for the same reason. One patient is 6 weeks' pregnant, the other is 36 weeks' pregnant. Are there any morally relevant differences between the two requests?

## The embryo/foetus is morally valuable because it is a potential human being

This view holds that the embryo is not morally valuable in and of itself. However because it can develop into a human child, assuming it is viable, it deserves moral concern. Killing an embryo is wrong because it deprives the child that would have potentially lived its existence. This view also generally holds that moral concern starts at conception. However:

- If it is potentially that important, are gametes deserving of moral concern as well? For example a couple that uses contraception is effectively preventing a number of potential children being realized.

## The embryo/foetus is morally valuable if it is a 'person'

This view holds that there is some characteristic or set of characteristics that make an entity a person, and thus of moral value. Common characteristics of personhood may include: consciousness (or perhaps *self-consciousness*), sentience, rationality, the ability to form future plans and the capacity to value one's own life. Various religious views may hold that embryos are not persons until the soul enters the body, which may be at conception or at a later stage. In this context, 'being *a person*' is not necessarily the same as 'being a *human being*'. Some humans may not qualify as persons, and some nonhumans may qualify as persons. Some of these characteristics develop in utero (i.e. sentience), while others do not develop until well after birth, and in the case of individuals with severe learning disabilities may never fully develop (e.g. self-consciousness, rationality).

This leads to questions as to how individuals who have not or will not develop into 'persons', and those who have lost their 'personhood' (i.e. coma, severe brain damage or dementia) are to be treated; what their status and moral value is and how their interests are best protected. Some characteristics may also include other animals: we have no reason to doubt that other mammals are able to feel pain in a similar way to humans and some higher primates may be self-conscious. But:

- Some would claim on the basis of these arguments that neonates are not persons, but parents are not able to lawfully kill their newborns. Depending on philosophical perspectives, cultural and religious beliefs and the legal system the answer to when personhood is attained varies widely.

## The embryo/foetus is morally valuable because it is valued by others

This view holds that embryos are morally valuable because they are the objects of moral concern to others. This means the value of the embryo is not *intrinsic*, but is conferred by others. Thus the wrong in killing an embryo, foetus or even an infant is not the wrong done to that entity, but is wrong because there exist individuals (e.g. the parents) who care for it and do not wish it to be harmed. There also exists a broader societal concern that the killing of such entities would diminish the concern for older children and human life in general. But:

- Does this mean it would be acceptable to kill newborns if no one around them cared? This idea appears to clash with the idea of a right-to-life for all humans from birth.

## The moral value of the embryo/foetus increases as it continues to develop

This view holds that the moral value of the zygote is less than that of the embryo, which in turn is less than that of the foetus and of the newborn. This view does not specify a particular stage of development that is of overriding importance, nor does this provide practical guidance on whether abortion at 12 weeks, 24 weeks or at term is morally acceptable. It is however reflected in the legislative stance around abortion in most jurisdictions, which permit abortion in early pregnancy but prohibit or severely restrict it as the pregnancy progresses to term. This view also fits with most peoples' intuitions: most people are sad when a miscarriage occurs, but are more affected the closer the pregnancy is to term.

## CONTRACEPTION

Legally this refers to any treatment that prevents fertilization of the human egg or implantation of the fertilized egg in the uterus (Fig. 4.2). This includes hormonal contraception, such as the pill and the Mirena coil, as well as nonhormonal contraception including condoms and the copper coil. Additionally, the legal definition of contraception also covers emergency contraception ('the morning after pill' and the copper coil).

Under the *National Health Service Act* 1977 (amended 2006), the Secretary of State for Health has a legal duty to ensure that reasonable requirements for contraceptive treatment and advice are met. Provision of contraception to children and Gillick competency is discussed in Chapter 3. The Fraser Guidelines are summarized in the following box. Sexual activity in children under 13 years is statutory rape, and this must be dealt with through the appropriate channels.

| ETHICS  |
| --- |
| FRASER GUIDELINES |
| In order to prescribe contraception to a child under 16, the clinician must be satisfied that: |

*(Continued)*

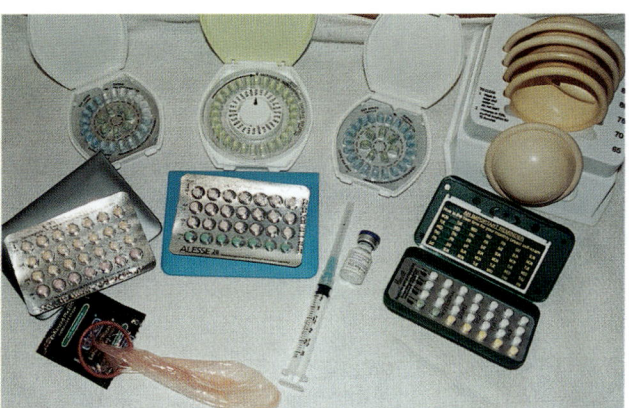

**Fig. 4.2** A selection of contraceptive devices including condoms, diaphragms, pills and injectable contraceptives.

1. The individual understands the given advice.
2. They cannot be persuaded to tell their parents or let the doctor tell them.
3. They are very likely to begin or to continue to have sexual intercourse with or without contraceptive treatment.
4. Their physical or mental health is likely to suffer unless they receive the advice or treatment.
5. The advice or treatment is in the individual's best interest.

## Legal divergence

In Scotland, the Fraser guidelines do not apply.

Instead, the *Age of Legal Capacity Act* 1991 is used, which applies similar criteria.

The legal definition of contraception can cause ethical issues for people who believe that life begins at conception, and thus that postconception contraception is a form of abortion. This led to the following case being brought:

### CASE 4.4  *R (SMEATON ON BEHALF OF SPUC) V. THE SECRETARY OF STATE ET AL.* (2002)

In 2002 the Society for the Protection of Unborn Children challenged government regulations allowing provision of emergency contraception ('the morning after pill' or the copper coil) without a prescription. Their argument was the medication caused a miscarriage since it prevented the implantation of the embryo into the womb and therefore should be subject to the same criteria as an abortion under the *Abortion Act* 1967. The government argued that the medication was a contraceptive. The judge ruled that a miscarriage only could occur after the fertilized embryo had implanted into the uterine lining, and thus that emergency contraception could be provided without meeting the criteria of the *Abortion Act* 1967. He also noted the societally harmful effects of subjecting emergency contraception to the same regulations as abortion.

Ethical objections to types of contraception tend to fall into three categories:

1. One argument goes that contraception is wrong because it interferes with a natural process (fertility) and promotes promiscuity, family breakdown and other deleterious social consequences by breaking the link between sex and reproduction.
2. The other main (consequentialist) argument is that no form of contraception is failsafe and that it may encourage more people to have sexual intercourse and increase the overall number of unwanted pregnancies, even though the individual risk is much lower. Additionally, many forms of contraception fail to protect the user against sexually transmitted diseases.
3. Despite significant developments in medicine, the responsibility to take the contraception and the burdens of side effects fall mainly on females—and males still have relatively few options.

Contrasting arguments may be deontological: at the ecological level, humankind has a duty to contain its population so as not to exceed available resources. Utilitarian arguments may include the idea that at an individual level prospective parents may wish to limit their family to a size they can support. A utilitarian viewpoint might consider that undesired pregnancy is a 'harm' and that therefore it is a benefit that sex can be enjoyed without pregnancy as a consequence.

There is a third key issue regarding the provision of contraception and contraceptive advice: Is the person using contraception in a position to give informed consent to (1) the contraception or (2) sexual intercourse? This is an issue regarding capacity rather than contraception and is considered in Chapter 3.

### HINTS AND TIPS

*Remember*: According to UK case law, pregnancy begins when the fertilized embryo is implanted in the womb. This means that the *Abortion Act* 1967 (amended 1990) does not apply to drugs that prevent implantation of the fertilized embryo.

## STERILIZATION

Sterilization is a medical treatment intended to make a person permanently infertile. In males this is often by vasectomy (Fig. 4.3), and in females it is often by hysterectomy or tubal ligation. Sterilization requires only the affected individual's consent and not their spouse or partner, however the decision will also affect their partner, especially if they want to have children. Sterilization can be ethically problematic:

- Some people who are sterilized may change their mind and regret the decision. Fully informed consent is therefore crucial. The question of how much one's present self can bind one's future self is particularly important. For this reason individuals over 30 years old, with existing children, are more likely to be successful when requesting sterilization.

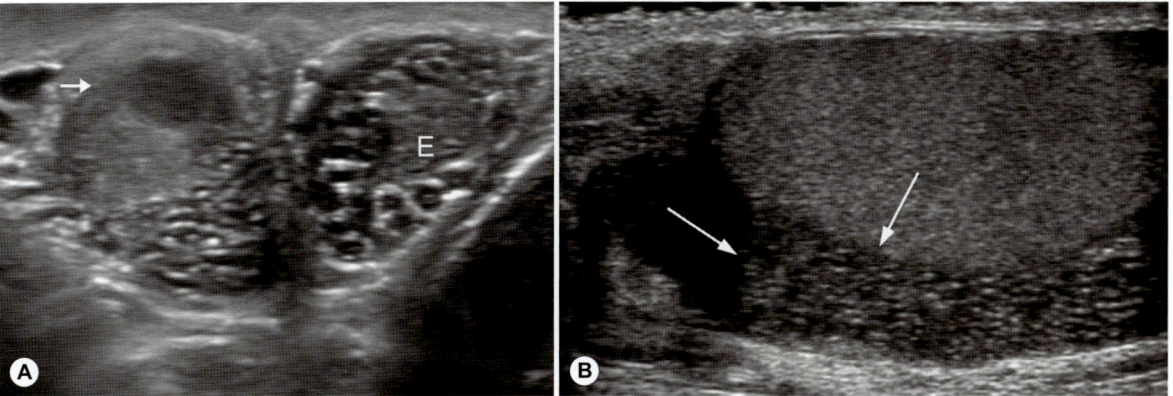

**Fig. 4.3** Postvasectomy changes. (A) Sperm granuloma. Transverse scan shows a heterogeneous mass (*arrow*) along the vas deferens and separate from the epididymis in a postvasectomy patient. (B) Postvasectomy changes in epididymis. Longitudinal image of the scrotum shows ectasia of the ductules of the epididymis (*arrows*) in a patient who had a vasectomy. Contraception needs to be used for 8–12 weeks postvasectomy and until confirmatory semen analysis.

- There have been instances in the past where particular groups, such as people with mental impairments, those with a history of substance misuse or people from ethnic minority backgrounds have been forcibly sterilized or sterilized without their knowledge and consent, in order to prevent them from passing on their 'defective genes' (this is a form of eugenics). In some cases this has been part of a programme to try and wipe out an ethnic group perceived to be undesirable.
- Coercing any type of person to be sterilized is generally seen as unacceptable.
- Should it be acceptable to sterilize a person lacking mental capacity if it is in their best interests or those of their existing or potential future children?
- Some religious groups consider sterilization to be a form of bodily mutilation that goes against the natural function of humans to reproduce, similar to the argument against contraception mentioned earlier.

## Failed sterilization

Some of the issues surrounding sterilization are illustrated by cases of 'failed sterilization'. These are considered as 'negligence' cases (see Chapter 1) in the civil courts. Key issues are as follows:

- Is consent fully informed?
- Can conception as a result of failed sterilization be considered a harm?

As with other medical negligence cases, information given must be in accordance with a *responsible body of professional practice*. In the case of sterilization, this means telling the patient that:

1. The operation is permanent and may be nonreversible.
2. There is a failure rate of the operation, that is while sterilization is effective, it is not an *absolute guarantee* of never conceiving.

Failure to give the information earlier and thereby not warning the patient of the foreseeable risk of pregnancy would be considered a 'breach of duty'. In the case of *McFarlane v. Tayside Health Board* (2000), where a female became pregnant after her husband had had a vasectomy, the court held that the benefits of parenthood must be offset against the financial costs. In the case of a subsequent abortion or pregnancy and delivery of a child with disability: the courts are more willing to consider the resulting discomfort and financial impact and are more prepared to award damages towards the maintenance and treatment of such children born as a result of failed sterilization. They are sometimes referred to as 'wrongful conception' and 'wrongful birth' cases; for example see *Khan v. Meadows* (2021).

> **HINTS AND TIPS**
>
> *Remember*: A failed sterilization operation on a male (if negligence is alleged) may result in a case being brought to court by the female who is his sexual partner.

## Sterilization and mental incapacity

As discussed in Chapter 3, lawful treatment for an adult lacking the relevant mental capacity can only be given if what is proposed is in their 'best interests'. Sterilization for 'best interests' appears more likely to be considered 'on behalf of' mentally incapacitated females than males. This is because pregnancy and indeed menstruation have been seen as potential harms for those with severe mental incapacity. By contrast, it is harder to argue that a male with significant mental incapacity gets a similar benefit from being sterilized. The sorts of things that law courts have considered when deciding what is in the patient's best interests include:

- The likelihood of pregnancy—that is, is the individual engaging or likely to engage in sexual intercourse?
- How well is the patient able to understand the concept of pregnancy and its relation to sex?
- Would the patient be able to cope with parenthood?
- Would this patient be able to use any other form of contraception?
- How would a sterilization operation affect the other medical problems of the patient—for example, will sterilization stop heavy periods from causing a patient distress?
- What other support is available to the patient?

---

**CASE 4.5** *THE MENTAL HEALTH TRUST & OTHERS V. DD & ANOTHER* (2015)

DD was a 36-year-old autistic female with a mild learning disability and an IQ of 70. She had had six previous pregnancies, and all of her children had been taken into care. The hospital petitioned the Court of Protection to have DD sterilized due to grave danger to her life and health from any future pregnancies and her lack of capacity to make decisions about contraception and pregnancy. Because potential pregnancy carried high risks, DD was unlikely to disclose if an intrauterine device (IUD) or intrauterine system (IUS) was expelled or removed and repeated insertion of an IUD/IUS or Depo-Provera injections would cause great professional intrusion into DD's life—the judge ruled it was in DD's best interests to be sterilized rather than have a long acting contraceptive.

---

## ABORTION

Abortion is the intentional termination of pregnancy with the resulting death of the embryo or foetus (Hope et al., 2008), normally by one of two methods—medical abortifacients or surgery. In contrast to many other practices discussed in this section, abortion is an ancient practice which, much like pregnancy, has become safer with the advent of modern medicine. While the Hippocratic Oath prohibits abortion, in both ancient Greece and Rome abortion and infanticide were practiced widely. As Christianity became more influential both were prohibited. Abortion remained illegal in most Western countries until the 1960s. The current limit of 24 weeks in the United Kingdom is higher than in many other European countries, such as Germany, France or the Netherlands where it is 12 weeks (Center for Reproductive Rights 2020). There are a wide range of moral and religious views on this topic.

## Legislation

In the United Kingdom, abortion is a criminal offence except in circumstances as defined in the *Abortion Act* 1967 (amended 1990). Key statutes pertaining to the law on abortion are as follows:

1. *Offences Against the Person Act* 1861, ss.58–59: these sections make illegal:
   a. The self-induction of miscarriage.
   b. A second person helping a female to procure an abortion.
   c. The supply or procurement of an abortifacient.
2. *Infant Life Preservation Act* 1929:
   a. Makes it illegal to destroy the life of a child capable of being born alive.
   b. The destruction of a 'child capable of being born alive' is not a criminal offence if this is done with the intention of saving the life of the mother.
3. *Abortion Act* 1967, amended by the *Human Fertilisation and Embryology Act* 1990, permits abortion with the approval of two doctors, one doctor in an emergency, under the following circumstances:
   a. The pregnancy is less than 24 weeks AND continuation of pregnancy would be a greater risk than termination, to the physical or mental health of the female OR any of her existing children.
   b. Termination is necessary to prevent grave permanent harm to the physical or mental health of the pregnant female.
   c. Continuation of the pregnancy would risk the life of the pregnant female.
   d. Substantial risk of the child being born with severe physical or mental 'handicap'.

The following are important with regards to the *Abortion Act*:

- There is no right to a termination, however the female may *refuse* a termination even at the cost of her life (see Chapter 3: Consent).
- Following amendments to the *Health and Social Care Act* 2022, both misoprostol and mifepristone may be taken at home.
- Neither the foetus nor the father nor any other partner have any rights under the *Abortion Act*.
- If consent is unable to be given, then a termination can be carried out as a best interest decision.
- If the foetus is born alive then all reasonable measures must be taken to save its life if it is in the child's best interests as the child has now gained independent legal personhood.
- Doctors have the right to conscientious objection with regards to participation in abortion. This does not apply in an emergency where the life or health of the pregnant female is at stake (ss4. 1–3). Where the doctor objects to

termination they must ensure that the patient has enough information to know that they can see another doctor, or if not practical the doctor must refer them on (General Medical Council 2023).

## Legal Difference

The *Abortion Act* (1967) does not apply in Northern Ireland. Instead, abortion is permitted under *The Abortion (Northern Ireland) (No. 2) Regulations 2020*, which also include provision for conscientious objection.

### CASE 4.6 *JANAWAY V. SALFORD HEALTH AUTHORITY* (1989): THE LIMITS OF CONSCIENTIOUS OBJECTION

Mrs Janaway was a medical secretary and a devout Roman Catholic. She objected to abortion and to having to type up abortion referral letters. Her employer fired her and she brought a judicial review, arguing that she was covered by the conscientious objection clauses of the abortion act and therefore did not have to type the letters. The case was dismissed because she was not directly involved in the abortion itself. The Court of Appeal and the House of Lords both upheld this.

## Ethical arguments for and against abortion

Ethical arguments for and against abortion revolve around the status of the foetus and the autonomy of the pregnant female or person. The status of the foetus and some of the arguments around it has been discussed earlier in this chapter. Often framed by two opposing positions, pro-life and pro-choice, no serious ethical conclusions can be drawn without considering the status, rights and situation of both the pregnant female or person and the foetus. In their most extreme and caricatured forms, both the pro-life and the pro-choice camps are guilty of failing to account for either (Fig 4.4).

The '*pro-life*' position: Holds that the life of the foetus is valuable because it is a human life, and thus a human person or potential person and therefore ought to be protected. This position encompasses a spectrum of views from those who believe abortion may be permitted in certain circumstances as a necessary evil, to those who believe that abortion is equivalent to murder as all human life is sacred and an embryo counts as a human life from the point of fertilization. Ethical arguments are often based around the rights of the foetus. Additional ethical arguments may be consequentialist,

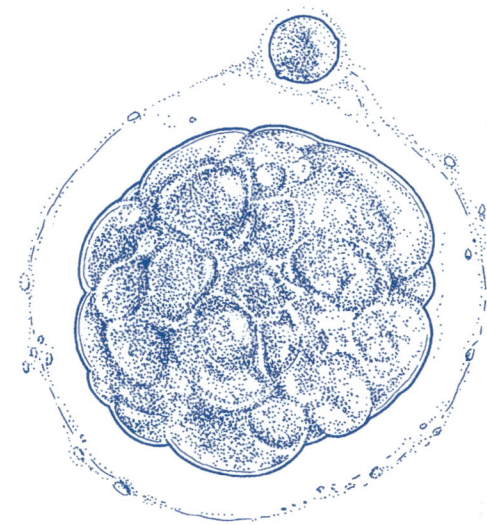

**Fig. 4.4** The morula stage of development. The status of the embryo/foetus is key to the abortion debate.

especially with regards to sex specific terminations or abortion on the grounds of anticipated disability, since these may cause societal harm.

### CASE 4.7 *CROWTER V. SECRETARY OF STATE FOR HEALTH AND SOCIAL CARE* (2022)

Heidi Crowter was a female with Down syndrome who along with Marie-Lea Wilson, the mother of a boy with Down syndrome, challenged the permissibility of abortion on the basis of serious foetal abnormality, particularly after 24 weeks, the usual time limit for abortion. They argued that abortion on the basis of anticipated disability was contrary to the European Convention on Human Rights (ECHR) and section 4 of the *Human Rights Act 1998*. If their argument was accepted, then Parliament would be required to reconsider the relevant section (1(1)(d)) of the *Abortion Act* 1967. The courts dismissed the first claim that was based on the rights of the foetus, as there are no legal rights for the foetus in English law nor under the ECHR. Their second claim, that abortion of these foetuses undermined the rights of living people with disabilities, was also dismissed.

The '*pro-choice*' position: Holds that ending a pregnancy is the choice of the individual involved. The value of the life of the foetus is not always seen as zero, but as being subordinate to the rights of the pregnant female or person to determine what happens to their own body. Like the pro-life position, there are a spectrum of views ranging from the classic dictum of 'safe, legal and rare' to believing it ought to be legal for any reason up to birth. Arguments for this position can come from consequentialist arguments, such as that lack of access to abortion increases the risk to the individual from unsafe terminations or from the pregnancy itself or that it may increase the poverty in which a family finds itself. Rights based arguments for this position include the idea that everyone has a right to autonomy over their own bodies (however this is not an absolute right) and as the foetus is either part of the pregnant individual's body, or separate but dependent on it, the pregnant individual has the right to choose what happens to the foetus as well. A famous argument for the right of self-determination is the violinist analogy by Judith Jarvis Thompson (1971).

### CASE 4.8 THOUGHT EXPERIMENT: THE UNCONSCIOUS VIOLINIST

The world's greatest violinist is dying of kidney failure. To save him the Society of Music Lovers kidnap you and connect you to him for the next 9 months, at which point he will have recovered. Would you be ethically justified in disconnecting yourself from him, even though he will die?

Ethical stances on abortion often change as the pregnancy progresses, which is reflected in law. Consider how the foetus develops throughout pregnancy and how this reflects on your own views. Some would argue that the physician's right to conscientiously object to an abortion in and of itself is an ethical issue, as it may lead to patients being unable to obtain a termination due to lack of willing doctors.

### CASE 4.9 *R V. CATT* (2013) AND *FOSTER V. R* (2023)—*OFFENCES AGAINST THE PERSON ACT*

Mrs Catt was a 36-year-old female who became pregnant. She had a past obstetric history that was complicated, including a child given up for adoption, a late term (23–25 weeks) abortion and two children whom she lived with after concealed pregnancies. She became pregnant and at around 23 weeks' gestation began visiting the Marie Stopes website looking at information around termination. She also searched the internet for information regarding illegal terminations and police involvement. She then attended a British Pregnancy Advisory Service (BPAS) clinic where it was estimated the pregnancy was 26 weeks and 3 days, and on the same day the hospital estimation was 29 weeks and 5 days, both beyond the limit for a termination. She ordered misoprostol online and took it at around 40 weeks' gestation. Because she made no contact with the midwifery department, they contacted Mrs Catt who lied that she had had a termination with Marie Stopes. She repeated the same to the police. The body of the foetus was never recovered. Eventually she was charged with child destruction and pleaded guilty.

Mrs Foster was a 44-year-old female who during the COVID-19 lockdowns obtained misoprostol and mifepristone over the telephone from BPAS. She was aware that she was beyond 24 weeks' pregnant and had known about the pregnancy since before the lockdowns began. She lied over the telephone that she was around 7 weeks' pregnant and was duly posted the abortifacients. At between 32 and 34 weeks of pregnancy, she took the medications and then made two emergency calls the same day. When the paramedics attended a second time, resuscitation of the child was attempted but failed. She later maintained to police and medical staff that she had been unaware of how advanced the pregnancy was. She pleaded guilty to the offence of administering poison with intent to procure a miscarriage.

## ASSISTED REPRODUCTION

Technically, assisted reproduction can refer to any method used to aid fertility. In this section three main groups of procedures are discussed: artificial insemination, IVF and surrogacy (Fig. 4.5). Mitochondrial donation (so-called three-parent babies) will most commonly occur with IVF but could theoretically occur with a surrogate pregnancy as well. Before the legislative framework and specific treatments can be discussed, it must be considered whether 'infertility' or 'sub-fertility' are illnesses. One approach is to consider whether a person or a couple have a *right* to have children. If we decide there is such a right, then the next question is whether the state (by way of the NHS) should fund or facilitate it. To begin with, we will examine the legislative framework for this area overall, and then the specific ethical and legal issues with each form of assisted reproduction.

### HINTS AND TIPS

*Remember*: Whether or not we believe people should have a right to assisted reproduction depends on whether we believe that there is a general right to have a child or whether infertility is an illness—AS WELL AS whether the particular method of assisted reproduction is ethically acceptable.

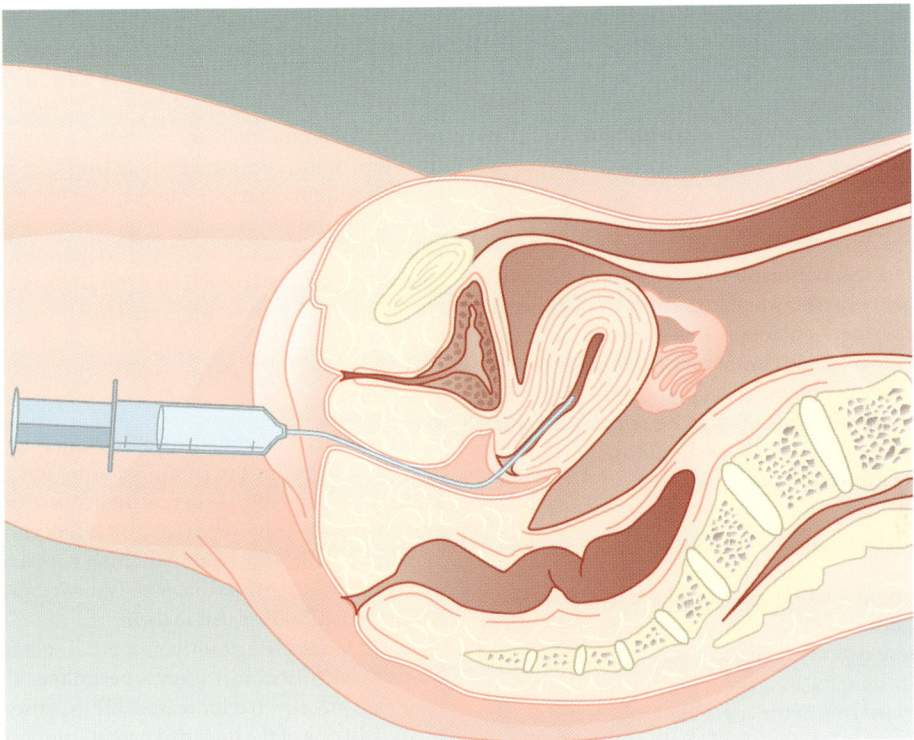

**Fig. 4.5** Illustration of the method of intrauterine insemination (IUI). Washed sperm are gently injected into the uterine cavity at the estimated time of ovulation. Untreated semen should not be used for IUI.

## Legislation

The most important pieces of legislation in this area are the *Human Fertilisation and Embryology Act* 1990 and the *Human Fertilization and Embryology (HFE) Act* 2008.

The HFE Acts govern:

1. The creation of embryos in vitro, that is outside the human body.
2. The storage and use of embryos and gametes.

This means it forms the basis for legislation on artificial insemination (in a clinic), egg donation and IVF. General principles include:

- Adequate consent must be obtained in writing from all parties.
- All parties must have been given the opportunity for counselling prior to any procedure.
- Mixing of human and animal gametes is strictly prohibited.
- No human embryo may be kept for research after 14 days or after the appearance of the primitive streak.
- No foetal germ cells may be used to provide fertility services.
- Eggs, sperm and embryos may be stored for up to 55 years but require renewed consent every 10 years. Donor eggs and sperm do not require re-consent. If patients consent to their eggs/sperm or embryos being used after their death, then they may be kept for 10 years after death.
- Egg/sperm donors may not be paid beyond reasonable expenses. There are age limits and they must be free of genetic disease.
- An individual may donate sperm to a maximum of 10 different recipients.
- Individuals born from egg/sperm donation over the age of 18 may apply for the details of the egg/sperm donor, if they were born after 1 April 2005.

The *Human Fertilisation and Embryology Act* 1990 (s.5) stipulates the creation of the Human Fertilization and Embryology Authority (HFEA): a body charged with the responsibility of:

1. Reviewing information about activities governed by the Act.
2. Granting licences to carry out activities specified in the Act.
3. Publicizing the services provided to the public.
4. Providing appropriate advice to licensed clinics.

The Act defines the following:

- An embryo is a live human embryo where fertilization is complete (i.e. has completed its first cell division).

- The mother is the gestational mother rather than the genetic mother.
- The father is either the spouse of the mother and the donor of the sperm, or spouse consenting to insemination, or father recognized by common law or father by adoption. There can only be one father.

## Artificial insemination

Also called Intrauterine Insemination, sperm is separated to use only the higher quality sperm, which can come from either the patient's husband/partner or a donor. This method can be used by single female, lesbian couples and some heterosexual couples. The chances of a successful pregnancy are lower than IVF. Ethico-legal problems with this tend to be related to gamete donation, for example how many times should an individual be permitted to donate gametes?

## In vitro fertilization

This is the fertilization of an egg outside of the human body. It requires the stimulation of ovulation in the female and the harvesting of eggs. These eggs are then incubated with the sperm in a petri dish, and in some cases a single spermatozoon may be injected under the covering of the egg. Finally, the fertilized egg (usually more than one) is transferred to the uterus. This may involve donated eggs and/or sperm. The ethical problems particular to IVF include:

- The production of excess embryos that must subsequently either be stored by cryopreservation or destroyed.
- The increased likelihood of multiple pregnancies and the subsequent increased demand for obstetric and neonatal services.
- The potential for embryo selection to avoid genetic disease, but also potentially to choose the sex or other characteristics of the embryos. Sex selection for nonmedical reasons is currently illegal in the United Kingdom.
- The potential for clinics to take advantage of couples desperate for a child, by giving them unrealistic hope.
- Discrimination in the provision of the service against poor, single or older patients.

## Mitochondrial donation

This is used in cases of severe mitochondrial disease and requires approval from the HFEA for each case. It is by definition, a form of IVF. There are two forms legal in the United Kingdom: Maternal Spindle Transfer, where the maternal nucleus is transferred into a donor ovum with the nucleus removed, and Pronuclear Transfer where the embryonic nucleus is transferred into a donor embryo with the nucleus removed. As mitochondrial DNA forms so little of the child's DNA, the donor is not deemed to be the genetic parent of the child. The child may, at 16 years, find out some nonidentifiable information about the donor. Ethical issues are perhaps more likely to arise in Pronuclear transfer as two embryos are created, with one being created simply to receive the donor nucleus. For those who believe that life and therefore moral concern begins at the point of conception, this causes additional issues. Examples include genetic contribution from three individuals raising questions about parental rights and pronuclear transfer leading to germline modification (to sperm, egg or embryo) altering the DNA of future generations (Dimond, 2015; Newson et al., 2016).

## Surrogacy

This can be either:

*Partial*: In which the surrogate's ovum is fertilized by the husband/partner from the commissioning couple either via IVF, artificial insemination or sexual intercourse so the surrogate not only carries the baby but has a genetic link with it.

*Full*: In which the commissioning couple provides both the ovum and the sperm, so that while the surrogate carries the child it is not genetically related to them.

In the United Kingdom, commercial surrogacy is prohibited; however, 'altruistic' surrogacy is permitted. This means the surrogate may be covered for reasonable expenses.

At least one of the intended parents must provide gametes for the child. The surrogate is legally the mother until an Act of Court granting custody to the 'commissioning' parents is completed. Until then, the surrogate is able at any time to stop the process.

In addition to the HFE Acts, the *Surrogacy Arrangement Act 1985* also governs this area.

The ethical problems of surrogacy include:

- It represents a separation of genetic, gestational and social parenting.
- It causes a pregnancy with the explicit aim of separating surrogate 'mother' and child.
- It raises the issue of the commodification of human life and the threat of 'baby selling'. This is particularly an issue where the commissioning parents travel abroad to jurisdictions that permit commercial surrogacy, where there is a significant financial imbalance between the commissioning parents and the surrogate and/or the legislation of that country tilts the balance of power towards the commissioning parents.
- It puts the surrogate through a pregnancy, which can lead to significant morbidity or mortality in order that other individuals can have a child genetically related to them.
- The vast majority of females do not want to be surrogates, are unable to be or ineligible to be, meaning that the majority of individuals who desire or can only have a child by surrogate are unable to do so, and in places that

permit commercial surrogacy only the wealthy are able to afford it.

- There are fears of the exploitation and/or coercion of individuals into being surrogates, especially abroad where commercial surrogacy is legal.
- The legislative framework in the United Kingdom allows the surrogate to change their mind at any point, but does not prevent the intended parents from refusing to take the child. Other legislative frameworks grant the intended parents greater power than the surrogate, increasing the risk of exploitation and/or coercion.

## Genetic counselling and screening

The United Kingdom has been at the forefront of advances in genetic medicine, which is discussed in Chapter 3. Clinical practice in fertility is governed mainly by the *Human Tissue Act* 2004 (applies in England, Wales and Northern Ireland), the *Human Tissue (Scotland) Act* 2006, the *Human Fertilisation and Embryology Act* 1990 and the *Human Fertilisation and Embryology Act* 2008. Some of the main ethical issues that may arise here include:

- Selection of embryos to be disease free.
- Genetic editing of embryos.
- In utero screening of embryos.
- Abortion of foetuses with specific genetic diseases:
  - In the case of severe foetal abnormality, abortion is allowed up to term. However what counts as a serious abnormality is not defined and may cause tensions between the parents and clinicians. In addition to the normal 'pro-choice' arguments, some would say that permitting abortion of foetuses with severe abnormalities allows individuals to have children (knowing they have that choice) where they would have otherwise chosen not to.
  - There is a concern that permitting abortion in anticipation of future disabilities may lead to marginalization and devaluing of people living with disabilities. This was the basis for *Crowter and Others v. Secretary of State for Health and Social Care* (2022).
- Obtaining informed consent
  - This is particularly relevant in the case of individuals with learning disabilities.
- Family planning.
- Confidentiality and disclosure of information.

## END OF LIFE

Care of the dying and care after death brings many ethical and legal considerations. All doctors will at some point be involved in the care of the dying, including as a junior doctor so as well as understanding the medical management of patients it is essential to understand the relevant ethical and legal frameworks. This section will cover the following areas:

- Advance planning, Do Not Attempt Cardiopulmonary Resuscitation (DNACPR), futility and withdrawal of Artificial Nutrition and Hydration (ANaH).
- Death, its definitions and certification of death.
- Physician-assisted suicide and euthanasia.
- Organ donation.

Ethical questions in this area not only include when it is appropriate to stop treatment, but whether hastening death is something that should take place in a clinical setting. The definition of death is another 'epistemological' question that has major implications, such as when efforts to maintain a body's vital functions can be withdrawn and whether organs may be taken from a body for use in transplants.

## Withholding and withdrawing life-sustaining treatment

In British law, an individual can refuse life-saving treatment or request for it to be withdrawn, assuming they have capacity. This includes if the withdrawal of treatment will result in their death, as illustrated by the case of *Re B* (2002). They cannot demand treatment that is not held to be in their best interests, as shown by the case of *R (Burke) v. GMC* (2005). Ethical and legal justifications for withholding or withdrawing a treatment are likely to be on the basis of:

- Refusal of consent, such as an advance decision.
- Futility.
- An argument that the burdens of the treatment are disproportionate to either the benefits or the likelihood of success.

The BMA, in line with the decisions of the courts, has produced guidance on withholding and withdrawing life-sustaining treatment including artificial nutrition and hydration. According to the guidance: use of nasogastric tubes, percutaneous gastrostomy and IV fluids are considered to be medical treatment. There is no obligation to provide treatment that will not benefit the patient and it is also permissible to withdraw treatment that is not benefitting the patient. These decisions will be made by one or more senior doctors. Where there is any disagreement regarding what is beneficial or the patient's wishes, it may be advisable to seek court approval before taking further action. Many of the court cases have been brought on behalf of individuals without capacity, especially children. For more on this see Chapter 3, Children, and Appendix I.

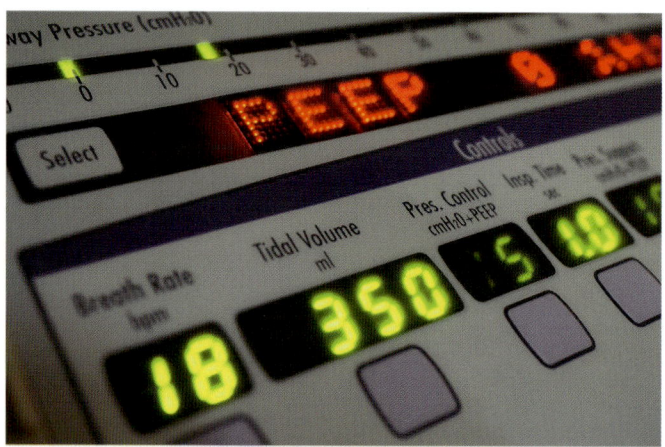

**Fig. 4.6** Control panel on a mechanical ventilator. A patient with mental capacity can refuse medical treatment, including life support measures.

### CASE 4.10  *RE B* (2002)

Miss B was a 41-year-old female who was paralyzed from the neck down and dependent on a ventilator (Fig. 4.6). She asked for the ventilator to be switched off. The medical team felt unable to comply on the basis that they felt she had a worthwhile life. The court held that Miss B was competent and well informed and therefore her refusal of ventilation had to be respected, even if this meant her death.

### CASE 4.11  *R (BURKE) V. GMC* (2005)

Mr Burke, a male with cerebellar ataxia, predicted that at some point in the future he would need artificial nutrition and hydration (ANaH) (Fig. 4.8). He was concerned that if he lost capacity a doctor would decide that ANaH was no longer in his best interests and he would die of thirst and starvation. He wanted to be able to demand these in advance. The court held that a patient has no right, whether he is competent or incompetent, to demand a treatment that is not in his best interests.

### CASE 4.12  *AIREDALE NHS TRUST V. BLAND* (1993)

Tony Bland (Fig. 4.7) was an 18-year-old Liverpool fan, who was injured at the Hillsborough football ground in April 1989 after being crushed in the crowd. He suffered a cardiac arrest and subsequent hypoxic brain injury. He was diagnosed as being in a permanent vegetative state and showed no signs of recovery. He was not ventilated, but was fed via a nasogastric tube. The hospital treating him sought court approval to discontinue nasogastric feeding, on the basis that this was a form of treatment and not in his best interests. His family were in agreement. The case was finally decided at the House of Lords, with the Law Lords holding that withdrawal of treatment (nasogastric feeding) was permissible in this case. They ruled that when carried out by medical professionals, there must be a duty to act for omission of treatment to be murder. In Mr Bland's case, withdrawal of tube feeding was an omission of medical treatment; tube feeding was not in the best interests of Mr Bland and therefore its withdrawal was permissible despite it inevitably leading to his death.

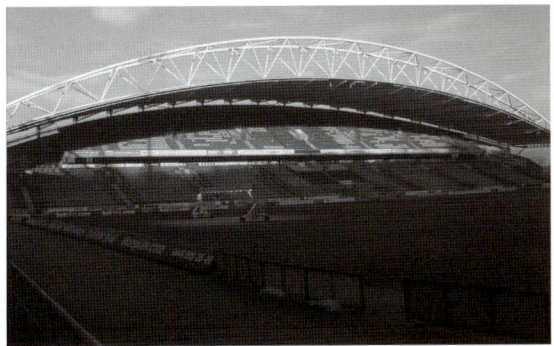

**Fig. 4.7** A modern football stadium. In spring 1989, 96 Liverpool fans were crushed to death in a Football Association Cup semifinal match between Liverpool and Nottingham Forest. This occurred at the Hillsborough Stadium in Sheffield and came to be known as The Hillsborough Disaster. Tony Bland was one of the football fans severely injured, and it led to the case of *Airedale NHS Trust v. Bland* (1993) being brought to the courts.

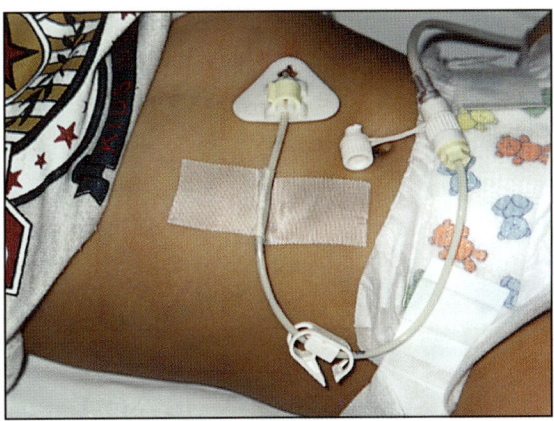

**Fig. 4.9** Percutaneous endoscopic gastrostomy tube for enteral feeding in a child.

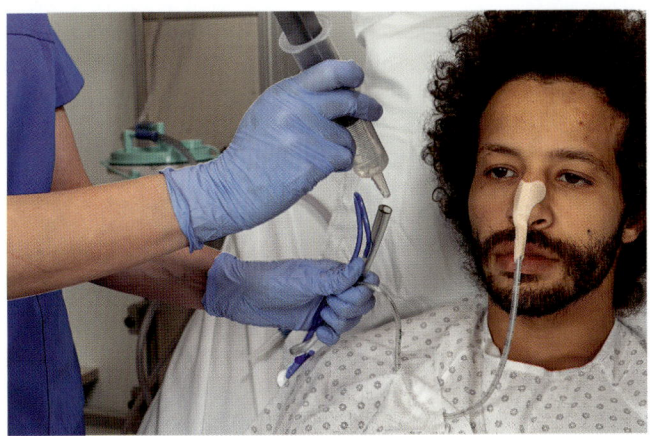

**Fig. 4.8** Nasogastric tube.

The case of *Airedale NHS Trust v. Bland* (1993) changed the landscape of practice around withdrawal of care. Prior to the legal ruling, withdrawal of ventilation or artificial nutrition and hydration in a patient was viewed as tantamount to murder. Key points of the Bland case were:

- This case confirmed the *act/omission distinction in law* (discussed later).
- Withdrawal of treatment is not a legally culpable omission *if in the patient's best interests*. Artificial nutrition can cause both discomfort and harm to a patient when used inappropriately.
- The case was decided on 'futility' of care, although some would argue feeding is never futile.

## Acts and omissions doctrine

The acts and omissions doctrine is well supported in case law and holds that there is a difference between an act and an omission. In the case of Tony Bland there was a difference between giving a medication to end his life (an action) and withdrawing artificial nutrition and hydration (an omission), even though the end result would be the same. Whether you accept this distinction will depend on the ethical theory you subscribe to; many consequentialists hold that there is no true difference between acts and omissions as the outcome is the same.

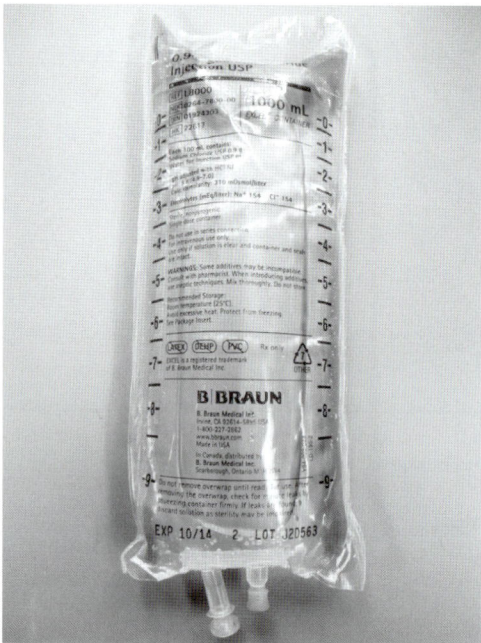

Fig. 4.10 Intravenous or subcutaneous fluid is a form of medical treatment.

## Treatment and basic care

Since the decision in *Airedale NHS Trust v. Bland* (1993), artificial nutrition and hydration (ANaH) are considered in law to be a form of treatment that can be withdrawn. Basic care, which includes oral feeding where appropriate as well as washing and maintaining the basic dignity of patients who are unable to do this for themselves, can never be withdrawn. Whether ANaH is treatment or basic care has been hotly debated in medical ethics circles for decades. However, classifying ANaH (Fig. 4.10) as treatment means that it can be given as part of treatment for conditions, such as severe anorexia nervosa.

## Do not attempt cardiopulmonary resuscitation decisions

The DNACPR order involves making an advance decision to withhold cardiorespiratory resuscitation from a patient in the event that they have a cardiac or respiratory arrest. DNACPR should be considered only when:

- Resuscitation is contrary to the informed wishes of a competent patient, that is, resuscitation is not *consented to*.
- Resuscitation is contrary to a valid *advance decision to refuse treatment*.
- Resuscitation is likely to be *futile*.
- Resuscitation is *not* in the best interests of the patient, that is, it is likely to cause a quality of life that is considered to be worse than death.

In many places DNACPR forms are being replaced or supplemented with ReSPECT forms in an attempt to provide more holistic end of life care (ReSPECT: Recommended Summary Plan for Emergency Care and Treatment). Although patients or relatives may not demand resuscitation, except in exceptional circumstances resuscitation should always be discussed with the patient and/or relatives prior to a DNACPR decision being made. The case of *R (on the application of Tracey) v. Cambridge University Hospital NHS Trust* (2014) has led to it being less defensible to put in place a DNACPR without patient involvement.

---

**CASE 4.13** *R (ON THE APPLICATION OF TRACEY) V. CAMBRIDGE UNIVERSITY HOSPITAL NHS TRUST (2014)*

Mrs Tracey was diagnosed with terminal lung cancer with an expected prognosis of 9 months. She was then involved in a car accident and sustained a high-level spinal cord injury. She was intubated and while in hospital developed pneumonia and deteriorated. Before the team attempted to extubate her they discussed a DNACPR decision and noted that Mrs Tracey wanted to be for full escalation and to be involved in discussions about her care. The team felt that her prognosis was extremely poor and that both Mrs Tracey and her family had unrealistic expectations about this. The consultant who placed the DNACPR order felt that he had discussed it with Mrs Tracey and her daughter and that she was in agreement. Her daughter later objected, feeling that neither her mother nor her family had known what the DNACPR decision entailed and would not have agreed to it if they did.

The DNACPR decision was then revoked. Mrs Tracey continued to decline and subsequently refused to discuss the matter any further. Eventually after discussion with the family, a second DNACPR was put in place. Mrs Tracey died shortly afterwards.

Her family brought a case against the hospital claiming that Mrs Tracey's article 8 rights had been violated by placing the first DNACPR decision against Mrs Tracey's wishes. The case was eventually brought to the Court of Appeals. The court ruled that Mrs Tracey's rights under article 8 had been breached, and that although patients could not demand cardiopulmonary resuscitation (CPR), there must be a strong presumption of involving the patient in these discussions. It was also ruled that wishing to spare the patient upset was not a good enough reason to not have a full discussion.

### COMMUNICATION

*Remember*: A DNACPR decision is not the same as withdrawing all treatment. It only relates to cardiopulmonary resuscitation. It can help to explain to the patient and/or family that other decisions like the potential for hospital admission or not, potential for escalation to intensive care or not and so on are separate decisions to be agreed, and that even with a DNACPR decision in place doctors still have a duty to make clinical assessments and offer treatments like pain relief or antibiotics if they are appropriate to the situation.

## Futility

Often given as a reason for a DNACPR decision or cessation of life-sustaining interventions, futility is often hard to define. In order to define futility it is often categorized further, for example in the following three ways by Jonsen et al. (2010) and adapted from Sokol (2009):

- Physiological: The intervention cannot physiologically achieve the desired effect; for example a shock in a nonshockable rhythm, such as asystole or Pulseless Electrical Activity. This is the least controversial form of futility.
- Quantitative: The intervention is very unlikely to achieve the desired effect; for example CPR in end-stage cancer, where it is highly improbable that the desired effect (e.g. return of circulation), will occur.
- Qualitative: Even if the intervention is successful, the outcome is so undesirable it is better not to attempt the intervention; for example continuing CPR after such a period of time where severe hypoxic brain injury is likely. This is the most controversial form of futility and is dependent on the views of the individuals involved. Not everyone considers life with severe hypoxic brain injury as a life not worth living.

It is often argued that futility must be goal specific: resection of a tumour with metastases may be futile in that it will not cure the patient, but may not be futile if it alleviates symptoms. Additionally the wishes of the patient and their quality of life must also be taken into consideration when thinking about futility, particularly qualitative futility.

## Neonates and children

here have been a number of cases where neonates or children with severe disabilities have had treatment withdrawn or withheld. The courts have tended to take the approach that aggressive treatment for children with severe disabilities need not be pursued, especially if there is only a short gain in life expectancy anticipated from treatment. The arguments for this tend to revolve around best interests and futility. These cases often generate lots of media attention and can be very difficult to navigate. See Chapter 3 Children and Appendix I with cases for self-directed study for more.

## PHYSICIAN-ASSISTED SUICIDE AND EUTHANASIA

Coming from the ancient Greek for a good death, euthanasia refers to the intentional ending of a patient's life, with the aim that this is of benefit to the patient. The act of euthanasia can be classified in relation to the following two factors (Huxtable, 2007):

1. The patient whose life is at stake:
   a. May want help dying = voluntary euthanasia.
   b. May not want help dying = involuntary euthanasia.
   c. May not be able to form or communicate a decision = nonvoluntary euthanasia.
2. Positive acts (active euthanasia) versus negative omissions (passive euthanasia).

   a. The terms 'physician-assisted suicide' and 'euthanasia' are often used interchangeably or with euthanasia being used as a shorthand for both. However strictly speaking, physician-assisted suicide is where the patient administers the lethal drug themselves, often by ingestion, and euthanasia is where the doctor or sometimes another health professional administers the lethal drug.

The evidence from jurisdictionhows that patients prefer euthanasia over PAS (Fig. 4.11). For example in Canada in 2022 there were 13,241 deaths due to euthanasia and PAS under the Medical Aid in Dying Programme. Of these, fewer than seven were PAS deaths, that is where the patient took the medication themselves (Health Canada, 2022).

Although the Hippocratic Oath prohibited euthanasia, it was practised in Graeco-Roman times before suicide more generally became prohibited under Christianity. At the end of the 19th and beginning of the 20th centuries, several countries including the United Kingdom saw campaigns for legalization of euthanasia and for the promotion of eugenics. The Nazis ran a programme of involuntary euthanasia targeting people with disabilities, which tainted the euthanasia and eugenics movements. In the United Kingdom, suicide was decriminalized in 1961, and a number of jurisdictions have legalized euthanasia and/or PAS.

## Legal status

Both PAS and euthanasia are currently illegal in the United Kingdom. Although the law makes no distinction between the two, ethically euthanasia differs from murder in that it is done with the intention of benefitting the individual who dies. If, either through an act or an omission a clinician causes the death of a patient, then they may face a variety of criminal charges including murder, attempted murder, manslaughter or aiding, abetting, counselling or procuring the suicide of another. In order for a murder charge to be brought against a clinician, there are two key factors to be considered:

• Did the clinician cause the patient to die? This includes hastening death by a few hours. However it can often be uncertain whether the patient died because of the doctor's actions or from natural causes.

• Did the clinician intend for the patient to die? This is closely related to the doctrine of double effect (see later).

Suicide was decriminalized by the *Suicide Act* 1961, later amended by the *Coroners and Justice Act* 2009. However, encouraging suicide or assisting in the suicide of another remains a criminal offence. The Director of Public Prosecutions has provided guidance to prosecutors around these laws, some of which are shown in Table 4.1.

There have been a number of attempts to legalize euthanasia or assisted suicide, but to date none have been successful.

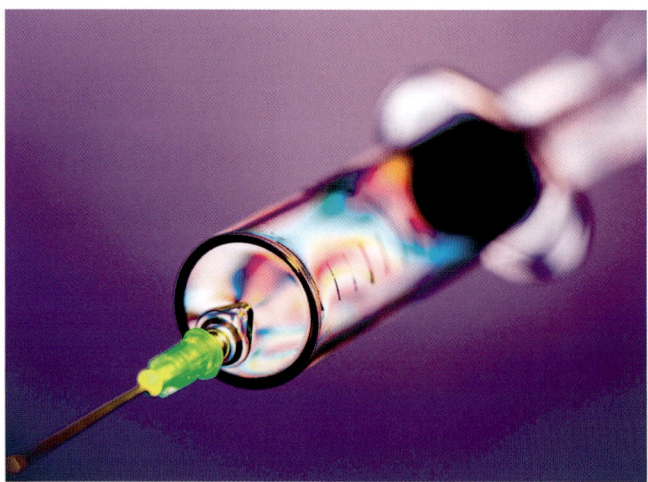

**Fig. 4.11** Despite repeated attempts, neither physician-assisted suicide nor euthanasia have been legalized at the time of writing in the United Kingdom.

**Table 4.1** Director of Public Prosecutions guidelines in cases of encouraging or assisting suicide

| Factors in favour of prosecution | Factors against prosecution |
|---|---|
| The victim was under 18 years of age. | The victim had reached a voluntary, clear, settled and informed decision to commit suicide. |
| The victim did not have the capacity, as defined by the *Mental Capacity Act* 2005, to reach an informed decision to commit suicide. | The suspect was wholly motivated by compassion. |
| The suspect was not wholly motivated by compassion; for example the suspect was motivated by the prospect that they or a person closely connected to them stood to gain in some way from the death of the victim. | The actions of the suspect, although sufficient to come within the definition of the offence, were of only minor encouragement or assistance. |
| The victim was physically able to undertake the act that constituted the assistance themself. | The suspect had sought to dissuade the victim from taking the course of action which resulted in their suicide. |
| The suspect was acting in their capacity as a medical doctor, nurse, other healthcare professional, a professional carer (whether for payment or not), or as a person in authority, such as a prison officer, *and the victim was in his or her care.* | The actions of the suspect may be characterized as reluctant encouragement or assistance in the face of a determined wish on the part of the victim to commit suicide. |

## Legal Differences

The *Suicide Act* 1961 does not apply in Scotland, as suicide was never a common law offence.

In Northern Ireland, the *Criminal Justice Act (Northern Ireland) 1966* serves the same function as the *Suicide Act* 1961.

Two important ethico-legal concepts in this area are the doctrine of double effect and the acts and omissions doctrine. The acts and omissions doctrine has been mentioned in a previous section of this chapter.

## Doctrine of double effect

The doctrine of double effect holds that an action that may shorten an individual's life is permissible, as long as that is not the aim and only a side effect. For example Mrs X has severe pneumonia complicating immobility after recently fracturing her hip and cannot be safely anaesthetized to undergo hip surgery: she is in a lot of pain and has a poor prognosis. Dr A wants to increase her morphine to control her pain. This may have the side effect of causing respiratory depression and shortening Mrs X's life. This was first notably mentioned in the case of *R v. Bodkin Adams* (1957).

### CASE 4.14  *R V. BODKINS ADAMS (1957)* — THE DOCTRINE OF DOUBLE EFFECT

Dr Adams was a GP who was tried for the murder of one of his patients who had made him a beneficiary of her will. The patient was an 80-year-old female who had had a stroke. Dr Adams prescribed her heroin and morphine and she subsequently died. Dr Adams was found not guilty and the judge held that as the aim of Dr Adams' treatment was to benefit the patient by relieving pain and suffering, the shortening of her life did not constitute murder.

## Acts and omissions doctrine, redux

As discussed earlier, the acts and omissions doctrine is well supported in case law and holds that there is a difference between acts and omissions. For example there is a difference between giving medication with the aim to end a patient's life (an act) and not doing CPR on a patient (an omission).

### CASE 4.15  *R V. COX* (1992) — AN EXAMPLE OF THE DIFFERENCE BETWEEN ACTS AND OMISSIONS

Dr Cox gave a patient of his, Mrs Lillian Boyes, an injection of potassium chloride after her repeated requests to die. The patient was 70 years old with severe rheumatoid arthritis and multiple other comorbidities. He was convicted of attempted murder and given a 1 year suspended sentence. The court found that there had been an intention to euthanise the patient, in part because the drug administered was not one with accepted painkilling or sedating effects. Because the patient had been cremated, the cause of death could not be proven; hence Dr Cox was charged with attempted murder. The Good Medical Practice (GMC) cautioned Dr Cox but allowed him to continue to practise on the condition that he undergo extra training in palliative medicine.

### CASE 4.16  *PRETTY V. THE UNITED KINGDOM* (2002)

Diane Pretty was in the latter stages of motor neurone disease when she brought a case against the government. She wanted to end her life to avoid dying what she saw as a painful and distressing death. However she was no longer in a position to do so and wanted her husband to be able to help her commit suicide. She sought assurance that he would not be prosecuted under the *Suicide Act* 1961. She argued her case on the grounds that her rights under articles 2, 3, 8, 9 and 14 of the European Convention on Human Rights had been violated. She eventually appealed to the European Court of Human Rights (ECtHR), after losing her previous appeals in the English Courts. The judges of the ECtHR agreed with the English Courts and ruled against her. They found that:

- Article 2 (the right to life) protected the right to life, not to die.
- Article 3 (the prohibition on torture or degrading treatment) did not extend to allowing a terminally ill individual to kill themselves by enlisting the help of another.
- Article 8 (the right to private life) was a qualified right, and that the interference in Mrs Pretty's private life was proportionate, given that the *Suicide Act* aimed to protect human life.

Mrs Pretty died a few days after she lost her case at the European Court of Human Rights.

## Ethical arguments for and against physician-assisted suicide and euthanasia

Outlined here are the main arguments for and against legislation of euthanasia in the United Kingdom, partially adapted from Hope et al. (2008) and limited to considerations of competent adults with a terminal illness and less than 6 months to live.

### The case for physician-assisted suicide and euthanasia

- Consistency
  - It is commonly accepted that it is possible to decide to kill oneself, so why should an individual who is physically unable to do so be denied the ability to exercise such judgement.
  - The law currently allows withdrawal and withholding of life-saving medical treatment (so-called passive euthanasia). If such a death is permissible then why should we also not permit active euthanasia, which would seem to cause less suffering than death from, for example, withdrawal of artificial nutrition and hydration?
- Principle-based arguments
  - Respect for a patient's autonomy in determining the time and manner of their death.
  - Beneficence prevents unnecessary suffering to the patient and their family.
  - Avoids the patient dying in an undignified manner.
- Other arguments
  - Allows protection of vulnerable patients by giving the State oversight of the process.
  - Removes the inequality that only rich patients can afford to travel abroad for euthanasia or physician-assisted suicide.

### The case against physician-assisted suicide and euthanasia

- Improvements and adequate investments in palliative care render euthanasia unnecessary if we accept that the main aim of euthanasia is to prevent suffering.
- Life is precious and valuable in and of itself, and we devalue it by permitting suicide.
- Weakens the taboo against suicide.
- Contrary to the aims of medicine which are to heal, prolong life and reduce suffering, not to cause death.
- May alter the relationship between doctors (and other health professionals) and their patients and degrade trust in the medical profession.
- Potential for an expansion of eligible patients beyond the original framework, also known as 'the slippery slope' argument (Case 4.16).

- Impossible to safeguard against abuses of the system and coercion/exploitation of vulnerable patients.
- Cheaper than high quality palliative care and may result in worse or less palliative care provision by governments or funding bodies trying to save money.

---

**CASE 4.17  THE SLIPPERY SLOPE**

The slippery slope argument is controversial and in the eyes of some individuals renders an argument invalid (see Chapter 1). However it is a powerful argument, so does the slippery slope exist?

**No**; in places like Oregan, legislation permitting PAS was passed in 1997. It has not been expanded in scope since then, suggesting that the slippery slope does not exist or is not inevitable.

**Yes**; places like Belgium, Holland and Canada have seen an expansion of their Assisted Dying laws since they were introduced; for example to remove the requirement for a prognosis of 6 months or less, include children or include patients with mental illness.

---

## DEATH

The questions of what death is and when it occurs are surprisingly difficult to answer. In English law there is no statutory definition of death, however there are generally two ways in which death is defined: cardiorespiratory death and brainstem death. In an environment free of modern medical care, one invariably leads to the other. It is only with modern intensive care facilities that this issue has arisen. Cardiorespiratory death is the death that most doctors are familiar with and verify. Brainstem death can only be diagnosed by senior consultant neurosurgeons, neurologists or intensive care doctors. Diagnosis has to be made by two doctors of appropriate training and seniority.

## Verification and certification of death

Verification and certification of death are two different tasks and are among the most important duties a doctor is asked to undertake. Steps for the verification of death are shown in the following CLINICAL NOTES box. Although certification of death is always a priority task it is important to be aware that families with certain religious beliefs or backgrounds (e.g. Jewish, Muslim) may require the dead to be buried within a certain timeframe, often within 24 hours.

## Death certification and when to notify the coroner

The main cause to write on the certificate (Fig. 4.12) is the single pathology directly leading to death. It is certified *to the best of the attending doctor's knowledge and belief*. The patient may have other comorbid conditions worsening the prognosis but not directly leading to death, for example type 2 diabetes mellitus, hypertension.

Studies of the accuracy of death certification have found up to one-third of death certificates contain major errors. Contributing factors include:

- Lack of training of doctors.
- Inadequate or misunderstood clinical information.
- Concealment of information that might distress family members.
- Omissions of information.
- Coding errors.

The certificate of death registration is essential for the funeral to proceed. A doctor has a statutory duty to complete this form and may do so if they have attended on the deceased at any point during their lifetime. This is a change from the previous requirement for the doctor to have attended the deceased in their final illness and seen the deceased in the last 28 days of their life (Department of Health and Social Care 2023).

Some deaths must be reported to the coroner by the doctor, summarized in the Notification of Deaths Regulations 2019:

- Death that may be linked to medical treatment, surgery or anaesthetic. This includes deaths from a recognized complication of a procedure, and where delayed diagnosis accelerated the trajectory to death.
- Death that may be linked back to an accident; however, long ago that happened.
- Death related to any previous occupation—*so take an occupational history.*
- Suicide and suspected suicide.
- Death linked to poisoning, intoxication or illicit drugs.
- Deaths within 24 hours of admission to hospital.
- Deaths when a doctor has not attended in the previous 28 days.
- When there is no doctor available who is in the position to issue a death certificate.
- When the cause of death is unknown or uncertain.
- Any unexpected death.
- Violent or traumatic deaths.
- Suspicious deaths.
- All deaths of people in police custody or detained under the *Mental Health Act*, even if due to natural causes.

When a death is reported to the coroner, the coroner may: certify the death on the basis of the information available or acquired, certify the death after ordering an autopsy (postmortem examination) or certify the death after holding an inquest.

**Coroners and Justice Act 2009**
Form prescribed by the Medical Certificate of Cause of Death Regulations 2024

## Attending Practitioner Medical Certificate of Cause of Death

For use by a Registered Medical Practitioner who has attended the deceased in their lifetime. This certificate is to be delivered by the relevant Medical Examiner as soon as practicable to the Registrar of Births and Deaths

Please refer to guidance for medical practitioners completing an MCCD on .GOV.UK

Unique ID:

Name of deceased (first, middle, and last) .................................................................

Date of birth DD/MM/YYYY ........................................................... Age

NHS number (if available) ...........................................................

Date of death as stated to me DD/MM/YYYY ...........................................................

Place of death ...........................................................

### CAUSE OF DEATH

The condition thought to be the underlying cause of death should appear in the lowest completed line of part I

| | Approximate interval between onset and death (These particulars not to be entered in the death register) |
| --- | --- |
| I (a) Disease or condition leading directly to death ........................................... | |
| (b) Other disease or condition, if any, leading to I (a) ........................................... | |
| (c) Other disease or condition, if any, leading to I (b) ........................................... | |
| (d) Other disease or condition, if any, leading to I (c) ........................................... | |
| II Other significant conditions contributing to the death but not relating to the disease or condition causing it ........................................... | |

*Circle the appropriate digit*

1.  The certified cause of death takes account of information obtained from post-mortem
2.  Information from post-mortem may be available later
3.  Post-mortem not being held
4.  This death was reported to the coroner whose duty to investigate under s1 CJA2009 was not engaged

*Circle the appropriate digit*

Was the deceased pregnant within the year prior to their death?

0.  Not applicable
1.  Pregnant at the time of death
2.  Pregnant 1–42 days before death
3.  Pregnant 43 days to a year before death
4.  Not pregnant
9.  Unknown

If the deceased was pregnant within the year prior to their death, did the pregnancy contribute to their death?

1.  Yes
2.  No
9.  Unknown

This death may have been due to, or contributed to, by the employment followed at some point by the deceased

Yes    No

I may be in a position to give, on application by the Registrar General, additional information as to the cause of death for the purpose of more precise statistical classification

**APC 1**
Form 66

**Fig. 4.12** Medical Certificate of Cause of Death (MCCD) — front of the form. (From https://www.legislation.gov.uk/uksi/2024/492/images/uksi_20240492_en_007 and https://www.legislation.gov.uk/uksi/2024/492/images/uksi_20240492_en_008. Public Domain.)

**Ethnicity**

Circle the digit of the ethnicity as it is recorded in the patient record. If there is no match with the list, or there is no ethnicity recorded, please circle '19. Not known.'

1. White: English, Welsh, Scottish, Northern Irish or British
2. White: Irish
3. White: Gypsy or Irish Traveller
4. White: Any other White background
5. Mixed or multiple ethnic groups: White and Black Caribbean
6. Mixed or multiple ethnic groups: White and Black African
7. Mixed or multiple ethnic groups: White and Asian
8. Mixed or multiple ethnic groups: Any other mixed or multiple ethnic background
9. Asian or Asian British: Indian
10. Asian or Asian British: Pakistani
11. Asian or Asian British: Bangladeshi
12. Asian or Asian British: Chinese
13. Asian or Asian British: Any other Asian background
14. Black, Black British, Caribbean or African: Caribbean
15. Black, Black British, Caribbean or African: African
16. Black, Black British, Caribbean or African: Any other Black, Black British or Caribbean background
17. Other ethnic group: Arab
18. Other ethnic group: Any other ethnic group
19. Not known

**Implantable medical devices**

Did the deceased have any implantable medical devices fitted during their lifetime?   Yes   No

If yes, provide details of the device and its location .......................................................................................

If yes, has the device been removed? ........................................

**For the attending practitioner to complete**

Full name ........................................ Qualifications (as registered by GMC) ........................ GMC number ....................

Declaration: I confirm that I attended the deceased before their death and that the cause of death is as stated in this certificate to the best of my knowledge and belief.

Signature ........................................ Date DD/MM/YYYY ...................

**For the medical examiner to complete**

Full name ........................................ Qualifications (as registered by GMC) ........................ GMC number ....................

Declaration: I am a duly appointed medical examiner and following scrutiny I confirm that the cause of death is as stated in this certificate to the best of my knowledge and belief.

Signature ........................................ Date DD/MM/YYYY ...................

**Fig. 4.12** Cont'd

## The Medical Examiner system

This is still relatively new and evolving in England and Wales and relates to all noncoronial deaths. Since April 2024 there has been a statutory requirement for all noncoronial deaths to be scrutinized by a Medical Examiner. Medical Examiners are senior doctors employed by hospitals who provide independent scrutiny of the causes of death, outside their usual clinical duties. The Medical Examiner has no previous connection to the deceased. The purpose of the Medical Examiner system is to:

- Increase public safeguards via independent medical scrutiny of all noncoronial deaths.
- Ensure appropriate referrals are made to the coroner.
- Provide a better service for the bereaved by direct liaison.
- Improve the quality of death certification and hence the quality of mortality data.

## Cremation

If the patient/family opts for cremation, then certain medical implants and devices present a dangerous explosion risk and need to be identified:

- **Any kind of battery**: For example pacemaker or implantable cardioverter-defibrillator (Fig. 4.13).
- **Radiation**: For example recent brachytherapy.
- **Pressurization**: For example Fixion intramedullary nails.

The doctor completing the Medical Certificate of Cause of Death (MCCD) is asked to identify and certify if such an implant or device is present or not. This replaces the need to complete a separate cremation form.

## Brainstem death

In order to diagnose someone on a ventilator as dead, the concept of brain death or brainstem death was developed. From a legal point of view in the United Kingdom, death is equated with irreversible loss of brainstem function as in the legal case *Re A* (1992).

The UK Medical Royal Colleges put forward criteria for brainstem death in 1976 (Anonymous, 1976, 1979). Hypothermia and drug intoxication must be ruled out as differential diagnoses, and the tests must be repeated; criteria include the absence of spontaneous respiration or brainstem reflexes. The doctor making the diagnosis must be a consultant and a second opinion must be sought from another doctor and both must be 5 years after full GMC registration. The official time of death is the time of completion of the second set of tests.

In the United States the term 'brain death' infers that the neocortex has also been destroyed: the concept of 'whole brain death'. 'The Harvard Criteria', a protocol for defining brain death, includes four major criteria for 'brain death':

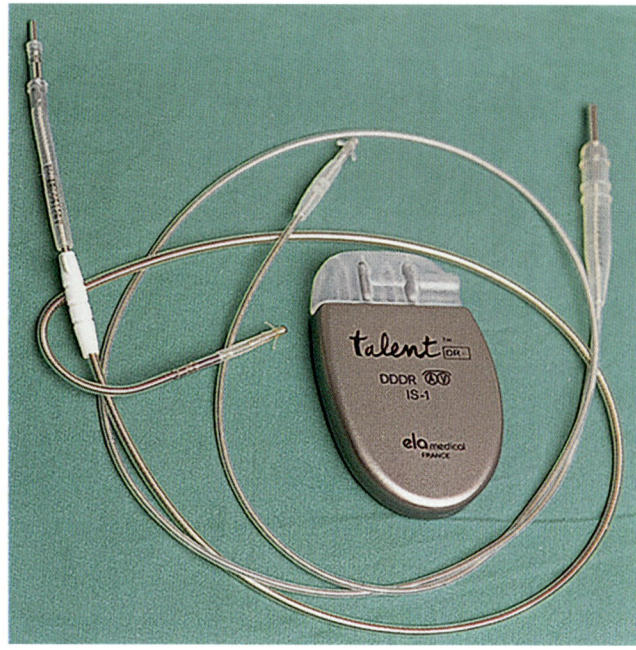

**Fig. 4.13** Permanent cardiac pacemaker unit. The doctor certifying death should identify any dangerous (explosive) devices in the body of the deceased.

1. Absence of cerebral responsiveness.
2. Absence of induced or spontaneous movement.
3. Absence of spontaneous respiration.
4. Absence of brainstem and deep tendon reflexes.
5. No patient meeting the Harvard Criteria has ever recovered.

Brainstem death—the UK version of brain death—is a compromise between two views:

1. That a person, or 'self', ceases to exist when they irreversibly lose the capacity for consciousness.
2. The human *organism* dies *only* when it ceases to function in an integrated way—biological death.

### HINTS AND TIPS

*Remember*: Brainstem death criteria are generally applied to patients who cannot be pronounced dead without switching off a ventilator, NOT to everyone who dies. Verification of death is usually done by junior doctors, specially trained nurses or other health professionals in the United Kingdom. But think—what makes you decide to pronounce one person dead and call the cardiac arrest team for someone else?

## Is brainstem death a sufficient condition for defining death?

McCullagh (1993) summarized the reasons for thinking of the brain as the organ critical to identifying the death of the individual. They include:

- After irreversible cessation of brain function, all other organ systems will inevitably cease to function.
- Unlike other organ systems, brain function, once lost, is irreplaceable.
- Irreversible loss of brain function is synonymous with permanent loss of consciousness.
- Loss of sentience is a feature of loss of brain function.
- The integrative function of the brain is lost if the brain ceases to function.
- Death on the basis of loss of brain function is doing no more than recognizing overtly the reason underlying the traditional diagnosis of death following cessation of the blood circulation. In other words, someone whose heart or lungs fail, dies when the brain dies—in theory the heart and lungs can be replaced.
- If a patient is brain-dead but their body is maintained on an artificial ventilator, then the cardiovascular, gastrointestinal and urinary systems continue to function. The body is warm, consumes oxygen and has a pulse. This is

not a 'dead body', even if the patient is categorized as dead. The patient as *a person* is dead but the body in some important senses is alive. A brain-dead, ventilated body is still recognized as a living organism.

## ORGAN TRANSPLANTATION

Organ transplantation is the process of transferring an organ or tissue from a donor to a living recipient. Donors can be living, brain-dead or dead after circulatory arrest. The demand for organs considerably outstrips the supply. This section discusses key legislation, types of organ donation, consent and supply/demand issues (Figs 4.14–4.15).

## Legislation

*Human Tissue Act* 2004. Passed in the wake of the Alder Hey inquiry (see Chapter 2), the *Human Tissue Act* created the Human Tissue Authority (HTA) to regulate activities involving human tissue and to ensure that adequate consent has been obtained. This includes postmortems, anatomical examinations, display of tissue from the deceased and the removal and storage of human tissue. Cell lines and hair and nails from living individuals are excluded from the Act. Live gametes and embryos are regulated under the *HFE Act* instead. New doctors and medical students may be familiar with the HTA as it has a role in regulating anatomical teaching. The HTA also considers potential living organ donors. The HTA has a statutory role in ensuring compliance with their guidelines. The *Human Tissue Act* 2004:

- Prohibits the sale of human material, thus making sale of organs illegal.
- Permits cold perfusion of cadaveric organs to improve the success of subsequent transplants.
- Does not affect the rights of coroners to conduct postmortems and retain tissue if they feel it necessary.
- Makes DNA theft illegal.

*Organ Donation (Deemed Consent) Act* **2019**. In 2019 this legislation was passed to change England to an opt-out organ donation system. This means:

- Individuals who do not wish to donate their organs must opt out.
- Anyone who has not registered their decision around organ donation will be assumed to have agreed to donate their organs.
- No organs will be taken without the family's consent however, regardless of the deceased's stance.
- The Act does not apply to children, patients with mental illness, prisoners or overseas visitors.

It remains to be seen what effect this has on the supply of organs.

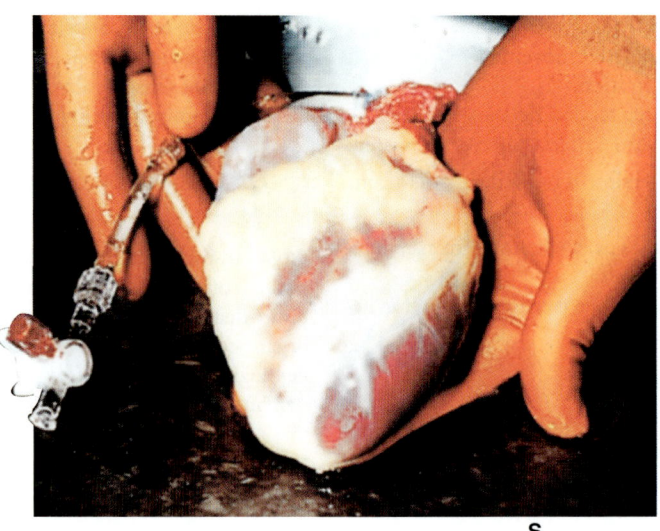

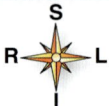

**Fig. 4.14** A human heart prepared for transplant.

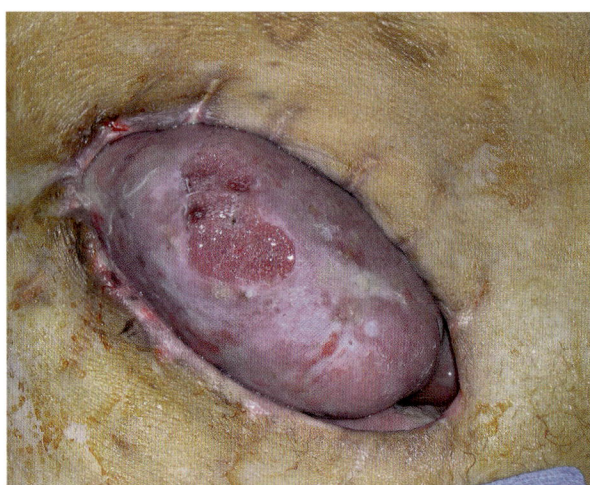

**Fig. 4.15** Intraoperative close-up view showing a viable and functional transplanted kidney.

**Legal Differences**

In Scotland, the *Human Tissue Act* (2004) does not apply, except for section 45, which regulates DNA analysis. Instead the relevant legislation is the *Human Tissue (Scotland) Act* 2006 and the *Human Tissue (Authorisation) (Scotland) Act* 2019, which also changed Scotland to an opt-out system of organ donation. The *Human Transplantation (Wales) Act* (2013) established an opt-out system in Wales. The *Organ Donation Deemed Consent Act* (2019) applies in England only and changed the organ donation process to an opt-out system. Northern Ireland introduced the *Organ and Tissue Donation (Deemed Consent) Act (Northern Ireland)* 2022, also an opt-out system.

## Types of organ donation

There are three broad categories of organ donors:

### Living

- These donors are most commonly family members or friends of the recipients, but may also choose to donate to an unknown individual. Only certain organs can be harvested from living donors, and the selection of donors is tightly regulated. It is illegal in most jurisdictions, except Iran, for living donors to sell their organs (Moeindarbari & Feizi, 2022).

### Brain-dead

- These are generally the most suitable organ donors, however there are a number of barriers to increasing donor numbers.
- They must have been declared brain-dead after brainstem testing (see previous).

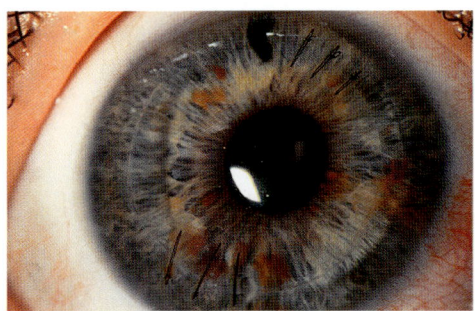

**Fig. 4.16** Treatment for postcorneal transplant astigmatism. Compression sutures were placed in the flat meridians (1:00 to 3:00 p.m. and 6:30 to 8:00 p.m.) and relaxing incisions were performed in the graft wound 90 degrees away.

## Dead after circulatory arrest

- These are patients who die in an anticipated manner, often after withdrawal of ventilatory support and where death occurs due to circulatory arrest.
- Corneas can be donated up to 24 hours after death, including after death in the community (Fig. 4.16).

## Current state of organ donation in the NHS

According to the NHS Blood and Transplant (2023) annual audit, 1980 patients met the brain death referral criteria and 5307 met the criteria for circulatory arrest. Seventy-nine per cent of suspected brain-dead patients were tested, and 68% of families consented or supported their relative's organ donation in brain-dead patients. Fifty-seven per cent of families consented in the case of circulatory death. Significantly fewer patients from Black, Asian or other ethnic minority backgrounds had consented for organ donation (35%). In the past year there has been a decrease in the consent rate for organ donors.

## Ethical issues in organ transplantation

There are a vast array of ethical issues raised in the field of organ transplantation, however one way to consider them is to split them into the following categories:

- Issues relating to the donor which can be split further into:
  - Cadaveric organ donation.
  - Living organ donation.
- Issues relating to the recipient.
- Broader societal issues.

**Issues relating to the donor—cadaveric organ donation**
- The epistemological issue of defining death, which often is a reason for family or public reluctance to donate.

- How long brain-dead patients ought to be kept ventilated after declaration of brain death before their organs are harvested.
- Whether it would be morally permissible to use brain-dead patients as a self-replenishing source of blood.
- The balance between finding suitable organ donors and ensuring that, if the families wish, patients with severe brain injuries are not prematurely removed from life support for the purpose of obtaining their organs and that families do not feel pressured into doing so.
- Should dying patients be intubated to allow the best chance of organ viability, even if it is of no benefit to the dying patient?
- Should organ donors be allowed to stipulate conditions attached to their donation? For example while requesting an organ goes to a family member or a friend is permitted, should patients be allowed to demand that it goes to a member of their ethnic or religious group?
- What tissues/organs should we be allowed to take? Does consent for organ donation include consent for harvesting of a patient's face or hands?

**Issues relating to the donor—living organ donation**
- How can we avoid coercion in the case of living donors? Coercion or significant pressure is far more likely in cases involving family members, especially where children are involved.
- Should parents be permitted to conceive so-called saviour siblings to provide organs or tissue for an already living child who is unwell?
- Should selling organs be permitted? The only jurisdiction that currently permits this is Iran, where a fixed price for a living kidney donation was introduced to try to tackle the shortage of willing donors.
- Should living donors be compensated? This might be financially or in other ways, like getting priority should they need a transplant in the future.

---

**CASE 4.18 THOUGHT EXPERIMENT: WHO SHOULD GET THE ORGAN?**

Decisions around selecting a recipient for an organ are complex, but mostly based on clinical need and likely outcome of the patient. However the role of other factors is controversial. Consider the following scenario:

You have a liver ready for transplant and five potential candidates. All have the same clinical level of need and are all likely to do well after the operation. Who do you prioritize?

- Alfred, 39, in recovery from alcohol dependence and with liver failure from previous alcohol abuse?

*(Continued)*

## CASE 4.18 — *Contd.*

- Benjamin, 42, a visiting tourist from South Africa?
- Charles, 57, a world-renowned surgeon?
- David, 34, a single parent with two small children?
- Edward, 22, an unemployed plumber?

Who you choose will often reflect the school of ethical thought you most sympathize with. Unless there is a reciprocal agreement with South Africa, Ben the tourist would not receive a liver ahead of any of the others. The majority of the public do not support giving organs to individuals where the organ damage is from alcohol or drug abuse.

**Issues relating to the recipient**
- Who gets an organ/how patients should be prioritised?
- How we can maximize or ensure patient compliance to give the organ the best chance of survival?

## Broader societal issues

How should society balance supply and demand and should we bring in new safety laws, for example around driving, even if it will reduce the supply of organs? Who in society should get an organ? Organs in the United Kingdom are prioritized to UK residents and citizens, but should there be other contributing factors beyond clinical need? For example should healthcare staff like doctors and nurses get priority or higher rate taxpayers? Should there be age limits or should we prioritize the young? A 19-year-old who receives an organ may benefit from many more years of life than a 60-year-old, but would this be considered ageist and unfair discrimination? NHS Blood and Transplant sets no maximum age limit for many organ transplants, but suggests that in most cases transplants are unlikely in individuals over 65 due to concerns about comorbidities. Should individuals or groups who are unwilling to donate their own organs be considered for receipt of an organ donation?

## CASE 4.19 THOUGHT EXPERIMENT: OPTING OUT OF ORGAN DONATION

Joan decides that she does not want to donate her organs and registers this under the opt-out legislation. She is then diagnosed with renal failure and requires dialysis. She is offered the option of being placed on the waiting list for a kidney transplant and accepts. She however would still be unwilling to donate her own organs. Should Joan receive a kidney? How would your view on this change if she refused for religious reasons?

Or belonged to a group that made up 5% of the population that accepted organ donations but refused to donate their own organs?

## CASE 4.20 THOUGHT EXPERIMENT: SELLING A KIDNEY

Should you be allowed to sell your kidney? Consider the following fictional case: Peter is a healthy 27-year-old. He wants to buy a house and needs some money for the deposit. He sees an advert for kidney donors and thinks that he should be allowed to sell his kidney.

Should Peter be allowed to sell his kidney? How would your answer change if Peter desperately needed the money to pay for a relative's medical bills?

## References

*Abortion Act* 1967, c. 87. https://www.legislation.gov.uk/ukpga/1967/87/contents

Academy of Medical Royal Colleges. (2008). *A code of practice for the diagnosis and confirmation of death.* https://www.aomrc.org.uk/wp-content/uploads/2016/04/Code_Practice_Confirmation_Diagnosis_Death_1008-4.pdf

*Age of Legal Capacity (Scotland) Act* 1991. c. 50. https://www.legislation.gov.uk/ukpga/1991/50/contents

*Airedale NHS Trust v. Bland (1993) AC 789.*

Anonymous. (1976). Diagnosis of brain death. Statement issued by the honorary secretary of the Conference of Medical Royal Colleges and their Faculties in the United Kingdom on 11 October 1976. *British Medical Journal, 2*(6045), 1187–1188. https://doi.org/10.1136/bmj.2.6045.1187.

Anonymous. (1979). Diagnosis of death. Memorandum issued by the honorary secretary of the Conference of Medical Royal Colleges and their Faculties in the United Kingdom on 15 January 1979. *British Medical Journal, 1*(6159), 332. https://doi.org/10.1136/bmj.1.6159.332.

Center for Reproductive Rights. (2020). *European abortion laws: A comparative overview.* https://reproductiverights.org/wp-content/uploads/2020/12/European-abortion-law-a-comparative-review.pdf

*Coroners and Justice Act* 2009, c. 25. https://www.legislation.gov.uk/ukpga/2009/25/contents

*Criminal Justice Act (Northern Ireland)* 1966. https://www.legislation.gov.uk/apni/1966/20/contents

*Crowter v. Secretary of State for Health and Social Care (2022) EWCA Civ 1559.*

Department of Health and Social Care. (2023). *An overview of the death certification reforms.* https://www.gov.uk/government/publications/changes-to-the-death-certification-process/an-overview-of-the-death-certification-reforms

Dimond, R. (2015). Social and ethical issues in mitochondrial donation. *British Medical Bulletin*, *115*(1), 173–182. https://doi.org/10.1093/bmb/ldv037.

*Foster v. R (2023) EWCA Crim 1196.*

General Medical Council. (2023). Good Medical Practice 2024. *GMC*: https://www.gmc-uk.org/-/media/documents/gmp-2024-final—english_pdf-102607294.pdf.

Gillon, R. (2001). Is there a 'new ethics of abortion'? *Journal of Medical Ethics*, *27*(Suppl 2), ii5–9. https://doi.org/10.1136/jme.27.suppl_2.ii5. (Accessed February 2024).

Health Canada. (2022). *Fourth annual report on medical assistance in dying in Canada 2022*. Ottawa, Canada. https://www.canada.ca/content/dam/hc-sc/documents/services/medical-assistance-dying/annual-report-2022/annual-report-2022.pdf.

*Health and Social Care Act* 2022, c.31. https://www.legislation.gov.uk/ukpga/2022/31/contents/enacted

Herring, J. (2010). Death and dying: *Law express: Medical law* (pp. 96–107) (2nd ed.). Pearson Education.

Hope, T., Savulescu, J., & Kendrick, J. (2008). *Medical ethics and law: The core curriculum* (2nd ed.). Elsevier.

*Human Fertilisation and Embryology Act* 1990, c. 37. https://www.legislation.gov.uk/ukpga/1990/37/contents

*Human Fertilisation and Embryology Act* 2008, c. 22. https://www.legislation.gov.uk/ukpga/2008/22/contents

*Human Tissue Act* 2004, c. 30. https://www.legislation.gov.uk/ukpga/2004/30/contents

*Human Tissue (Authorisation) (Scotland) Act* 2019, asp 11.https://www.legislation.gov.uk/asp/2019/11/enacted

*Human Tissue (Scotland) Act* 2006, asp 4. https://www.legislation.gov.uk/asp/2006/4/contents

*Human Transplantation (Wales) Act* 2013, anaw 5. https://www.legislation.gov.uk/anaw/2013/5/contents/enacted.

Huxtable, R. (2007). *Euthanasia, ethics and the law: From conflict to compromise*. Routledge-Cavendish.

*Infant Life (Preservation) Act* 1929, c. 34. https://www.legislation.gov.uk/ukpga/Geo5/19-20/34/section/1

*Janaway v. Salford Health Authority (1989) AC 537.*

Jonsen, A., Siegler, M., & Winslade, W. (2010). *Clinical ethics* (7th ed.). McGraw-Hill.

*Khan v. Meadows (2021) UKSC 21.*

Mactier, H., et al. (2020). Perinatal management of extreme preterm birth before 27 weeks of gestation: A framework for practice. *Archives of Disease in Childhood - Fetal and Neonatal Edition*, *105*(3), 232–239. https://doi.org/10.1136/archdischild-2019-318402.

McCullagh, P. (1993). Brain Dead: *Brain absent. Brain donors*. John Wiley & Sons Ltd.

*McFarlane and Another v. Tayside Health Board (Scotland) (2000) 2 AC 59.* https://publications.parliament.uk/pa/ld199900/ldjudgmt/jd991125/macfar-1.htm

*Mental Capacity Act* 2005, c.9. https://www.legislation.gov.uk/ukpga/2005/9/contents

Moeindarbari, T., & Feizi, M. (2022). Kidneys for sale: Empirical evidence from Iran. *Transplant International*, *35*, 10178. https://doi.org/10.3389/ti.2022.10178.

*National Health Service Act* 1977.

Newson, A. J., Wilkinson, S., & Wrigley, A. (2016). Ethical and legal issues in mitochondrial transfer. *EMBO Molecular Medicine*, *8*(6), 589–591. https://doi.org/10.15252/emmm.201606281.

NHS Blood and Transplant. (2023). *Organ and tissue donation and transplantation annual activity report*. https://nhsbtdbe.blob.core.windows.net/umbraco-assets-corp/30198/activity-report-2022-2023-final.pdf

Notification of Deaths Regulations 2019, No. 1112. https://www.legislation.gov.uk/uksi/2019/1112/regulation/3/made

*Offences Against the Person Act* 1861, c. 100. https://www.legislation.gov.uk/ukpga/Vict/24-25/100/contents (Accessed February 2024)

*Organ Donation (Deemed Consent) Act* 2019, c. 7. https://www.legislation.gov.uk/ukpga/2019/7/notes/division/3/index.htm

*Organ and Tissue Donation (Deemed Consent) Act (Northern Ireland)* 2022, c. 10. https://www.legislation.gov.uk/nia/2022/10/contents

*Paton v. British Pregnancy Advisory Service Trustees (1979) QB 276.*

*Pretty v. The United Kingdom (2346/02) (2002) ECHR.* https://hudoc.echr.coe.int/eng#%7B%22itemid%22:%5B%22001-60448%22%5D%7D

*Re A (1992) 3 Med LR 303.*

*Re B (Adult: Refusal of Medical Treatment) (2002) 2 FCR 1.*

*R. (Burke) v. GMC and Others (2005) EWCA Civ 1003.*

*R (on the application of Tracey) v. Cambridge University Hospital NHS Trust (2014) EWCA Civ 822.* https://www.judiciary.uk/wp-content/uploads/2014/06/tracey-approved.pdf

*R v. Bodkin Adams (1957) Crim LR 365.*

*R v. Catt (2013) EWCA Crim 1187.*

*R v. Cox (1992) 12 BMLR 38.*

*Re F (in Utero) (1988) Fam 122.*

*R (Smeaton on behalf of SPUC) v. The Secretary of State et al (2002) 2 FCR 193.*

Sokol, D. K. (2009). The slipperiness of futility. *BMJ*, *338*, b2222. https://doi.org/10.1136/bmj.b2222.

*Suicide Act* 1961. c. 60. https://www.legislation.gov.uk/ukpga/Eliz2/9-10/60

*Surrogacy Arrangements Act* 1985, c. 49. https://www.legislation.gov.uk/ukpga/1985/49

The Abortion (Northern Ireland) (No. 2) Regulations 2020. https://www.legislation.gov.uk/uksi/2020/503/contents/made

*The Mental Health Trust & Others v. DD & Another (2015) EWCOP 4.* https://www.bailii.org/ew/cases/EWCOP/2015/4.html

Thomson, J. (1971). A defense of abortion. *Philosophy and Public Affairs*, *1*, 47–66. https://users.manchester.edu/Facstaff/SSNaragon/Online/texts/235/Thomson,%20Defense%20of%20Abortion.pdf.

## Further Reading

British Medical Association. (2023). *Organ donation*. https://www.bma.org.uk/advice-and-support/ethics/end-of-life/organ-donation

British Transplantation Society. (2023). *UK guidelines on transplantation from deceasaed donors after circulatory death*. https://bts.org.uk/transplantation-from-deceased-donors-after-circulatory-death/#Introductionandneedfortheguideline

Crown Office & Procurator Fiscal Service. (2024). *Our role in investigating deaths*. https://www.copfs.gov.uk/about-copfs/our-role-in-investigating-deaths/

Director of Public Prosecutions. (2014). *Suicide: Policy for prosecutors in respect of cases of encouraging or assisting suicide*. https://www.

cps.gov.uk/legal-guidance/suicide-policy-prosecutors-respect-cases-encouraging-or-assisting-suicide

Glover, J. (1977). Causing death and saving lives. Pelican Books.

Harris, J. (1994). *The value of life*. Routledge.

Harris, J. (Ed.), (2001). *Bioethics*. Oxford University Press.

Harris, J., & Holm, S. (Eds.). (1998). *The future of human reproduction*. Oxford University Press.

Human Fertilisation and Embryology Authority. (2022). *Treatments*. https://www.hfea.gov.uk/treatments/

Human Tissue Authority. (2024). *Codes of practice*. https://www.hta.gov.uk/codes

Kellar, R. (2021). *Supreme Court revisits wrongful birth claims: An extended look – Robert Kellar QC and Owain Thomas QC*. https://ukhumanrightsblog.com/2021/06/24/supreme-court-revisits-wrongful-birth-claims-an-extended-look-robert-kellar-qc-and-owain-thomas-qc/.

*MacLennan v. MacLennan 1958 S.C. 105; 1958 S.L.T. 12.*

McHale, J., Fox, M., & Murphy, J. (1997). *Health care law: Texts and materials*. Sweet & Maxwell.

National Institute for Health and Care Excellence. (2011). Organ donation for transplantation: improving donor identification and consent rates for deceased organ donation. *Clinical guideline [CG135] Updated 21 December 2016*. https://www.nice.org.uk/guidance/cg135/chapter/1-Recommendations.

National Institute for Health and Care Excellence. (2023). *Scenario: Emergency hormonal contraception*. https://cks.nice.org.uk/topics/contraception-emergency/management/management/

NHS Blood and Transplant. (2023a). *Consent and authorisation*. https://www.odt.nhs.uk/deceased-donation/best-practice-guidance/consent-and-authorisation/

NHS Blood and Transplant. (2023b). *POL274/8 - Living donor kidney transplantation*. https://nhsbtdbe.blob.core.windows.net/umbraco-assets-corp/31150/pol274.pdf

NHS Blood and Transplant. (2024). *Organ donation laws*. https://www.organdonation.nhs.uk/uk-laws/

*R v. Human Fertilisation & Embryology Authority, ex parte Blood (1997) 2 All ER 687.*

Redfern, M., Keeling, J. W., & Powell, E. (2000). *The Royal Liverpool children's inquiry report*. The Stationery Office. https://assets.publishing.service.gov.uk/media/5a74a0b5e5274a410efd121e/0012_ii.pdf.

Sokol, D. K. (2009). The death of DNR: Can a change of terminology improve end of life care? *British Medical Journal, 338*, b1723. https://doi.org/10.1136/bmj.b1723.

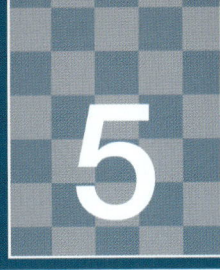

# Public health 5

This chapter summarizes key concepts in public health alongside important ethical and legal issues. The emphasis is on populations constituted of diverse individuals.

## THE NATURE OF PUBLIC HEALTH: CULTURE, EVENTS, POLITICS, THEORIES, PRINCIPLES AND VALUES

It is commonly said the main aims of public health are to protect and improve population health and to reduce health inequalities, perhaps creating a sense of objectivity analogous to any claims of objectivity in clinical medicine. Public health arguably aims to define, influence and create action towards *what is valued as 'good health'* at a population level by a sufficient consensus of stakeholders. It is a meeting point for different schools of thought and, like clinical medicine, reflects the social culture in which it is practised. In the United Kingdom it is unnecessary to have a medical qualification to be a consultant in public health.

Interpretative influences come from the voice of clinical medicine, politics, economics and academic disciplines considering behaviour, sociology and epidemiology. International relations are relevant, demonstrated by the COVID-19 pandemic crossing borders and with differential access to vaccines and treatments between higher- and lower-income nations. The ethics of public health continue to emerge as distinct from those of clinical medicine, originally gaining pace in light of the 1980s HIV-AIDS epidemic and the rise of screening programme. The UK National Screening Committee was created in 1996.

The So-called Western culture translates into liberal political currents which emphasize individualism, autonomy and self-determination, along with neutrality of the state and pluralistic conceptions of what entails 'a good life'. An idiom encapsulating this is the saying *you do you*. This value system is not ubiquitous, as some cultures inherently place more value on communal life (Hofstede 2001). A permeating tension in public health ethics is striking the balance between individual autonomy and conceptions of the communal good. Action is more likely where individual interest aligns with the common good but can still be stymied by problems like addiction. The more 'liberal' a culture, the more resistance to mandatory compliance with public health interventions can be expected since interventions tend to be perceived as infringements on individual freedom of choice. Besides

the consent-compulsoriness continuum is the added reality of finite resources. Who makes the decisions about deploying finite human, physical and economic resources for public health, including research, and how are decisions made? Debate continues around the extent to which public health researchers should be involved in influencing policy: does it compromise scientific rigour, or is it part of an applied academic role?

Health can be defined as an absence of disease, a presence of well-being or in other ways; Seedhouse (2001) suggests health is not an end in itself but instead just one among various means necessary to fulfilling life goals. Health can be defined in terms of self-awareness and actionable autonomy, which is even less 'biomedical'. Such viewpoints help to understand pluralistic public health practices and differential acceptability and uptake of public health interventions. Excessive exercise of state powers favouring singular approaches runs the risk of creating ill-feeling by exposing value conflict on the nature of 'health'.

### ETHICS

#### PUBLIC HEALTH ETHICS—KEY POINTS

- Public health is value based, necessitating debate around what is valued as 'health'.
- 'Western cultures' and 'liberal politics' are expressions commonly applied where individualism, autonomy and self-determination are highly valued.
- A key ethical tension in public health is balancing individualism with public benefit.

Holland (2023) proposes public health problems be approached by seeking and periodically renegotiating a 'reflective equilibrium' between ethical theories, principles and the nature of a particular situation.

## Theories

Different theories can inform arguments for and against the approach to public health problems. There is no 'right' theory.

The ethical theory most commonly associated with public health is utilitarianism, a branch of consequentialism. Consequentialism broadly says the value of an action is assessed by its consequences, the route there being a lesser concern. Among the difficulties with consequentialism are the uncertain long-term consequences of many public health interventions. For example, COVID-19 lockdowns limited short-term virus spread, but longer term consequences on mental and emotional health and postpandemic waiting lists in the National Health Service (NHS) should also be factored in. Utilitarianism broadly seeks to maximize 'good'. Since interpretations of 'good' are subjective, health can be defined in various ways, and even if there were a settled definition, then health is still only one type of 'good' and not automatically the most valuable in a given situation. How do we measure the pleasure or sense of community a person may find in smoking or drinking alcohol? (Figs 5.1–5.3) Utilitarian calculations are only as good as the data we value as worthwhile, and find practical, to put into them. A common criticism of utilitarianism is it ends up being impersonal and taking a narrow biomedical view of what constitutes health when in reality few people desire an impersonal life. Utilitarianism can accommodate redefinitions of 'good' if a culture is willing to redefine it and recognize that people make trade-offs against different types of well-being. Public health practice seeks a sufficient consensus around both 'good' and 'health' to facilitate action at scale. Sufficient consensus is not objective either since it depends on which stakeholders are invited or have the energy to participate.

Deontological theories broadly say that an action itself can be right or wrong, good or bad, irrespective of the outcome. A deontological perspective likely asserts that a public health policy risking an individual to benefit a community is only justifiable where anyone would agree to be the individual at risk: the universalisability principle is met. So it might be argued that forced vaccination of an individual against their consent is 'wrong' at a fundamental level. Virtue ethics focuses on the moral character and intentions underpinning actions, perhaps espousing traits like kindness, courage, patience, open mindedness and

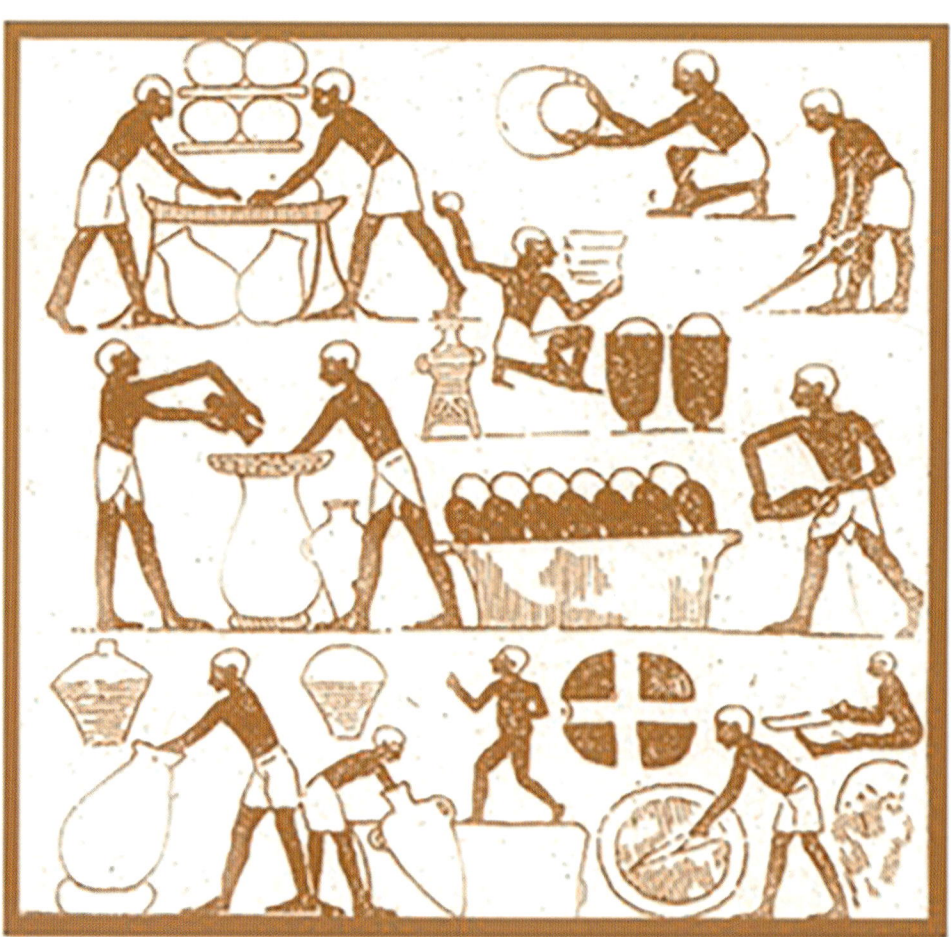

**Fig. 5.1** People have been brewing beer and making wine for millennia, and the history of people smoking is probably of a similar length.

prudence. Public health policies that promote human flourishing (eudaimonia) and foster virtuous dispositions are likely to be favoured. Virtue ethics does not tell us which virtue(s) to prioritize. Views on desired virtues can vary with time, circumstance and culture.

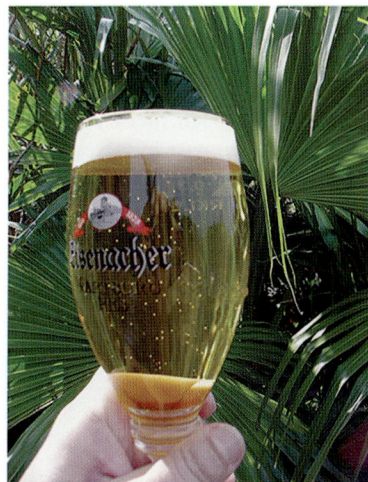

**Fig. 5.2** Do you know anyone who ever enjoyed a drink of beer?

## Principles

Which principles shall we prefer? It is again a debate for a given situation.

Holland (2023) characterized the 'four principles' of ethics in clinical medicine as being of limited use in public health. Autonomy simply favours one pole of the individualism–communitarianism continuum, while beneficence, nonmaleficence and justice can be argued at either pole of that continuum—for the individual or the community. The principle of *freedom* can also often be argued on either side: should an injecting drug user be free to access a safe injecting facility or needle exchange, or should people in society be free of the fear of crime and antisocial behaviour that is associated with drug use?

*Mill's harm principle* can be useful: State intervention that infringes on individuals is justified to avoid harm to others. We still require debate about what constitutes sufficient 'harm' to warrant the degree of intervention, and this entails making value judgements. Does an 'increased risk' meet the definition of 'harm'? Notifiable diseases are example situations where the risk to others is socially accepted and legally supported as justifying the notification and subsequent actions.

Childress et al. (2002) proposed certain conditions to consider as potential justifications for overriding individual liberty:

- Effectiveness
- Proportionality

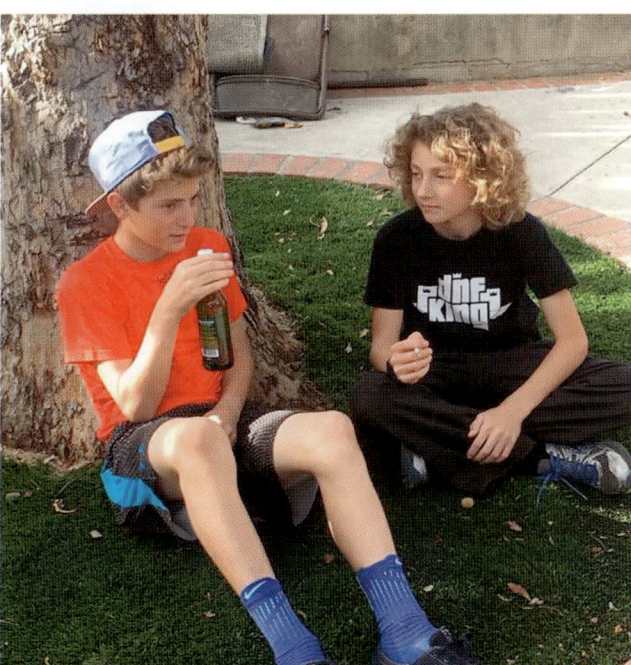

**Fig. 5.3** One child holds an alcoholic drink and one a cigarette. These can become 'gateway substances' to illicit products. Yet many adults use alcohol or cigarettes without recourse to other substances. How much right does public health practice have to 'intervene' in people in these areas?

- Necessity
- Least infringement
- Public justification

Upshur (2002) offers a similar list of principles to consider which include:

- Least restrictive or coercive means: For example education and discussion before regulation.
- Reciprocity: The state proportionately compensates people for the inconvenience of public health impositions.
- Transparency: To uphold trust in public health institutions.

Other principle frameworks are debated, and some socially accepted principles appear to be:

- Precautionary principle: Action to avoid a serious potential threat in conditions of scientific uncertainty.
- Equity principle: Fair resource allocation to factor against socioeconomic disadvantage.

Taking just the last example of the equity principle, it sounds good, but in reality there is no easy consensus on how to identify the inequalities that are unjust, how to intervene or when other principles become more important. Public health interventions are sometimes apt to improve measures of population health while widening certain measures of inequality.

The principle of least infringement (least restrictive or coercive means) is captured in the Nuffield Council on Bioethics (2007) Intervention Ladder. It climbs through the following steps: do nothing, provide information, enable choice, guide choice by changing the default policy, guide choice by incentives, guide choice by disincentives, restrict choice and eliminate choice. Generally speaking, higher steps need stronger justification. In the light of awareness of a problem, doing nothing sometimes needs a strong justification as well.

---

**CASE 5.1  WHAT WAS VALUED: COVID-19 LOCKDOWN**

Lockdown was effective in reducing the rate of virus transmission, and arguably necessary in the public interest to prevent an overwhelming demand on hospital resources. Early in the pandemic, the risk of severe illness was recognized and also as well as conditions of scientific uncertainty. The UK government followed the proportionality and precautionary principles and the reciprocity principle by offering part-payments of salaries for people unable to go to work. Lockdowns were mostly bad for well-being and difficult to fully enforce. The social restrictions in place formally at any given time varied in their extent of application, but policy and reality were both expressions of what was valued.

---

## PUBLIC HEALTH ACTIVITIES AND 'BIG DATA'

Public health practice aims to maintain and improve health and reduce the causes of illness through organized efforts at a societal level (Winslow, 1920):

- Health protection: Air quality (Fig. 5.4), water quality, food standards, infectious disease control, environmental hazards and chemical incidents.
- Health promotion: Improving living conditions and reducing inequalities through, for example, smoking cessation initiatives and improving access to physical activity (Fig. 5.5). Health education is generally socially acceptable,

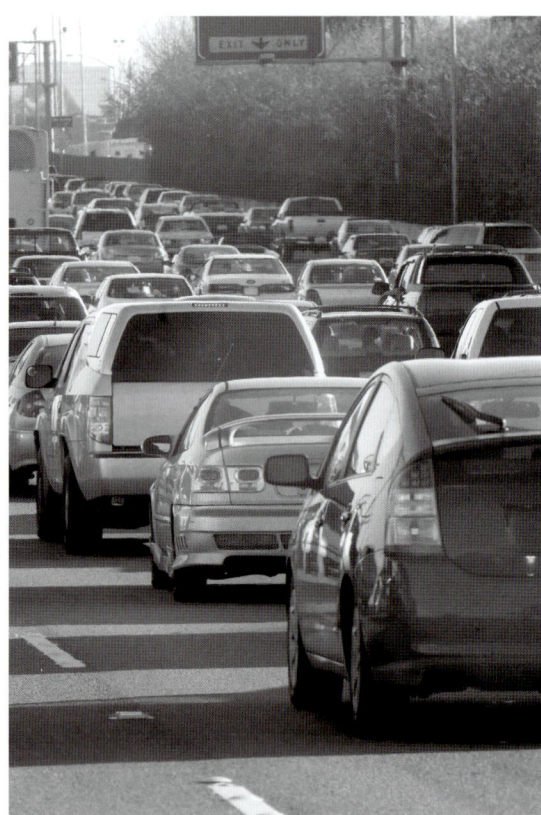

**Fig. 5.4** Environmental epidemiology is the study of the effect on human health of physical, chemical and biological factors in the external environment. Air pollution caused by vehicle emissions and other sources contributes to many health concerns, including the increasing prevalence of respiratory problems such as asthma. In 2013 Ella Adoo-Kissi-Debrah, aged 9 years and with a background of severe asthma, became the first person in the United Kingdom to have air pollution given as the cause of death on the death certificate following a coronial inquest.

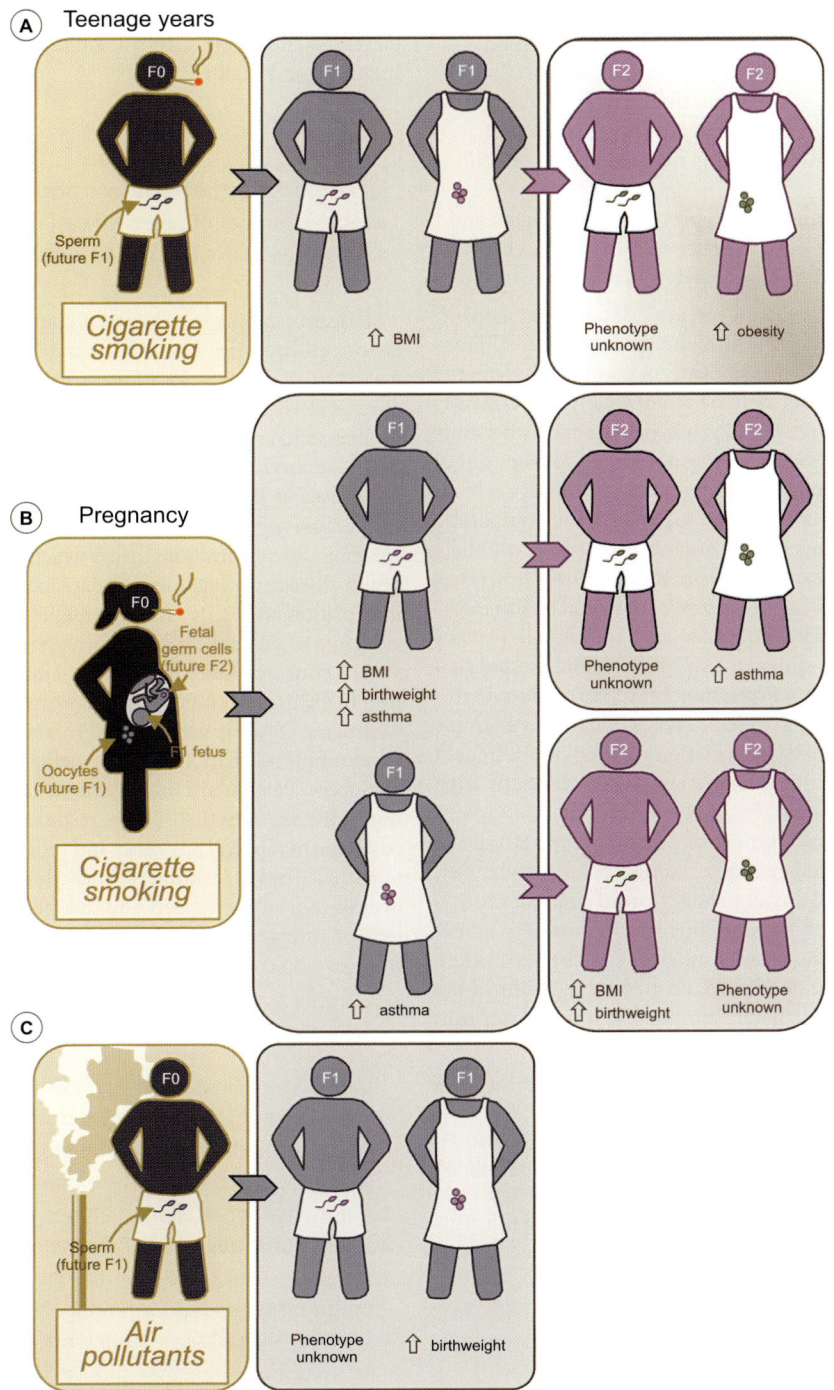

**Fig. 5.5** Sexually dimorphic multigenerational effects of toxicant exposure in humans. Cigarette smoking (*tan-coloured background*) in an F0 (A) male or (B) pregnant female leads to sexually dimorphic effects on the health of their F1 children and F2 grandchildren. (C) Direct effects of paternal air pollutant exposure on the birthweight of their daughters. F0, *Parental generation*; F1, *first filial generation*; F2, *second filial generation*.

so long as it is not pushy or judgemental because it tends to increase the autonomy of individuals to make informed choices. This is an example of 'soft paternalism'—in contrast to 'hard paternalism', which is interfering with people against their will and without consent but allegedly in their best interests. The latter is often poorly received and/or difficult to fully enforce.

- Health services: Actions that support effective, efficient and accessible overall services. The later sections in this chapter consider health services in general terms.

Large-scale operational and research datasets are considered fundamental to public health and epidemiological practice. 'Big data' sets are not automatically of good quality: quality data are essential for practice to be scientifically and ethically sound. The exercise of individual privacy rights can undermine data quality and generalizability if too many people opt out of sharing health data. Sophisticated digital re-identification techniques continue to undermine trust in personal data remaining anonymised, and many health organizations have publicly apologized for data leaks and data sharing breaches (Das, 2023). The tension between disclosure of personal health information for public health purposes and individual privacy rights is an important ethical dilemma. It can be argued that blanket laws like the *Data Protection Act* (2018) fail to distinguish privacy risks between different types of data, for example sensitive personal financial information with no public benefit and low sensitivity health information with potentially high public benefit when pooled.

Different conceptual frameworks influence what type of data are prioritized: for example biomedical, lifestyle, cultural, behavioural and social production of disease models will produce different types of public health data (Krieger & Zierler, 1996). One conceptual framework is not better than another in general, but one approach may be superior in the context of a given public health problem if it translates into actionable policy.

Underdetermination refers to the problem that public health evidence can be used to support various hypotheses and that data interpretation is value laden. Competing value positions are exactly that: not necessarily right or wrong. A response is to think about the purpose of public health, to enable the pursuit of what is valued as good population health. This does not address the central question of what is valued or how that is determined.

## Changing patterns of disease

Life expectancy at birth in the United Kingdom:

- In 1901: males—47 years; females—50 years
- In 2022: males—78 years; females—82 years (Office for National Statistics, 2024)

Most of these gains in life expectancy are attributable to increased childhood survival. Some of the additional years are spent in 'good health'.

> **HINTS AND TIPS**
>
> *Life expectancy* helps assess population health. It is the average number of years we can expect an individual of a given age to live if current mortality trends continue.

Disease patterns vary between countries. More economically developed countries have higher burdens of noncommunicable degenerative diseases, for example cardiovascular and metabolic diseases like diabetes and obesity, respiratory diseases, cancers, mental illness and arthritis. In developing economies the main causes of death are also cardiovascular and respiratory diseases, with infectious diseases like malaria, tuberculosis and HIV continuing as major causes of mortality and morbidity. This corresponds with the epidemiological transitions theory which links changing patterns of health, disease, demographics and socioeconomics (Omran, 2005). Information on UK death certificates is pooled together and provides important public health information.

The concept of intergenerational justice is our moral obligation to ensure that our current actions do not compromise the well-being of future generations. This is a key concept in light of, for example, climate change as well as concerns about scarce resources. Particular considerations include ageing with high morbidity burdens that require resources, and rising healthcare costs due to medical advances and more choices being available to patients and practitioners. Lifestyle choices contribute to the overall morbidity burden and can be considered through the lens of intergenerational justice, as illustrated in the case of Frances who continues to smoke.

> **CASE 5.2  FRANCES WANTS TO KEEP SMOKING**
>
> Frances is a 24-year-old living with her partner and their 2-year-old son. She cut down during her pregnancy to 10 cigarettes daily but did not stop entirely, and the pregnancy and delivery were uneventful. When she has brought her son at different times to the GP surgery for vaccinations, the topic of smoking cessation has been brought up, but she does not really want to stop. Her grandmother smoked for most of her life and lived to her early 1990s. Most of her work colleagues smoke and so does her partner, though they do not smoke in the house since their son has been born. Frances has mild asthma and occasionally requests a salbutamol inhaler prescription.

*(Continued)*

**CASE 5.2 —** *Contd.*

The patient and the clinician likely both know that smoking cessation is desirable, for the patient and child and if there are future pregnancies. Excessive emphasis by the clinician(s) may risk a deteriorating professional relationship with the patient and disengagement from other aspects of health provision. *How will you balance the knowledge and expectations that come from a public health perspective with the values and best interests of the individual patient?*

If an individual is at liberty to smoke and access state-funded care for smoking-related diseases, then arguably the state has grounds for upstream interventions to prevent or discourage smoking. Around 45% of British smokers state a clear desire to quit, ~38% are not sure either way and ~16% have no intention to quit (Office for National Statistics, 2023).

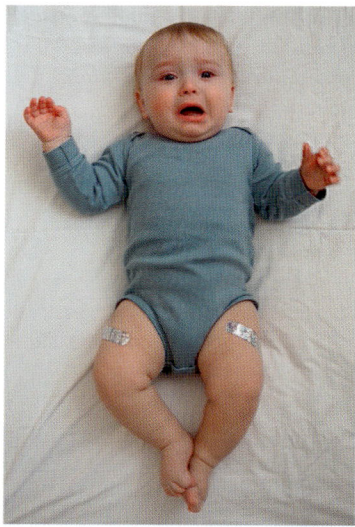

**Fig. 5.6** Young children are often upset straight after vaccination, which is an intervention to reduce the child's risk of suffering from serious infectious illness. Immunization against common serious pathogens means childhood death or lasting disability following infection is now a relatively uncommon event in the United Kingdom. Hopefully, this little one was soon picked up and comforted!

## PREVENTION

We will turn attention now to the first of three key activity areas in public health: prevention (Kisling & Das, 2023).

- Primordial prevention: risk factor reduction aimed at whole populations

    This is typically achieved through laws and national policy and a focus on environmental and social conditions. It can include measures like better sanitation or cleaner air and improving access to physical recreation spaces.
- Primary prevention: to stop disease developing in at-risk populations or healthy individuals

    It may need strategies to remove, destroy or anticipate agents that cause disease. Targeted immunization programmes are relevant. Primary prevention interventions generally need to have low levels of risk to individuals (Fig. 5.6).
- Secondary prevention: detect disease early and act to cure or prevent progression

    The most important example is screening programmes coupled to effective interventions. Disease is typically subclinical or asymptomatic at this stage.
- Tertiary prevention: to reduce damage from existing disease

    For example, encouraging smokers with chronic obstructive pulmonary disease or lung cancer to quit. This level of prevention has little effect on overall disease levels in the population. Harm reduction strategies like those around illicit drugs may work at this level, for example needle exchange and

opiate substitute prescribing, but for some patients these interventions function at the secondary prevention level and may facilitate some health promotion as well.

## Immunization and Communicable diseases

Effective immunization achieves primary prevention against an infectious disease agent through administering a vaccine which provokes immune memory. *Herd immunity* means immunity of a group or community:

- Typically 90% to 95% of people need to be vaccinated to break the chain of community transmission, the level of coverage needed varies by pathogen.
- Allows vulnerable people who cannot be vaccinated to benefit from lower risks of infection (e.g. those with immune compromise, on immunosuppressant treatments, newborns and frail older people).
- No vaccine is 100% effective, and all approved vaccines have some side effect/risk profile, and these are weighed against the risks from serious infection. The UK Government offers a Vaccine Damage Payment, which may be claimed by a person who becomes severely disabled as a result of a vaccination.
- Vaccine uptake in the United Kingdom is generally high, although some regions and some communities have low

uptakes (Torracinta, Tanner, & Vanderslott, 2021). Low vaccine uptake is associated with:

- Socioeconomic deprivation and minority ethnic groups (access issues).
- Socioeconomic affluence (conscious vaccine rejection).
- Children of mothers with alcohol or substance use disorders.
- Mobile families.
- Birth order, large families.
- Children with chronic illnesses.
- Attitudes of parents/caregivers.
- Misleading information on risks (e.g. measles, mumps and rubella (MMR) and autism—this had a 'long tail' of effect after media coverage declined).
- Lack of professional confidence in vaccine advocacy.

The UK immunization schedule includes children from 8 weeks of age who are unable to consent for themselves, teenagers who may have become competent to consent (tetanus, diphtheria and polio; meningococcal groups ACWY and human papillomavirus) and adults aged over 65 years (pneumococcal, influenza and shingles).

Some vaccine hesitancy and refusal can be managed with education when the behaviour is based on misinformation or misplaced belief. A level of refusal exists beyond this, raising the issue of the right to refuse a medical intervention for any reason (e.g. due to consideration of the risks, for political reasons) or for no reason. Some nations mandate vaccination while others take a slightly softer line of making school places conditional on evidence of vaccine status. Following the principle of least infringement a lower level than this can be effective, requiring parents to declare the vaccination status of their children at school enrolment. Child vaccination raises a particular quandary, since until children develop sufficient competence to consent, their health decisions are caught between the potential authority of the state and their parents. There is a stronger case for mandatory vaccination in certain settings entered by choice, such as the health professions.

Mill's harm principle might be used to argue for vaccination since nonvaccination increases the risks of harm to others including those who are medically unable to take a vaccine. Holland (2023) points out that vaccine refusal perhaps does not harm others since causing harm is different from refusing to benefit someone.

Free-riding here means benefitting from the risks others take in being vaccinated without making the contribution of being vaccinated oneself and assuming there are no medical contraindications to vaccination. A utilitarian could say that when herd immunity requires 90% to 95% population coverage and the desired outcome of breaking the chain of transmission is met, the 5% to 10% of free-riders are of no consequence. A deontologist more likely sees antivaccine free-riders as unethical irrespective of the consequences. A virtue ethicist might accommodate the potential motive of a parent to protect a child from a perceived risk as a reason for vaccine refusal.

A moral 'duty not to infect' others is an ethical idea specific to the realm of infectious diseases and focuses on individual responsibility rather than state interference. It is not universally agreed at a fundamental level that such a duty exists for infectious diseases in general. A variation on this emphasizes the context of the individual(s) involved, including the seriousness and/or impact of the infectious disease and the chance of catching the diseases elsewhere anyway. There have been successful prosecutions in England under the *Offences Against the Person Act* 1861, as grievous bodily harm, for 'reckless transmission' of HIV (Terrence Higgins Trust & National AIDS Trust, 2010).

### Legal Difference

The *Offences Against the Person Act* 1861 does not apply in Scotland. Instead there is a common law offence of Culpable and Reckless Conduct.

### CASE 5.3  MMR VACCINE HESITANCY

Jane is the mum of a healthy 1-year-old called Celia and is expressing hesitancy about arranging her MMR vaccination which is due. How would you approach the conversation with Jane?

Suggestions: Explore Jane's current understanding, previous experiences with any other children she has or stories she has heard from people that she knows; ask if she has any specific questions or concerns; ask if she would like you to explain the evidence around MMR vaccination and the risks from measles, mumps and rubella infection in unvaccinated people; explain that while you encourage vaccination now this is not a once-only opportunity, and catch-up vaccination is an option including at the time Celia develops the capacity to make her own decisions.

### CLINICAL NOTES

### NOTIFIABLE DISEASES (HEALTH PROTECTION (NOTIFICATION) REGULATIONS 2010)

Reasonable clinical suspicion of a notifiable disease (Figs 5.7-5.11) is all that is required. The aim is to detect disease outbreaks and epidemics as rapidly as possible, so in this particular context the accuracy of diagnosis is of secondary importance.

*(Continued)*

Inform the local authority (local council) proper officers about:

Acute encephalitis

Acute infectious hepatitis

Acute meningitis

Acute poliomyelitis

Anthrax

Botulism

Brucellosis

Cholera

COVID-19

Diphtheria

Enteric fever (typhoid or paratyphoid fever)

Food poisoning

Haemolytic uraemic syndrome

Infectious bloody diarrhoea

Invasive group A streptococcal disease

Legionnaires disease

Leprosy

Malaria

Measles

Meningococcal septicaemia

Monkeypox

Mumps

Plague

Rabies

Rubella

Severe acute respiratory syndrome

Scarlet fever

Smallpox

Tetanus

Tuberculosis

Typhus

Viral haemorrhagic fever

Whooping cough

Yellow fever

Report other diseases that may present significant risks to human health under the category 'other significant disease'. While it is good practice to tell the patient, you do not need their consent to make the notification because ultimately their general right to confidentiality is limited by the (potential or actual) presence of serious and addressable risks posed to others in the community.

The scale of a communicable disease can vary from an individual infection to:

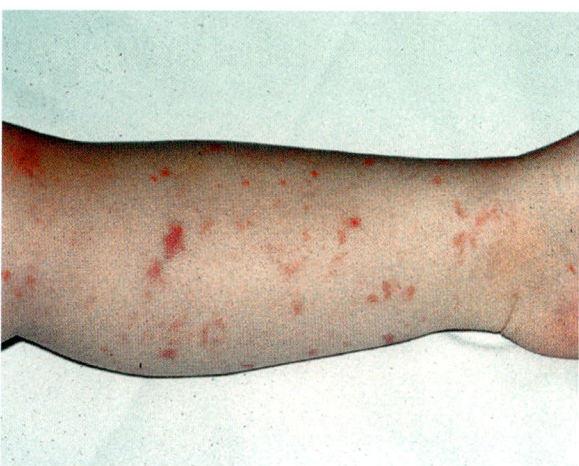

**Fig. 5.7** An early purpuric rash in meningococcal septicaemia. Meningococcal septicaemia is a notifiable disease in the United Kingdom. (Courtesy Meningitis Research Foundation.)

- *Outbreak*: Restricted to a local increased incidence of disease, for example in a town.
- *Endemic*: The disease incidence that is continuously present in a population.
- *Epidemic*: Increased disease incidence in a population above the endemic rate.
- *Pandemic*: Epidemic crossing international boundaries affecting large numbers.

In England, Government offices (e.g. Department of Health and Social Care, Office for National Statistics) collate surveillance data and distribute reports for information and action. Sources of surveillance data include:

- Statutory notifications of notifiable disease
- Laboratory reports (e.g. positive swabs)
- Royal College of General Practitioners sentinel reporting system
- Hospital Episode Statistics data
- Death certificates
- Vaccine uptake
- Sickness absence
- Special systems, for example:
  - HIV reporting, voluntary to the Communicable Disease Surveillance Centre
  - British Paediatrics Surveillance Unit
  - Creutzfeldt–Jakob Disease Surveillance Unit

## COVID-19

COVID-19 was a new disease-causing virus first identified in Wuhan, China, in December 2019 (Fig. 5.11). It spread rapidly and has been the most impactful worldwide pandemic since the 1918 to 1920 flu (the Great Influenza Pandemic, or 'Spanish

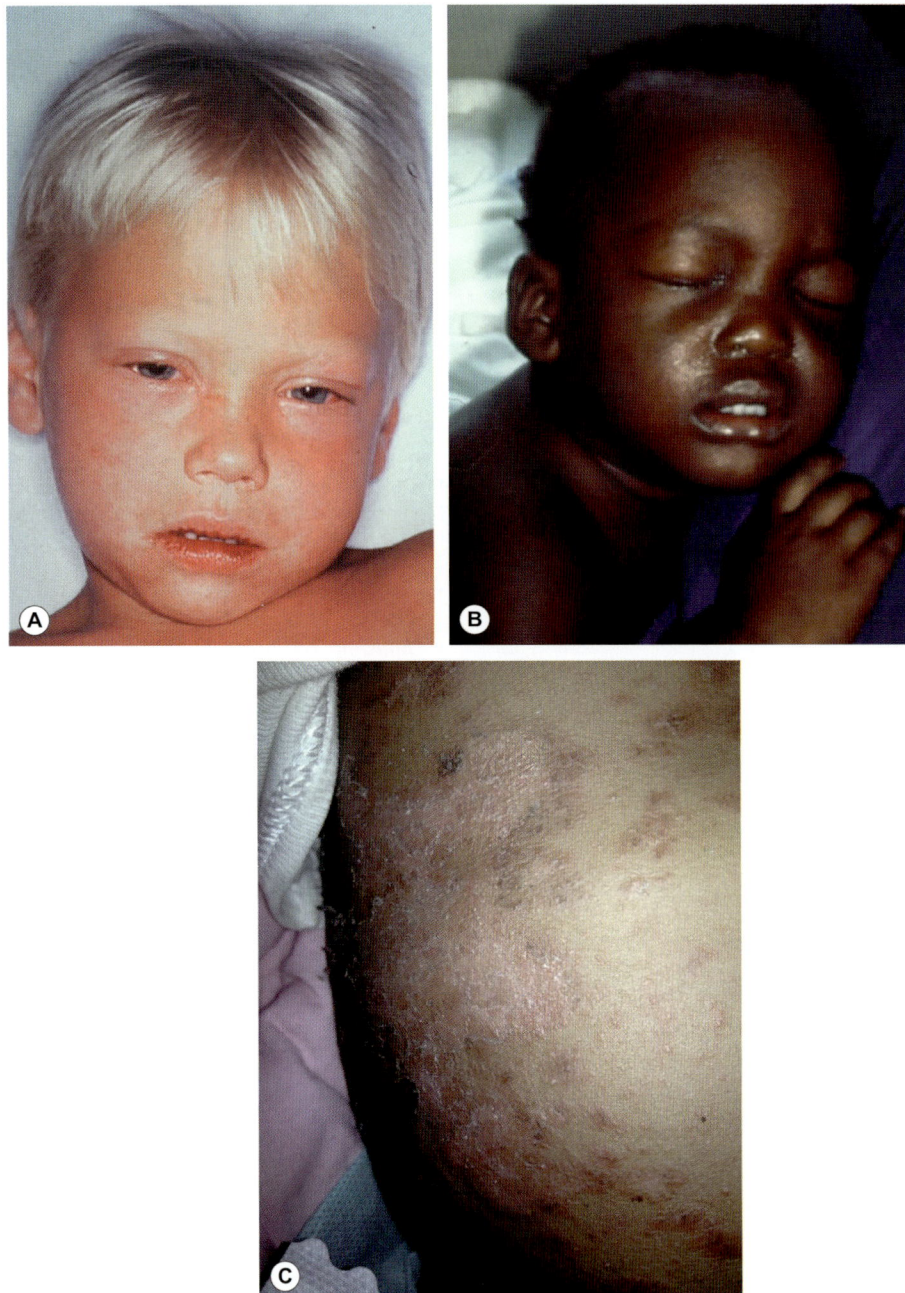

**Fig. 5.8** Measles is also a notifiable disease. The rash can vary. (A) Classic erythematous rash, conjunctivitis and coryza; (B) the rash is difficult to perceive on dark skin, but the patient has typical conjunctivitis and coryza; (C) prolonged desquamating dermatitis in a malnourished child with measles.

Flu'). Seasonal vaccination is available from the NHS for people at the highest risk, and personal protective equipment is worn proportionate to the estimated level of clinical risk.

During the peak of the COVID-19 pandemic, a range of emergency legislation was enacted in the United Kingdom, including the *Coronavirus Act* 2020. Restrictions on the freedom of movement were in place to control the spread of disease and prevent unmanageable demand on health services; financial support was made available to those prevented from working and the extent of remote, online working (including teaching and learning) increased considerably and rapidly.

Doctors and other health professionals initially worked in an atmosphere of uncertainty about the nature of the disease, including the risks to themselves, with no known effective treatments. Emergency efforts were made to produce, obtain and supply large quantities of personal protective equipment (e.g. face masks, visors, aprons, gloves). Clinical practice combined with well scaled and funded research led to the identification of symptomatology, clinical signs, risk factors for severe illness, development and availability of testing, discovery and development of effective treatments and the swift development of vaccines.

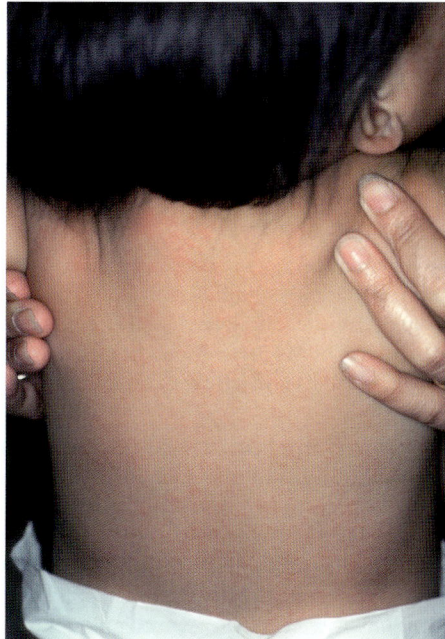

**Fig. 5.9** Rubella is a notifiable disease.

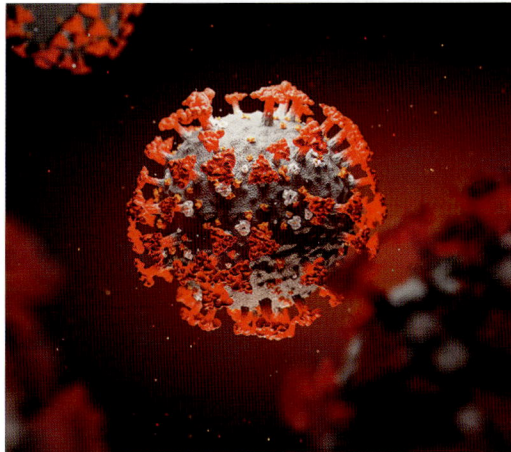

**Fig. 5.11** COVID-19 virus, seen using an electron microscope. The virus was so named by the World Health Organization. How did COVID-19 affect your life?

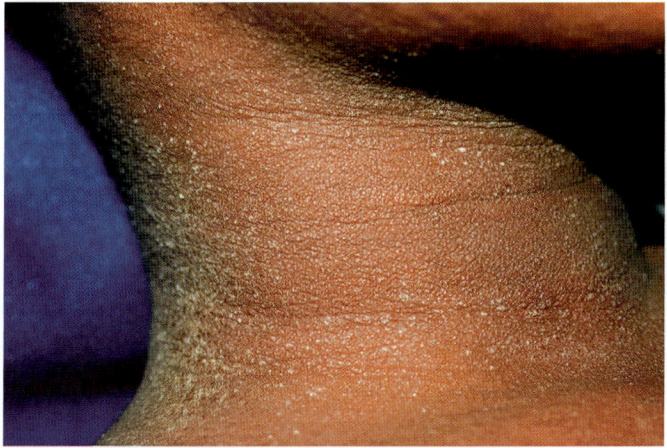

**Fig. 5.10** Scarlet fever is a notifiable disease. Note the early desquamation; the rash can feel rough like sandpaper.

## Screening

Screening means investigating people without symptoms to detect conditions that can be treated more effectively at an early stage. It is a form of secondary prevention.

**HINTS AND TIPS**

*Remember*: Screening tests are usually not diagnostic, they are inexpensive and easy to do. People with 'positive screening' tests are at high(er) risk of having the condition and are offered further testing to confirm or refute a diagnosis.

The World Health Organization guidelines for screening are based on Wilson and Jungner's work from 1968:

1. The condition screened for is an important health problem.
2. The natural history is well understood.
3. There is a detectable early stage.
4. Treatment at an early stage is more effective than at a later stage.
5. There is a suitable, valid test for the early stage.
6. The early-stage test is acceptable to people.
7. Intervals for repeating the test are determined.
8. The health service has the capacity to handle the extra workload (staff, space, equipment).
9. Benefits outweigh risks.
10. Costs are balanced against the benefits.

## Biases complicating the evaluation of screening programmes

- Selection bias: People who participate in screening often differ from those who do not.
- Lead-time bias: When screening identifies disease earlier than would otherwise happen, the patient appears to survive with the condition longer, but in fact they die at the same time as they would have and just *live longer in the knowledge of their diagnosis*.
- Length bias: For conditions that were going to have a long preclinical stage anyway, they may be detected early but by nature were always going to have a more favourable prognosis. Again, the patient simply lives longer in the knowledge of their diagnosis.

## Possible harms of screening

Screening is a medical intervention in people who are not ill and who usually have not asked for it.

- False-positive screening can cause unnecessary anxiety about having a serious condition.
- Follow-up diagnostic testing carries risks (e.g. colonoscopy has an associated bowel perforation rate of <1:1000).
- False-negative results give false reassurance.

## Mass, targeted and opportunistic screening

*Mass screening:* Involves the whole population or a large sub-group (e.g. bowel, breast-Fig. 5.12).

*Targeted screening:* Involves selected groups where there are increased risks to the patient or others from the condition (e.g. health workers for hepatitis B, food handlers for *Salmonella*).

*Opportunistic screening:* When a person presents to the doctor for another reason (e.g. checking blood pressure, cholesterol). Opportunistic screening or case finding has advantages: over 90% of people visit their GP surgery over a 2-year period so it can be cost-effective and detect a large proportion of cases. The disadvantage is the reliance on GPs to regularly test for the condition(s) even when the patient presents with other problems: overall workload can make this impractical.

**CLINICAL NOTES**

**NHS SCREENING PROGRAMMES IN 2024**
**Pregnancy**
- Infectious diseases: hepatitis B, HIV, syphilis.
- Trisomies: Down syndrome, Patau syndrome and Edwards syndrome.
- Haemoglobinopathies: sickle cell disease and thalassaemia.

*(Continued)*

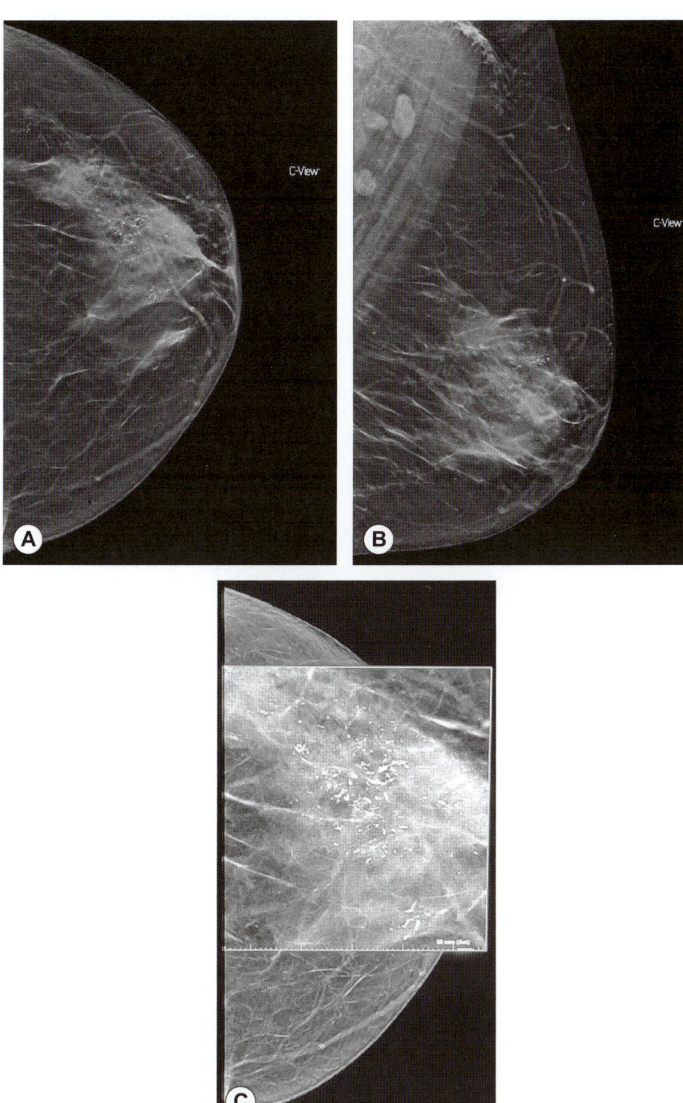

**Fig. 5.12** Digital screening mammogram of a 53-year-old (only the left breast is shown here). There are grouped fine pleomorphic calcifications in the upper outer quadrant. Vacuum-assisted biopsy under stereotactic guidance revealed invasive ductal cancer.

**CLINICAL NOTES — *Contd.***

- Physical anomalies: 'the 20-week scan' by ultrasound.
- Retinal screening in pregnancy for those with type 1 or 2 diabetes mellitus.

**Newborn**

- Clinical examination soon after birth and at 6 weeks: includes eyes, heart, hips and testes.

- Hearing.
- Blood spot test for nine rare conditions (sickle cell, cystic fibrosis, congenital hypothyroidism, six inherited metabolic diseases—phenylketonuria, medium-chain acyl-CoA dehydrogenase deficiency, maple syrup urine disease, isovaleric acidaemia, glutaric aciduria type 1, homocystinuria.

**Diabetic retinopathy**

- Annually from age 12.

*(Continued)*

## CLINICAL NOTES — *Contd.*

### Cervical cancer

- People aged 25 to 49 years and registered with a GP as female are invited every 3 years.[1]
- People aged 50 to 64 years and registered with a GP as female are invited every 5 years.[1]

### Breast cancer

- People aged 50 to 70 years and registered with a GP as female are invited every 3 years.[1]
- Over 70s can self-refer.

### Bowel cancer

- Everyone aged 60 to 74 is offered a home test kit every 2 years.
- Over 75s can self-refer every 2 years.

### Abdominal aortic aneurysm (Fig. 5.13)

- People registered with a GP as male are invited during the year they turn age 65.[1]
- Over 65s can self-refer.

[1]For further discussion on the current intersection of screening and transgender, see Chapter 3.

## CASE 5.5 SCREENING FOR PROSTATE AND OVARIAN CANCER

These are important health problems and there are currently no UK mass screening programmes. Blood prostate-specific antigen (PSA) levels are commonly raised in benign conditions of the prostate, and in some prostate cancers PSA levels are normal. Follow-up diagnostic testing is invasive, expensive and the scale needed would create a large demand for the overall service. Similar principles apply to blood testing for cancer antigen 125 for ovarian cancer.

### Pause for thought

You are waiting at a bus stop as you go about your life and see a large advert stating that one in eight males will get prostate cancer. You happen to know that screening is currently ineffective for this condition, whereas in some cases it can be aggressive many patients with prostate cancer in fact eventually die of other causes. You wonder how many people might see the advert and ask their GP about PSA testing or start worrying about their dad. What may be motivating this 'educational' advert, and are there any benefits for people in general? What are the disadvantages?

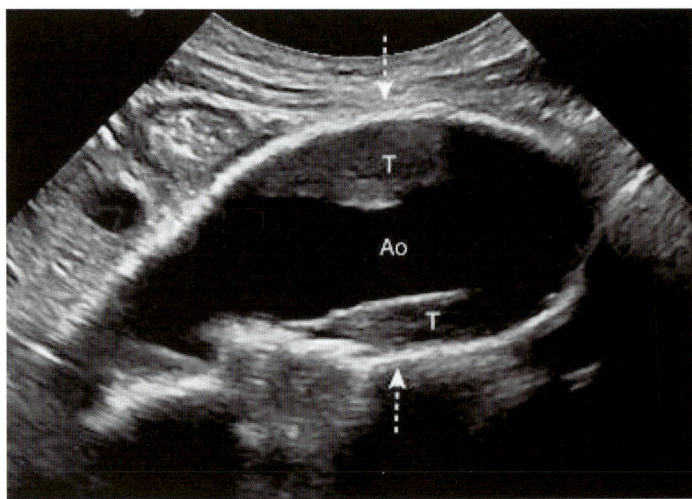

**Fig. 5.13** Abdominal aortic aneurysm. Sagittal view of the aorta displays a fusiform dilation of the abdominal aorta of 4.3 cm (between *dashed arrows*). The aneurysm contains an echogenic mural thrombus (*T*), and the remaining patent aortic lumen (*Ao*) with flowing blood is anechoic. For aneurysms of 4 to 5 cm in diameter, the risk of rupture increases to almost 25%.

Key ethical issues around screening will continue to include consent, confidentiality, discrimination, stigmatization and psychological distress. Screening offers the benefits of early detection of serious disease set against the intrusion, inconvenience and unpleasantness of being tested and waiting for results among people who do not think they are ill. One view sees this as the medicalisation of asymptomatic normal life; does the 'reassurance' of a negative test truly help someone who was simply going about their life as usual? Competent adults may feel disempowered about refusing screening, as refusers may be stigmatized. Positive screening tends to set off a series of diagnostic tests and treatments that can give rise to feelings of loss of control in someone who has been made into a patient, who previously felt well. In other situations, such as foetal screening leading to termination of pregnancy, it is debated 'who benefits' from screening including whether it is positioned to reduce the birth incidence of conditions associated with disability and what message this sends about disability discrimination. In the example of Down syndrome, people can go on to live reasonably independent lives. Preconception screening, such as for cystic fibrosis carrier status, is arguably ethically superior to antenatal screening since there is no question about the foetus being screened as a means to an end. Although there are no mass UK population programmes for preconception screening at present, scientific advances will likely create new screening possibilities for heritable monogenic, polygenic and chromosomal disorders. In preconception screening information is provided in advance to potential parents to facilitate reproductive choice. Screening should be scientifically based in terms of the sensitivity and specificity thresholds and screening intervals and eligibility. In reality, other influences also come to bear, such as political requirements, to be seen to be doing something about high profile conditions—a reflection of public perceptions about a given condition and the extent of available resources to maintain a screening service. The UK National Screening Committee (2022) criteria are a modern development on those of Wilson and Jungner and take into account the developments in genetic medicine. However, they still take a predominantly utilitarian approach to what is desirable and might be criticized as overly biomedical.

---

**CASE 5.6 TESTING FOR AN INCURABLE CONDITION**

If population screening became available for a currently untreatable or incurable condition, it could benefit you in the sense of helping you and/or your family plan for the future or help the wider society and perhaps facilitate research which improves the prospects for understanding and treating the condition in future; would you want the potential 'burden' or 'freedom' of knowing your status or the 'uncertainty' or 'normality' of not knowing?

---

## HEALTH PROMOTION

We turn to health promotion as the second of three key activity areas in public health practice. Effective health promotion relies on several factors: **P**ublic, **E**mployers, **V**oluntary groups, **A**dvertising, **M**edia, **P**rimary and secondary schooling, **L**ocal authority, **I**ndustry, **G**overnment, **H**ealth services and **T**raining (mnemonic PE VAMP LIGHT). Health services, including the NHS, are only one element among many.

### Behavioural modification

The ethics of behavioural modification as an approach to health promotion dance along the lines of empowerment, persuasion and counter-manipulation or coercion. Specific advice, like the 'back to sleep' campaign to reduce the risk of sudden infant death syndrome, is generally less controversial than targeting personal preferences. Personal preferences are strongly influenced by upbringing, culture, background wealth and other factors not under individual control. Hence Holland (2023) emphasizes the importance of avoiding tones of 'victim blaming' in behavioural modification campaigns. Behaviours are only freely chosen in the light of appropriate insight, which positions education as an empowering complement and potentially a counter-manipulation alongside ongoing macro-environmental influences on people. It can be asked if public communication campaigns create stigma—such as around HIV or obesity—and a potential for misuse for political purposes can be recognized. Are 'scare tactics' ever justified? Soft paternalism is a paradigm of intervention that recognizes the current actions of a person may be misaligned with their genuine preferences. However, from a population perspective it is difficult to determine someone like this from someone wilfully making an unwise health choice. Soft paternalism seeks to create autonomy and voluntary change, often through information and education.

The extent of value placed on liberalism in the prevailing culture is relevant. As with many areas of public health, behavioural modification often addresses people who are not patients and who have not asked for help (Fig. 5.15). Empowerment strategies are typically seen as ethical in liberal cultures, but of limited effectiveness. Coercive or restrictive strategies are typically seen as unethical but more effective, at least as defined by the attainment of a narrowly defined end. As in the case of COVID-19 lockdown rules or illicit drug laws, coercive strategies can also be impossible or difficult to enforce.

Policies like manipulating food prices and levies on cigarettes ostensibly aim to promote healthier population behaviours. They can also disproportionately burden people who are the most socioeconomically disadvantaged and vulnerable in society and widen health inequalities. For example, such people are more likely to smoke. How much state interference in influencing the environment is reasonable? What about advertising restrictions; the rights of the advertiser to promote their business and the rights of adults and children to be protected from manipulative advertising? Should environmental interventions be regarded as population research—as often they have not been tried before, or can they be defended on the grounds of intended or expected benefit?

It is established that financial incentives are at best only effective in short-term behavioural change for patients (Jochelson, 2007), and the ethics of these are sometimes highly questionable. Many current population health issues are either underpinned or significantly sustained by an individual component of addiction. Smoking, alcohol, illicit drug use and gambling are all examples. It is unclear to what extent population health promotion interventions really address the complex underlying biopsychosocial roots of addiction.

Health promotion in the individual patient consultation can be considered through the lens of a stages of change model (Fig. 5.14 gives one example, though there are many others including COM-B (Capability-Opportunity-Motivation→Behaviour) and Theoretical Domains Framework. Patients are at different stages of making changes, including not being ready at all. We have a duty to use knowledge and insights from a public health perspective within the consultation, and we also must treat patients as individuals.

The concept of 'behavioural nudging' involves presenting the opportunity or choice of making a small change or adjustment in a favourable way, with the idea that incremental changes can accumulate towards a desired benefit or aim. Within the medical consultation, it may be relevant to take an interest in the specifics of the patient's life and help the patient to identify what they value and why, and where small behavioural changes are desired and possible. Nudging at the population level has been typed as 'liberal paternalism' (Thaler and Sunstein, 2021): a lens that claims there is a minimal infringement of individual liberty in presenting choices, that inevitably have to be made anyway and are susceptible to other influences like commercial marketing, in a way that instead makes it easier to choose an option that favours desired public health outcomes. Whether this choice framing is pragmatic or manipulative depends on your philosophical disposition. Other potential criticisms include the shallow nature of the approach—nudging does not address underlying behavioural motivations or inequalities.

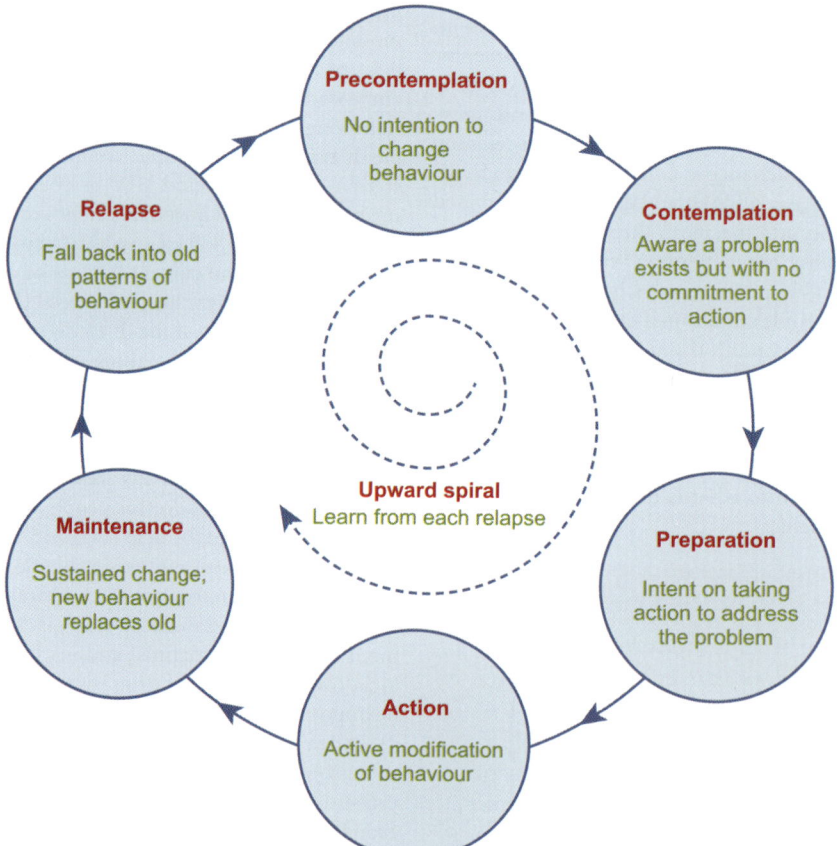

**Fig. 5.14** Stages of change model. (Adapted from Prochaska, J., & DiClemente, C. (1983). Stages and processes of self-change of smoking: Toward an integrative model of change. *Journal of Consulting and Clinical Psychology*, *51*(3), 390–395.)

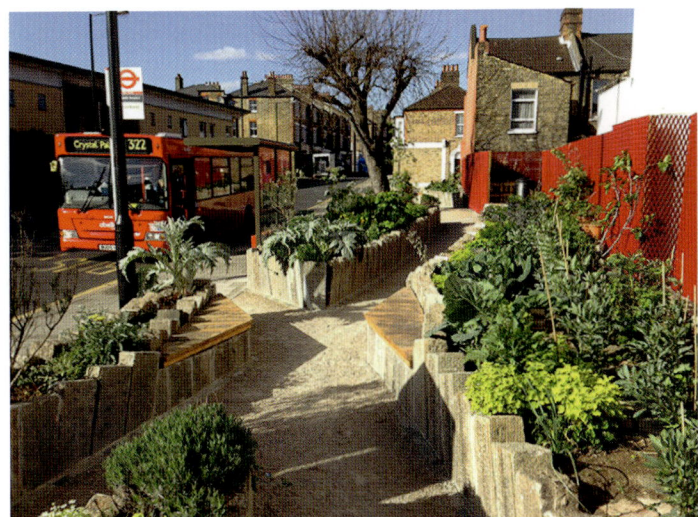

**Fig. 5.15**  The Edible Bus Stop, London, by The Edible Bus Stop consultancy brings alternative methods of greening streets.

---

**CASE 5.7  FINANCIAL INCENTIVES FOR GENERAL PRACTICE ORGANIZATIONS TO MODIFY BEHAVIOUR?**

**THE QUALITY AND OUTCOMES FRAMEWORK (QOF)**

Since 2004 QOF has been a voluntary annual incentive programme for NHS GP surgeries in England, Wales and Northern Ireland. There are currently five domains in England: Clinical, Public Health (blood pressure, obesity, smoking), Public Health—Additional Services (cervical screening), Public Health—Vaccination and Immunization, and Quality Improvement. QOF Indicators are developed and reviewed by the National Institute for Health and Care Excellence (NICE). NICE has a broader role advising on cost-effective health and social care interventions, as a quasi-autonomous nongovernmental organization. An NHS GP surgery scores 'QOF points' according to achievement in various domains, which are then monetized. For example (NICE, 2024): *The percentage of babies who reached 8 months old in the preceding 12 months, who have received at least 3 doses of a diphtheria, tetanus and pertussis containing vaccine before the age of 8 months.*

QOF is an upstream policy decision at the service contracting level which has some influence in the spheres of prevention and health promotion. It also creates large amounts of data since the vast majority of the population are registered with an NHS GP. What do you see as the pros and cons of NHS GP Surgeries attracting additional income for selected areas of clinical practice?

## HEALTH SERVICES

We now turn to the third and final thread of activity in public health, health services in the broad sense.

## Distributive justice

Distributive justice in general means the perceived fairness of an allocation or entitlement to access resources relative to other people in a society. 'Postcode lottery' has been used to describe regional variations in both the type and quality of NHS services (Fig. 5.16). If we say resources are best allocated according to local priorities, then, for example, if local priorities mean people in Oxford do not get a service that is available in London—a dissatisfied person in Oxford might use a phrase like 'postcode lottery' to describe the perceived unfairness of being denied something because of where they live. The meaning of postcode lottery has broadened in recent years to reflect that where a person lives impacts on their health through a wide range of factors. Direct providers of clinical services to patients have limited impact on many of the factors influencing the variation in health from place to place.

'Rationing' implies there are insufficient resources to meet the wants or needs of everyone, and that, however fairly resources are allocated, someone will always be dissatisfied. Distinguishing wants from needs is an ongoing debate. For example the need for healthcare in the United Kingdom is largely addressed by the state and funded by taxes, which raises the question of what is a healthcare need. Is founding a family a healthcare need on the grounds that infertility treatments are delivered by health professionals? Who should address this need

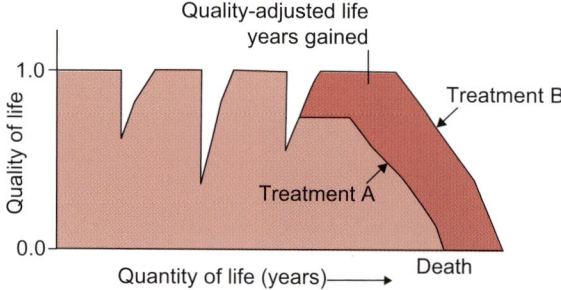

**Fig. 5.16** A schematic representation of the impact of two treatments (A and B) on a chronic disease that is characterized by episodes of relapse and remissions. The area under the curves represents the total number of quality-adjusted life years (QALYs) associated with each treatment. The gain in QALYs from treatment B is the shaded area between both curves.

and to what extent should taxpayers pay? Many social interventions also improve health, such as measures to reduce air pollution, access to green spaces and long-term care for older adults or people with disabilities needing assistance with daily living. In England these are not considered health services.

## Ethics of commissioning

'Commissioners' of NHS health services identify the needs of a defined population, identify health service providers to meet the need, contract with those providers and evaluate performance of the services. Important principles include:

- Conflicts of interest: Commissioners should not be able to commission a service that they also provide; any other conflicts of interest are declared.
- Transparency: Decision-making processes are explained publicly.
- Patient and public involvement: Balanced with expertise about the nature of clinical services that are possible.
- Cost–utility: Affordability and maximizing benefit for the population.

---

**CASE 5.8 PUBLIC PARTICIPATION IN HEALTH SERVICE COMMISSIONING**

In 1989 the *Basic Medical Service Act* was passed in the State of Oregon (United States). The Act required employers to cover employees for health insurance and extended state health insurance for the unemployed from 42 to 100% of costs. Universal coverage was balanced with a democratically informed and explicit system of healthcare rationing.

---

Around 700 medical conditions were paired with treatments, and a state Health Services Commission decided on priority setting. In doing so they used measures of cost-utility analysis and input from community meetings and 'citizens juries'. Two ethical approaches to distributive justice—cost–utility and public participation—were embraced transparently in a new way (Spicer, 2010).

## Principles of healthcare resource allocation

Healthcare needs are ideally met in proportion to the prevalence of population needs (Fig. 5.17). Within treatment areas, resources are prioritized according to the extremity of need and those with similar levels of need have an equal chance to access healthcare (Berney et al., 2005). Some further principles include:

- Resources are not provided for ineffective healthcare.
- Lifestyle does not determine access to healthcare.
- Public advise on but do not determine policy.
- Rationing is made explicit. Where a treatment is not provided on the NHS, a clinician who considers the case of their patient to be exceptional can apply on behalf of the patient for an Individual Funding Request. These may or may not be granted (NHS England, 2023).

NHS funding overall comes from general taxation, and while almost everyone pays some amount of tax or buys some taxable products the amount of tax contributed varies. This broadly corresponds with the principle of vertical equity since people with more resources available also contribute more. Funds are applied in the NHS using the principle of horizontal equity, which broadly corresponds to equal treatment for equal need.

In emergency or disaster situations in particular, other approaches to deploying resources are sometimes taken. For example, military personnel with lesser levels of health need may be returned to combat more quickly by being treated first and this may be overall advantageous—an example of 'reverse triage'. This approach can be broadened to consider situations of resource constraint, to argue for a focus on those most likely to benefit from treatment rather than the sickest.

## Utilitarianism and quality-adjusted life years

Quality-adjusted life years (QALYs) are a utilitarian approach to cost-effectiveness. 'The essence of a QALY is that it takes one year of healthy life expectancy to be worth 1 and regards a

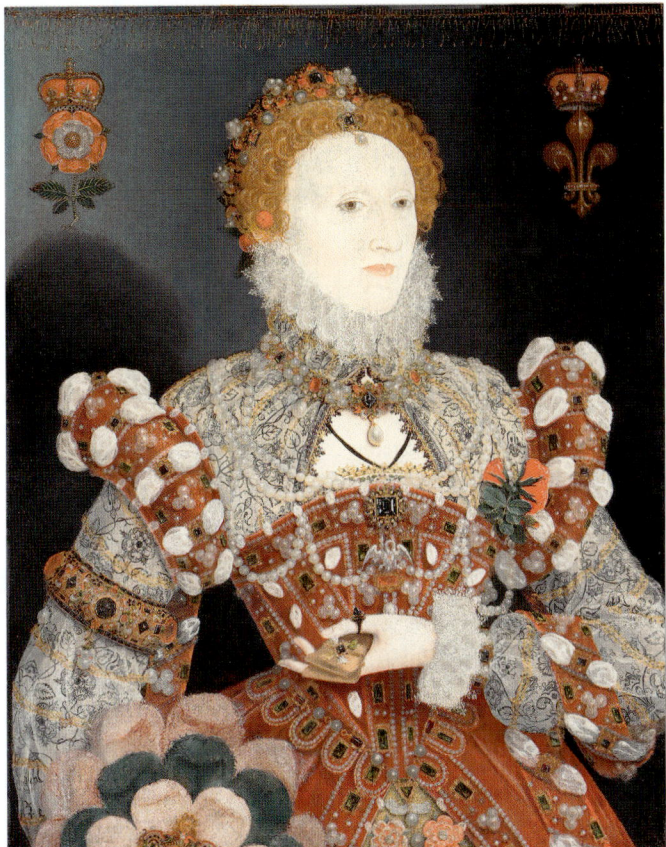

**Fig. 5.17** The *Poor Law Relief Act* (1601) was introduced by the Government of Queen Elizabeth I, after the dissolution of the monasteries under Henry VIII had removed the main source of social security for people unable to support themselves. The essence of this system was only replaced after World War II (1939–45) with the modern welfare state in the United Kingdom.

year of unhealthy life expectancy as worth less than 1. Its precise value is lower the worse the quality of life' (Williams, 1985). QALYs provide a mechanism by which different types of health benefits can be compared, with some degree of objectivity. The National Institute of Health and Care Excellence (NICE) in the United Kingdom currently tends to approve new treatments costing no more than £20,000 to £30,000 per QALY gained, which is an example of QALYs being used in resource allocation decisions (Gandjour, 2020).

Two major criticisms of QALYs are:

1. They favour people who are younger and healthier. So there are concerns about justice for older people and younger people with long-term disabilities.
2. They are difficult to calculate practically and reliably. Quality of life is subjective to the individual, varying with who is asked and how the question is asked. Can we really compare the quality of life between conditions, for example blindness, kidney failure and learning disability?

A phrase commonly attributed to Albert Einstein recognizes not everything that can be counted counts, and not everything that counts can be counted.

**CASE 5.9 QALYS AND DOUBLE JEOPARDY**

Tom and Harry are both 20 years old and suffer identical injuries in a car crash. Tom was previously well, and Harry has a background of being blind. Assuming they both go on to live to the same age, the same treatment for their injuries will create more QALYs for Tom. The QALY system assumes that Harry's blindness means he cannot be restored to as good a level of health. Harris (1995) called this problem double jeopardy. Harry already has the disability of blindness, and this disability under the QALY system can adversely affect the priority assigned to him in receiving treatment for an unrelated condition.

## 'Distributive justice' before the NHS

It is worth contextualizing the present-day challenges with resource allocation and rationing against a longer historical timeline (see also Chapter 1). In the 1800s UK hospitals were considered dangerous and low-status places due to a lack of anaesthesia and aseptic techniques, and they were run by charities or local authorities. The *Poor Law* system from the early 1600s continued, catering for the needs of the poorest people and unemployed. Patients had to be 'deservingly poor' to qualify for treatment. Those who could afford it could pay to consult a qualified doctor.

David Lloyd George (then Chancellor, later Prime Minister) introduced the UK *National Health Insurance Act* 1911. The government here extended the role of the existing Friendly Societies and Trade Unions that offered health services to some workers—by introducing a 'National Health Insurance' scheme for GP services. Taxes were taken from pay to fund GP services for that person (not for the whole family). Hospital services were not included. The old paper-based notes in UK General Practices are still called 'Lloyd George notes' because of their origins. Universal population coverage was rolled out as the NHS in 1948 after the Second World War. The Poor Laws were superseded by the modern welfare state.

## Birth of the NHS

Hospitals became state controlled as part of the wartime Emergency Medical Service. The Beveridge (1942) report established the principles for a postwar 'welfare state'. Negotiations between the government and the British Medical Association led to the *National Health Service Act* (1946). Effective health promotion and improved public health were anticipated to lead to falling costs for health services.

## Evolution of the NHS

The NHS has proved relatively dynamic and has seen continuous reform:

1. *Hierarchical (1948–79)*: Totalitarian control by officials, politicians and some senior doctors: an example of 'top–down' regulation.
2. *Market (1979–97)*: Introduction of internal market mechanisms: while the state remained the single payer, so-called 'purchasers' (later renamed 'commissioners') held budget allocations and were distinguished from 'providers'—this intended to encourage efficiencies by creating the opportunity for competitive tendering for contracts—this started with tendering for NHS domestic/cleaning services.
3. *Network (1997–present)*: Amalgamating the pros and cons of (1) and (2) above. Encouraging collaborations and partnerships within the system.

The NHS remains free of charge at the point of delivery and this principle is enshrined in the NHS Constitution. Certain limited exceptions are sanctioned by Parliament: for example each prescription item in England costs the patient £9.65 in 2024 unless an exemption is applied by virtue of age or a qualifying condition. Demand for a free service is not inevitably endless. The amount demanded of a 'free at the point of delivery' service like the NHS is determined at the point where a person sees no additional benefit to be gained from seeking further attention.

Sometimes the term 'health tourism' is used to describe people travelling to the United Kingdom for healthcare. Generally speaking, GP and primary care services are free to all. Secondary care services are only free to people 'ordinarily resident' in the United Kingdom; this means overseas visitors are liable to being charged. Refugees and asylum seekers are exempt from charges for secondary care services, and other exceptions to charging also apply.

## Private providers in the NHS

Involving private companies in state-funded health services raises a conflict of duties and interests in the United Kingdom. The primary legal duty of UK company directors is to act 'for the benefit of the members [of the company] as a whole' (Companies Act 2006, *s*.172). Nonfinancial considerations are made secondary. Other concerns include:

- Private companies paying dividends to shareholders, taking money away from patient care or investment in training and research.
- As NHS hospitals lose patients to commercially run providers, students and junior doctors get fewer opportunities for practical training.
- The private sector is involved in building and running some NHS hospitals in England under a scheme called the Private Finance Initiative; the NHS pays over a period of 25 to 30 years, but costly contracts have left many hospitals with challenging levels of debt.

Most general practices are and always have been independent contractors to the NHS operating as Partnerships further to the *Partnership Act* 1890, with the GP Partners also bound by professional codes of conduct. Recent years have seen several changes: non-GPs being allowed to become Partners, a range of other organizational forms emerging including non-profits and Community Interest Companies and larger registered patient list sizes. Currently, an average practice list is ~10,000 patients. Larger organizations may be better able to implement quality and safety processes, but there may be trade-offs with staff disengagement and reduced continuity of care, which typically leads to increased secondary care demand.

## Care in the community

Driving forces for community care include:

- Less hospital beds per capita—Numbers have been falling for a long time due to improved techniques and policies that allow shorter stays in hospitals and to reduce costs. There has been an increase in the use of day surgery. The United Kingdom has one of the lowest ratios of hospital beds per capita in Europe, approximately 1:416 people (British Medical Association, 2022).
- Patients often prefer treatment out of the hospital when possible.
- Community care often offers good value for money and more flexible services.
- Technological advances make opportunities for remote assessment, monitoring and treatment.

## Different systems for organizing and funding healthcare

A healthcare system can be considered among four types (Field 1973; Fitzpatrick 2003):

1. **Pluralistic, for example the United States**
   - Several nonintegrated methods of providing funds, for example insurance, fee-for-service with medical monopoly resulting in high cost-per-capita.
   - Access can be problematic for those who cannot afford it.
   - Facilities owned by private groups or the state.
   - Tend to have a relative lack of public health initiatives.
2. **Health insurance, for example Canada, Japan**
   - Third party gathers resources in the form of compulsory insurance.
   - Tends to offer good access for patients and reduced waiting times.
   - Insurers may favour cheaper providers or procedures; premiums can vary with age; insurance policies may not cover all eventualities.
3. **Health service, for example United Kingdom and Sweden**
   - The state owns *most* facilities and services are mostly free-to-all at the point of use with relatively favourable cost-per-capita.
   - Independence of doctors, despite most of their income coming from the government.
   - Waiting times can be long.
4. **Socialized health system, for example the former USSR**
   - The state owns *all* facilities, everyone is equal and there is no other option.
   - Nearly all healthcare professionals are employed by the government.
   - Lack of responsiveness and a challenge to keep up with technological advances.

## Health inequalities and healthcare inequalities

Health inequalities describe how factors like age, sex, gender, ethnicity, origin, nutrition, housing, location, education, employment, financial well-being and social class are associated with variability in health outcomes Fig. 5.18. A large enough healthcare system can provide some or all of the data that suggest or evidence of the existence of health inequalities and social injustices. Social determinants often affect health outcomes more than healthcare itself (Fig. 5.18). Healthcare inequalities relate to the variability in health outcomes that are introduced by the system of healthcare provision. Scobie and Morris (2020) reported that people living in the most deprived areas of England experience worse access, quality of care and poorer health outcomes than people living in the least deprived areas. These include spending longer in A&E and having a worse experience of making a GP appointment.

NHS England currently has an inequalities strategy called *CORE 20 PLUS 5,* which aims to focus attention towards: the *most deprived 20%* of the national population as defined by the Index of Multiple Deprivation; *PLUS* groups including ethnic minority communities, people with a learning disability, autistic people, people with multiple long-term health conditions, other groups that share protected characteristics as defined by the *Equality Act* 2010, coastal communities where there may be small areas of high deprivation hidden among relative affluence, groups experiencing social exclusion known as inclusion health groups (for example people experiencing homelessness, drug and alcohol dependence, vulnerable migrants, Gypsy, Roma and Traveller communities, sex workers, people in contact with the justice system, victims of modern slavery); and *five specific clinical areas*. The five clinical areas are (1) maternity, (2) severe mental illness, (3) chronic respiratory disease, (4) early cancer diagnosis and (5) hypertension and hyperlipidaemia case finding and optimal management. Considered altogether, this inequalities strategy seems likely to encompass a large fraction of the entire population (Figs 5.19 and 5.20).

---

**CASE 5.10  HARM REDUCTION: UNDERAGE SEX AND ILLICIT DRUG USE**

Teenage pregnancy and substance misuse (Figs 5.19-5.20) are both associated with health inequalities. Harm reduction policies related to illegal activities like illicit drug use and underage sex are examples where restrictive policies including the law continually prove to be unenforceable. The Fraser Guidelines are an example of a harm reduction approach around contraceptive prescribing in under 16 years (see Chapter 3). With illicit drug use, abstinence often proves ineffective due to the

*(Continued)*

The main determinants of health

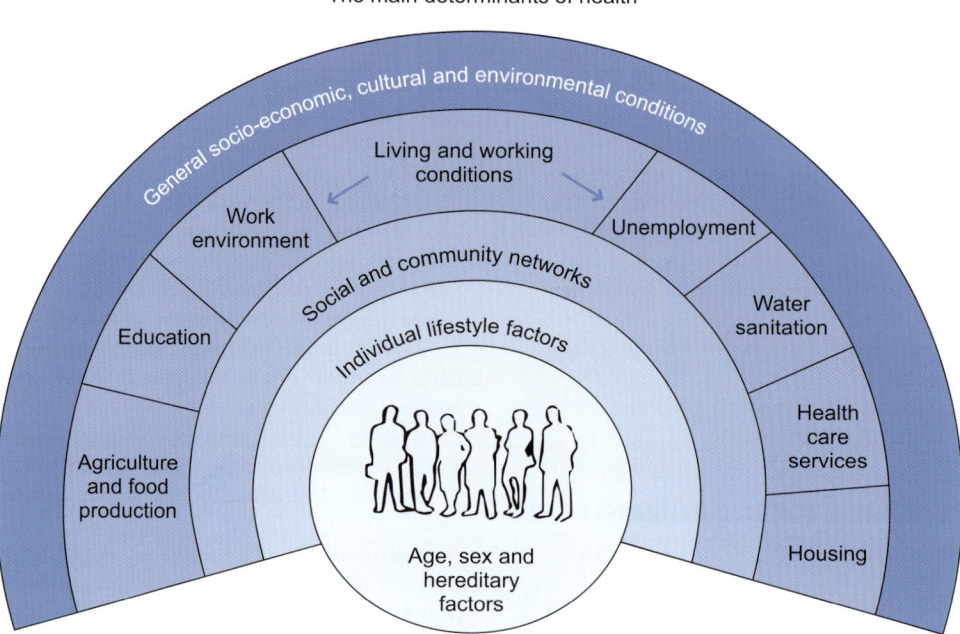

**Fig. 5.18** Biological, behavioural and social influences on health. While healthcare services can and do introduce inequalities and are right to address, there are many more significant influences on health inequalities that the system of healthcare—including public health practice—either can only minimally influence or not address at all.

**CASE 5.10 —** *Contd.*

nature of addiction. Various needle exchange programmes, supervised injection facilities and substitute prescription programmes exist. It is argued that harm reduction approaches might bring a drug user into an environment that puts them in contact with health professionals with the consequence of nudging them towards abstinence. Christie, Groarke and Sweet (2008) argue for harm reduction policies on utilitarian and virtue ethics grounds, particularly compassion. Deontologists are more likely to see harm reduction here as inherently wrong, particularly if they regard legislation as a significant barometer. It can be questioned whether harm reduction policies significantly undermine the law, or whether, for example, the benefits of medical prescribing of substitute opioids or hormonal contraception to females aged under 16 outweigh this—respectively by reducing the personal and social complications of substance misuse or underage pregnancy. Similarly it may be questioned whether teaching safe injection or prescribing underage contraception sends a mixed message by ultimately facilitating the continuation of risky and illegal behaviours.

Improvements in life expectancy in recent decades have disproportionately benefitted people with more privileged demographic profiles. Hence while there have been widespread advances in technology and changes in the standard of living, health inequalities along the socioeconomic gradient have continued to widen. The amount of time that people spend in poor health (morbidity) has also increased. Healthy life expectancy in England varies by over 18 years between the most and least deprived groups, from approximately 52 to 70 years of healthy life (The King's Fund, 2021). The UK Office for National Statistics (2024) reported small falls in total life expectancy across the United Kingdom, to 78.6 years for males and 82.6 years for females, with data impacted to some extent by the COVID-19 pandemic. Even before the pandemic The Marmot Review 2010 and its follow-up in 2020 had already reported that, for the first time in a century, life expectancy had not increased when considered overall across the United Kingdom; for the poorest females in society, life expectancy had already fallen by 10% (Marmot et al., 2010, 2020). In particular:

- These data reiterate the north/south health divide.
- Increased mortality rates for males and females aged 45 to 49 years may be related to so-called 'deaths of despair' from suicide, drugs and alcohol abuse, as seen in the United States.
- Child poverty has increased to 22% in comparison with Europe's lowest of 10% in Norway, Iceland and the Netherlands.
- There is a housing crisis and a rise in homelessness.

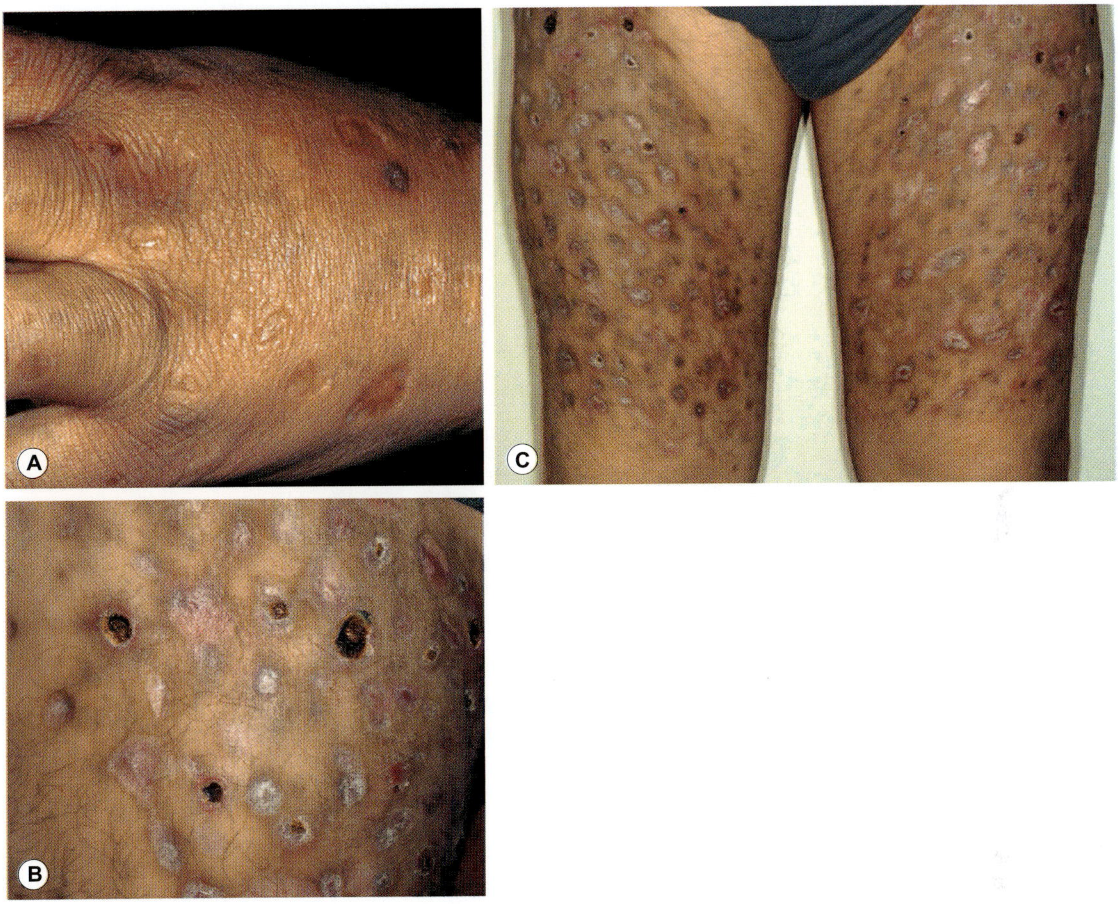

**Fig. 5.19** 'Skin popping' scars. (A–C) Multiple circular depressed scars, some with rims of postinflammatory hyperpigmentation, admixed with circular haemorrhagic crusts overlying ulcerations. Cocaine was injected into the thighs.

The historic Acheson (1998) and Black et al. (1980) reports favoured *materialist* explanations as most significant—implying the association between social deprivation and health is explained to a significant extent by differences in wealth. Further study has lent support to this. This means the health of patients is significantly determined by such things as lack of clothes and food, poor housing (damp, cold, overcrowded, located in areas with high air pollution and without suitable outdoor play spaces for children) and poor access to education and healthcare. House prices tend to increase in areas with good schools so children from poorer families become less able to use education as a route out of the cycle of poverty. Tudor-Hart (1971) introduced the concept of the 'Inverse Care Law', which claims that healthcare is least available where it is most needed. There are also *behavioural differences* between social groups, for example more smoking and less breastfeeding in more deprived populations. Marmot considers that wealth, power and status are all relevant: financial position alone does not explain all the variance; the degree of control a person has over their own work and life is important as is the social position a person inhabits.

---

**ETHICS**

**THE INVERSE CARE LAW**

Dr Julian Tudor-Hart was a GP in Wales who introduced the concept of the 'Inverse Care Law' in the 1970s. This states healthcare is least available where it is most needed, that is in areas with more socially deprived people. Others have suggested that even where healthcare and other services are available, they are less accessible and/or underused.

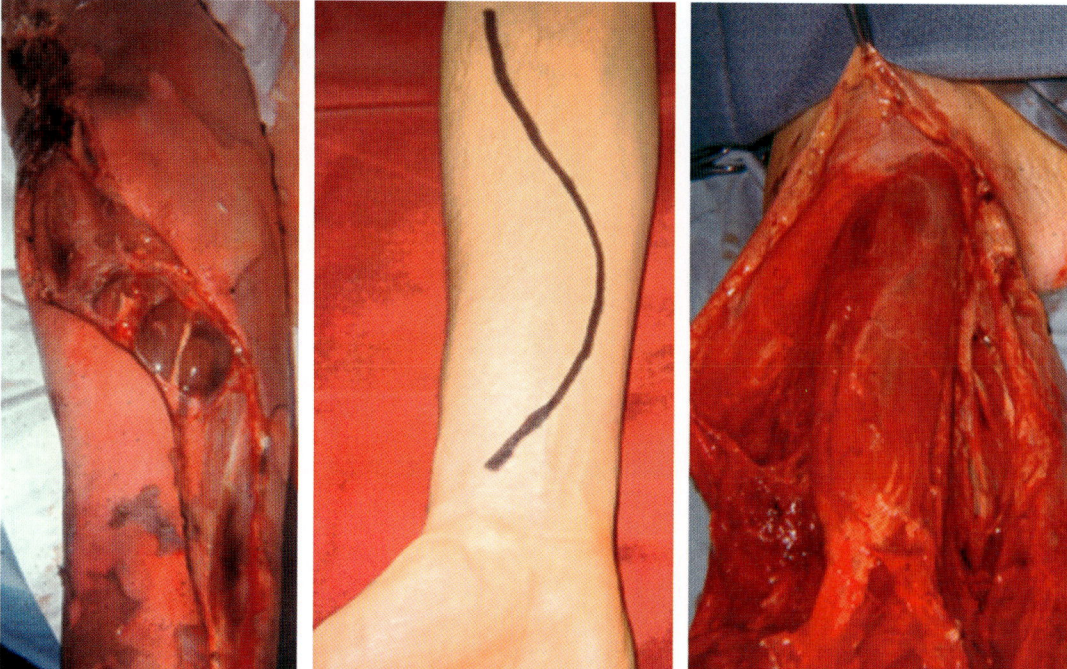

**Fig. 5.20** Injection of contaminated 'mixed jive' heroin into the forearm subcutaneous tissues led to extensive soft tissue necrosis, involving the forearm and distal arm with associated compartment syndrome. Extensive soft tissue debridement and extension of the forearm fasciotomy incision proximal to include the anterior compartment of the arm resulted in limb salvage and a good long-term result. The classic incision for a fasciotomy of the anterior arm is shown.

---

### HINTS AND TIPS

#### THE CYCLE OF POVERTY

In the Victorian era—mid-19th to early 20th centuries—it was said 'poverty caused disease which caused poverty'. While the welfare state mitigates this to an extent, experiencing disadvantage in one area of life is associated with disadvantage in others.

- How reasonable is it to encourage a person to change their preferred habits or behaviours for an expected health benefit?
- Various social and environmental factors are associated with better health—to what extent should these be funded from a state health budget?
- What health services are essential? Who should make rationing decisions?

### CLINICAL NOTES

#### KEY QUESTIONS IN PUBLIC HEALTH ETHICS

- When does or should individual autonomy become limited by population health concerns?
  - For example, smoking in public places only became illegal in the United Kingdom in the late 2000s.
  - For example, the right to decline vaccinations.
- Does population screening that prevents ill health for small numbers of people justify the medicalisation of normal life for everyone?

### References

Acheson, D. (1998). (Chairman) *An independent inquiry into inequalities in health report.* London: The Stationery Office.

Berney, L., et al. (2005). Ethical principles and the rationing of health care: A qualitative study in general practice. *British Journal of General Practice, 55*(517), 620–625.

Beveridge, W. (1942). *Social insurance and allied services.* London: The Stationery Office.

Black, D., et al. (1980). *Inequalities in health: Report of a research working group.* London: Department of Health and Social Security.

British Medical Association. (2022). *NHS hospital beds data analysis.* BMA. https://www.bma.org.uk/advice-and-support/nhs-delivery-and-workforce/pressures/nhs-hospital-beds-data-analysis#:~:text=2020%20data%20or%20latest%20available&text=The%20average%20number%20of%20beds,%2C%20by%20contrast%2C%20has%207.8

Childress, J. F., et al. (2002). Public health ethics: mapping the terrain. *Journal of Law, Medicine and Ethics*, 30(2), 170–178.

Christie, T., Groarke, L., & Sweet, W. (2008). Virtue ethics as an alternative to deontological and consequential reasoning in the harm reduction debate. *International Journal of Drug Policy*, 19, 52–58.

*Companies Act* 2006.

*Coronavirus Act* 2020.

Das, S. (27 May 2023). NHS data breach: trusts shared patient details with Facebook without consent. *The Guardian*. https://www.theguardian.com/society/2023/may/27/nhs-data-breach-trusts-shared-patient-details-with-facebook-meta-without-consent

*Data Protection Act* (2018).

*Equality Act* 2010.

Field, M. G. (1973). The concept of the "health system" at the macrosociological level. *Social Science and Medicine*, 7(10), 763–785. https://doi.org/10.1016/0037-7856(73)90118-2.

Fitzpatrick, R. (2003). 'Organizing and funding health care' In G. Scambler (Ed.), *Sociology as applied to medicine* (5th ed., pp. 292–307). Edinburgh: Saunders.

Gandjour, A. (2020). Willingness to pay for new medicines: A step towards narrowing the gap between NICE and IQWiG. *BMC Health Services Research*, 343. https://doi.org/10.1186/s12913-020-5050-9. (2020).

Harris, J. (1995). Double jeopardy and the veil of ignorance—A reply. *Journal of Medical Ethics*, 21, 151–157.

Health Protection (Notification) Regulations 2010.

Hofstede, G. (2001). *Culture's Consequences. Comparing values, behaviours, institutions, and organisations across nations* (2nd ed.). London: Sage Publications.

Holland, S. (2023). *Public health ethics* (3rd ed.). Cambridge: Polity Press.

Iacobucci, G. (2022). COVID-19: Government abandons mandatory vaccination of NHS staff. *British Medical Journal*, 376, o269. https://doi.org/10.1136/bmj.o269.

Jochelson, K. (2007). *Paying the patient: Improving health using financial incentives*. London: King's Fund.

Kisling, L. A. & Das, J. M. (2023). Prevention strategies. In: *StatPearls*. StatPearls Publishing. https://www.ncbi.nlm.nih.gov/books/NBK537222/.

Krieger, N., & Zierler, S. (1996). What explains the public's health?—A call for epidemiological theory. *Epidemiology*, 7(1), 107–109.

Marmot, M., et al. (2010). *Fair Society, healthy lives: Strategic review of health inequalities in England post-2010*. London: The Marmot Review.

Marmot, M., et al. (2020). *Health equity in England: The Marmot review 10 years on*. London: Institute of Health Equity.

*National Health Insurance Act* 1911.

*National Health Service Act* (1946).

NHS England. (2023). *Individual funding requests for specialised services: A guide for patients. Version 2*. Publication reference: PR2085. NHS England.

NICE. (2024) NICE Quality and Outcomes Framework indicator. Available at: https://www.nice.org.uk/standards-and-indicators/qofindicators/.

Nuffield Council on Bioethics. (2007). *Public health: Ethical issues*. London: Nuffield Council on Bioethics.

*Offences Against the Person Act* 1861.

Office for National Statistics. (2023). *Dataset: Adult smoking habits in Great Britain*. Newport: Crown.

Office for National Statistics. (2024). *Statistical bulletin. National life tables—Life expectancy in the UK: 2020 to 2022*. Office for National Statistics. https://www.ons.gov.uk/peoplepopulationandcommunity/birthsdeathsandmarriages/lifeexpectancies/bulletins/nationallifetablesunitedkingdom/2020to2022.

Omran, A. R. (2005). The epidemiologic transition. A theory of the epidemiology of population change. *The Milbank Quarterly*, 83(4), 731–757. https://doi.org/10.1111/j.1468-0009.2005.00398.x.

*Partnership Act* 1890.

*Poor Law Relief Act* (1601).

Scobie, S. & Morris, J. (2020) *Quality and inequality: digging deeper. QualityWatch briefing*. Nuffield Trust and the Health Foundation: Available at https://www.nuffieldtrust.org.uk/resource/quality-and-inequality-digging-deeper.

Seedhouse, D. (2001). *Health: The foundations for achievement* (2nd ed.). Chichester: John Wiley & Sons.

Spicer, J. (2010). Oregon and the UK: experiments in resource allocation. *London Journal of Primary Care*, 3(2), 105–108. https://doi.org/10.1080/17571472.2010.11493312.

Terrence Higgins Trust & National AIDS Trust. (2010). *Prosecutions for HIV transmission. A guide for people living with HIV in England and Wales*. London: National AIDS Trust.

Thaler, R. H., & Sunstein, C. R. (2021). *Nudge: The final edition. Updated edition*. New York: Penguin Books an imprint of Penguin Random House LLC.

The King's Fund. (2021). *Health Inequalities in a nutshell*. The King's Fund. https://www.kingsfund.org.uk/projects/nhs-in-a-nutshell/health-inequalities#the-deprivation-gap.

Torracinta, L., Tanner, R., & Vanderslott, S. (2021). MMR vaccine attitude and uptake research in the United Kingdom: A critical review. *Vaccines (Basel)*, 9(4), 402. https://doi.org/10.3390/vaccines9040402.

Tudor Hart, J. (1971). The Inverse Care Law. *The Lancet*, 297(7696), 405–412. https://doi.org/10.1016/S0140-6736(71)92410-X.

UK National Screening Committee. (2022). *Guidance. Criteria for a population screening programme*. https://www.gov.uk/government/publications/evidence-review-criteria-national-screening-programmes/criteria-for-appraising-the-viability-effectiveness-and-appropriateness-of-a-screening-programme.

Upshur, R. E. (2002). Principles for the justification of public health intervention. *Canadian Journal of Public Health*, 93(2), 101–103.

Williams, A. (1985) 'The value of QALYs'. *Health and Social Service Journal*, (Centre 8 Suppl.), 3–5.

Wilson, J. M. G., & Jungner, Y. G. (1968). *Principles and practice of screening for disease*. Geneva: World Health Organization.

Winslow, C. E. (1920). The untilled fields of public health. *Science*, 51(1306), 23–33. https://doi.org/10.1126/science.51.1306.23.

**Further Reading**

Council for International Organizations of Medical Sciences. (2009). *International ethical guidelines for epidemiological studies*. Geneva: CIOMS.

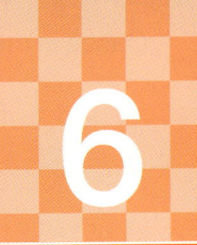

# Cases in medical ethics and law

## FOUNDATIONS OF PROFESSIONALISM

## Case 6.1: Senior consultant's data falsification presents an ethical dilemma for medical student

### Scenario summary

Alex, a final-year medical student in the United Kingdom, is on a clinical rotation at a busy hospital. While assisting Dr Thompson, a senior consultant renowned for his contributions to the hospital's reputation, Alex discovers that Dr Thompson is deliberately falsifying patient data. Dr Thompson is altering medical records to reflect better patient outcomes—such as reduced complication rates and shorter hospital stays—to improve hospital statistics and meet administrative targets. Alex faces a moral and professional dilemma: whether to report the misconduct, risking his future career prospects, or to remain silent.

### Legal aspects related to the case

- **General Medical Council (GMC) Guidance:** According to the GMC's *Good Medical Practice* (2024), doctors must be honest, trustworthy and act with integrity. Falsifying patient records breaches these fundamental duties. In a notable case, Dr Jane Barton faced serious professional consequences after the GMC found her actions misleading and dishonest.
- **Duty to Report Concerns:** Doctors are required to take prompt action if they believe patient safety is compromised (GMC, 2024). Medical students, though not fully licensed, are expected to adhere to similar standards. Under the GMC's Duty of Candour (2015, 2024), healthcare professionals are obligated to report errors or misconduct that could harm patients.
- **Public Interest Disclosure Act 1998 (PIDA):** Offers legal protection for workers who disclose information about malpractice, wrongdoing or health and safety risks. Protects against unfair dismissal or victimization as a result of the disclosure. In *Day v. Health Education England & Others* (2017), the Court of Appeal extended whistleblowing protections to include doctors in training.
- **Fraud Act 2006:** Falsifying patient data to improve hospital statistics may constitute fraud under Section 2 (Fraud by False Representation). Dr Thompson could face criminal charges if found guilty of dishonestly making a false representation with intent to gain or cause loss. In *R v. Patel* (2008), a dentist was prosecuted for falsifying treatment records to receive payments.
- *Data Protection Act* **2018 and General Data Protection Regulation (GDPR):** Personal data must be accurate and kept up to date. Altering patient records compromises data integrity, violating data protection laws. The Information

Commissioner's Office (ICO) can impose penalties on organizations and individuals for such breaches.
- **Clinical Governance and National Health Service (NHS) Policies:** NHS guidelines emphasize maintaining precise and truthful patient records for patient safety and care continuity. NHS Trusts may conduct internal investigations leading to disciplinary actions against staff who falsify records.

### Ethical issues raised

- **Integrity and Honesty:** Honesty is a cornerstone of medical ethics, essential for trust between patients, doctors and society. The Declaration of Geneva emphasizes the commitment to act with conscience and dignity.
- **Patient Safety and Welfare:** Falsified records can lead to inappropriate care decisions, medication errors or missed complications. Misrecording allergy information could result in a patient receiving a drug they are allergic to, causing harm.
- **Duty to Report Misconduct:** Failing to report compromises ethical standards and may contribute to a culture of negligence. The Bawa-Garba case highlighted the importance of systemic openness and individual responsibility in reporting concerns.
- **Moral Distress and Professional Identity:** Moral distress, a psychological response, may affect Alex if he feels powerless to take ethical action. This could cause cynicism or an erosion of professional values.
- **Confidentiality and Trust:** Alex must consider patient confidentiality when reporting, ensuring disclosures are made appropriately. GMC guidelines provide frameworks for responsible reporting without breaching confidentiality.

### Clinical issues

- **Accuracy of Medical Records:** Records inform ongoing treatment plans, referrals and multidisciplinary communication. Incorrect recording of a patient's medication could lead to dangerous drug interactions.
- **Clinical Governance and Quality Improvement:** Accurate data are vital for auditing outcomes, improving services and patient safety initiatives. The Mid Staffordshire NHS Foundation Trust public enquiry revealed that misleading data contributed to systemic failures.
- **Implications for Public Health Data:** Falsified statistics can affect funding decisions, resource distribution and healthcare policies. Inflated success rates may divert resources from departments needing improvement.
- **Team Dynamics and Professional Relationships:** Misconduct erodes trust, leading to a toxic work environment, decreased morale and impaired teamwork. Effective collaboration relies on mutual respect and honesty.

- **Fear of Reprisal and Career Impact:** Concerns over negative repercussions, such as poor references or victimization. Balancing personal welfare against ethical duties is challenging. In Dr Raj Mattu's case, after raising concerns about patient safety, he faced prolonged suspension and legal battles.
- **Education and Training:** Senior doctors serve as role models; unethical behaviour negatively influences trainees. The hidden curriculum impacts medical students' professional development.

## Potential implications

- Alex has an ethical duty to protect patients and uphold the integrity of the profession.
- Alex's understanding of the protections under the *Public Interest Disclosure Act* 1998 may alleviate his fears of reprisal. Alex should seek guidance from a trusted mentor, medical school advisors or a senior colleague on how to proceed.
- Alex must ensure patient confidentiality is preserved. Providing information through appropriate channels minimizes the risk of unintended disclosure.
- Reporting the issue may prompt an investigation that leads to organizational improvements, strengthening clinical governance and data integrity.
- Dealing with such a situation can be stressful. Accessing support services, such as counselling or peer support groups, can help Alex manage any emotional impact.

# Case 6.2: Ethical concerns in trial of new treatment

## Scenario summary

Dr Emily Lewis, a clinical researcher at a UK university hospital, is offered significant funding by PharmaCo to conduct a drug trial for 'Immunex', a new medication for a serious chronic condition (e.g. rheumatoid arthritis) that already has effective treatments. The proposed study includes a placebo-controlled arm, meaning some participants would discontinue their current effective therapy to receive a placebo. Dr Lewis is enticed by the potential benefits but is concerned about the ethical implications of exposing patients to harm.

## Legal aspects related to the case

- **Declaration of Helsinki (2013):** Emphasizes that new interventions must be tested against the best proven interventions. Placebo-controlled trials are acceptable only when no current effective treatment exists or for compelling scientific reasons. Paragraph 33 states, 'The benefits, risks, burdens and effectiveness of a new intervention must be tested against those of the best proven intervention(s)'.
- **International Conference on Harmonization Good Clinical Practice (GCP) Guidelines (1996):** Ensures the rights, safety and well-being of trial subjects are protected. Requires that anticipated benefits justify the risks. Section 2.3 emphasizes that 'the rights, safety and well-being of the trial subjects are the most important considerations'.
- **UK Medicines for Human Use (Clinical Trials) Regulations 2004:** Mandates that all clinical trials must be approved by a Research Ethics Committee (REC) and adhere to GCP standards. Conducting a trial without REC approval is illegal and may result in sanctions.
- **EU Clinical Trials Regulation EU No 536/2014:** Reinforces the obligation to minimize risk and burden to participants. Emphasizes informed consent and the risk–benefit assessment. Article 28 requires that the anticipated benefits justify the risks.
- **Informed Consent Laws:** Participants must be fully informed about the study, including risks, benefits and alternatives. Failure to obtain proper consent could result in legal action for battery or negligence.
- **Common Law Duty of Care:** Researchers owe participants a duty of care. Exposing participants to unnecessary harm may constitute a breach of this duty. In *Chester v. Afshar* (2004), the House of Lords held that failure to inform a patient of risks invalidated consent.

## Ethical issues raised

- **Risk of Harm to Participants (Nonmaleficence):** Withdrawing effective treatment exposes participants to disease progression and suffering. Ethical principles mandate avoiding harm.
- **Lack of Clinical Equipoise:** Clinical equipoise requires genuine uncertainty about the best treatment. Existing effective treatments mean that withholding them is unethical.
- **Informed Consent and Therapeutic Misconception:** Participants may believe they will receive therapeutic benefit, compromising informed consent. They may not fully grasp the implications of being in the placebo group.
- **Exploitation and Undue Influence:** Financial incentives may pressure researchers to compromise ethical standards. Conflicts of interest may arise, potentially biasing the study design and conduct.
- **Professional Integrity and Responsibilities:** Researchers must prioritize participant welfare over personal or institutional gain. Upholding ethical standards maintains public trust in medical research.
- **Compliance with the Declaration of Helsinki:** Noncompliance could discredit the research and harm

professional reputation. Journals may refuse to publish studies that do not adhere to these principles.

## Clinical issues

- **Study Design Flaws:** Ethical and methodological concerns arise when effective treatments are available. An active comparator trial would be more appropriate, comparing the new drug to the standard treatment.
- **Patient Selection and Vulnerability:** Removing effective therapy can lead to worsening conditions. In chronic diseases, disease progression may cause irreversible damage during the trial period.
- **Risk–Benefit Assessment:** Uncertain benefits of the new drug do not outweigh the known risks of stopping effective treatment. Participants in the placebo group received no direct benefit.
- **Regulatory Approval and Compliance:** Ethics committees and regulatory bodies are unlikely to approve the study. Proceeding could result in wasted resources and legal sanctions.

## Potential implications

- Conducting a placebo-controlled trial when effective treatments are available raises significant ethical issues.
- Withdrawing effective therapy from participants may violate the principle of nonmaleficence (do no harm) by exposing them to unnecessary risk of disease progression and suffering.
- This poses a direct threat to patient welfare and may undermine trust in the research process.
- Negative outcomes for participants could also have broader implications for clinical practice by discouraging patient participation in future clinical trials and damaging the reputation of the research institution.

## Case 6.3: Religious beliefs conflict with medical student's clinical duties in abortion care

### Scenario summary

Sarah, a devoutly religious medical student, is on her Obstetrics and Gynaecology rotation. She is assigned to assess Emma, a 24-year-old female seeking a termination of pregnancy. Sarah's personal beliefs are strongly against abortion. She feels conflicted about participating in the consultation, torn between her religious convictions and her professional responsibilities to provide unbiased, compassionate care.

### Legal aspects related to the case

- *Abortion Act* 1967 (as amended by the *Human Fertilisation and Embryology Act* 1990): Contains a Conscientious Objection Clause (Section 4), allowing

healthcare professionals to refuse participation in terminations due to personal beliefs, except when it is necessary to save the female's life or prevent grave permanent injury. Sarah has the legal right to opt out of participating in the procedure.

- **GMC Guidance on Personal Beliefs and Medical Practice (2013a & 2024):** Doctors must not allow personal beliefs to adversely affect patient care. They must ensure patients have sufficient information to exercise their right to see another practitioner. Sarah should inform her supervisor promptly to avoid delaying Emma's care.
- *Equality Act* 2010: Prohibits discrimination based on protected characteristics, including sex and pregnancy. Healthcare professionals must not discriminate against patients requesting lawful treatments.
- *Human Rights Act* 1998: Article 9 protects freedom of thought, conscience and religion. However, this right is qualified and does not permit professionals to neglect their duties.
- **Medical School Policies and Fitness to Practice Regulations:** Medical schools may require students to demonstrate competencies in certain areas, including understanding termination procedures. Failure to meet learning objectives may impact Sarah's progression.
- **NHS Trust Policies:** Trusts typically have policies to accommodate staff conscientious objections while ensuring patient care is not affected. Protocols exist for reassigning patient care responsibilities.

### Ethical issues raised

- **Patient Autonomy and Rights:** Emma has the right to make informed decisions about her health without judgement. Ensuring Emma feels supported and respected during a vulnerable time is crucial.
- **Nonmaleficence and Beneficence:** Sarah must ensure her actions do not cause harm, including emotional distress or delayed care. A dismissive attitude could negatively impact Emma's well-being.
- **Professionalism and Duty of Care:** As a medical student, Sarah is expected to provide care impartially and uphold professional standards. Balancing personal beliefs with the duty to treat or facilitate care is essential.
- **Respect for Colleagues and Teamwork:** Effective communication is necessary. Informing the team promptly allows for smooth reassignment, maintaining team efficiency and preventing unexpected burdens on colleagues.
- **Conflict Between Personal Beliefs and Professional Duties:** Navigating situations where personal beliefs may conflict with professional responsibilities requires seeking guidance to manage these conflicts appropriately.

- **Impact on Patient Trust and Public Perception:** Negative experiences can erode patient trust in healthcare services. Emma feeling judged could discourage her from seeking future care.

## Clinical issues

- **Continuity and Timeliness of Care:** Ensuring Emma receives care without unnecessary postponement is essential. Timely interventions are important in time-sensitive procedures like terminations.
- **Referral and Alternative Arrangements:** Sarah should promptly inform her supervisor to arrange for another clinician. For instance, saying, 'I have a conscientious objection to this procedure; could a colleague see Emma to ensure she receives care without delay?'
- **Educational Requirements and Competency:** Sarah may need to find alternative ways to meet curriculum requirements, such as engaging in ethical discussions or observing procedures without direct involvement.
- **Communication Skills:** Conveying information to Emma without expressing personal judgements is crucial. Ensuring Emma feels respected and heard promotes a positive patient experience.
- **Support Systems and Professional Development:** Utilizing mentorship, counselling or ethics committees can help Sarah navigate her personal beliefs and professional duties. Discussing concerns with a tutor or pastoral care services is beneficial.
- **Impact on Team Dynamics:** Open communication prevents misunderstandings and maintains team harmony. Colleagues appreciate honesty and clarity in roles and responsibilities.

## Potential implications

- Sarah's conscientious objection is legally protected under the *Abortion Act* 1967, allowing healthcare professionals to opt out of participating in terminations due to personal beliefs, except in emergencies where the female's life is at risk.
- However, she must ensure patient care is not compromised by promptly informing her supervisor so alternative arrangements can be made. Failure to do so could breach the *Equality Act* 2010 if it results in discrimination against the patient.
- Sarah must balance her personal beliefs with her professional duty to prioritize patient welfare. While her moral integrity is important, she is obligated to respect the patient's autonomy and right to make informed decisions about her health.
- Ethical principles of nonmaleficence (avoiding harm) and beneficence (acting in the patient's best interest) require her to ensure her objection doesn't cause undue delay or emotional distress to Emma.

## Case 6.4: Medical student asked to obtain surgical consent despite insufficient training

### Scenario summary

Laura, a third-year medical student in the United Kingdom, is on her surgical rotation. During a busy day in the operating theatre, Dr Andrews, a senior surgeon, asks Laura to obtain consent from Mr Patel, a patient scheduled for a laparoscopic cholecystectomy (gallbladder removal). Laura has observed the procedure but has not been fully trained in obtaining informed consent for surgeries. She feels unsure about explaining the risks, benefits and alternatives adequately. Laura is concerned that if she refuses, it might reflect poorly on her professionalism and affect her assessments.

### Legal aspects related to the case

- **Informed Consent Requirements:** Under UK law, obtaining valid informed consent requires that patients are made aware of any material risks involved in a proposed treatment and of reasonable alternatives. This follows the precedent set by *Montgomery v. Lanarkshire Health Board* (2015) UKSC 11. The person obtaining consent must be suitably qualified and competent to explain these risks.
- **Role of Medical Students:** Medical students are not licensed practitioners. According to the GMC guidance, students must work within their competence and under supervision (*Good Medical Practice*; GMC, 2024). They should not undertake tasks for which they are not trained or feel adequately prepared.
- **Delegation and Responsibility:** The GMC states that doctors must delegate appropriately (GMC, 2024). Dr Andrews should ensure that anyone he delegates tasks to has the necessary knowledge and skills.
- **Potential Legal Consequences:** If consent is not properly obtained, and the patient suffers harm or alleges they were not informed appropriately, legal action for negligence or battery could be taken against the healthcare professionals involved and the institution.

### Ethical issues raised

- **Patient Autonomy and Informed Consent:** Respecting patient autonomy is fundamental. Laura may lack the necessary expertise to provide Mr Patel with comprehensive information, potentially compromising his ability to make an informed decision.
- **Professional Integrity and Competence:** Laura has an ethical duty to recognize her limitations. Proceeding despite her uncertainty may violate the principle of *nonmaleficence* (do no harm).

- **Supervision and Accountability:** Dr Andrews has an ethical responsibility to ensure tasks are delegated appropriately. Asking a medical student to obtain consent for a procedure they are not fully trained on may be inappropriate.
- **Education and Training:** While gaining experience is important, it should not come at the expense of patient safety or ethical standards.
- **Potential Impact on Patient Trust:** If Mr Patel later discovers that consent was obtained by someone not fully qualified, it could undermine his trust in the healthcare team.

## Clinical issues

- **Quality of Consent:** Comprehensive consent involves explaining the procedure, potential risks (e.g. infection, bleeding, injury to bile ducts), benefits and alternative treatments. Laura may not provide complete information, affecting the validity of the consent.
- **Patient Safety:** Inadequate consent could lead to Mr Patel being unprepared for possible complications, impacting his postoperative care and recovery.
- **Educational Opportunity:** This situation highlights the importance of appropriate clinical supervision and the need for students to speak up when feeling unprepared.

## Potential implications

- Laura should communicate her concerns to Dr Andrews, expressing that she does not feel fully competent to obtain consent independently.
- Dr Andrews can use this as a teaching opportunity by either guiding Laura through the process or having her observe while he obtains consent.
- Ensuring that consent is obtained properly protects patient rights and upholds professional standards, maintaining trust in the healthcare system.

# Case 6.5: Medication error under system pressures results in harm to paediatric patient

## Scenario summary

Dr James Miller, a junior doctor in his first year of postgraduate training, is working a double shift due to severe staff shortages at a busy UK hospital. The hospital is experiencing systemic issues, including inadequate staffing, faulty IT systems and overwhelming patient loads. Exhausted and under pressure, Dr Miller inadvertently prescribes ten times the recommended dose of a medication for a paediatric patient, Emily, who is admitted with sepsis. The error is not detected promptly, and Emily suffers significant harm as a result. Dr Miller is devastated, recognizing that systemic failures contributed to his mistake. He fears disciplinary action and legal repercussions.

## Legal aspects related to the case

- **Duty of Care and Negligence:** Healthcare professionals have a legal duty to provide care that meets established standards. A breach of this duty, resulting in harm, can constitute negligence.
- **Gross Negligence Manslaughter:** In rare and severe cases, such as in *R v. Adomako* (1994) UKHL 6, individuals may face criminal charges if their negligence is deemed grossly negligent manslaughter.
- **The *Bawa-Garba* Case:** In *Bawa-Garba v. GMC* (2018) EWCA Civ 1879, Dr Hadiza Bawa-Garba, a paediatric registrar, was convicted of gross negligence manslaughter after systemic failures and her own errors led to a child's death. This case highlights how individual clinicians may be held legally accountable, even when systemic issues are present.
- **Organizational Responsibility:** Under the *Health and Social Care Act* 2008 (Regulated Activities) Regulations 2014, healthcare institutions have a legal obligation to ensure safe staffing levels and systems that support safe care.
- **Duty of Candour:** Both individual practitioners and organizations have a statutory duty to be open and honest with patients when things go wrong (GMC and NMC, 2015).

## Ethical issues raised

- **Nonmaleficence and Beneficence:** Dr Miller's primary ethical obligation is to do no harm. Systemic pressures compromised his ability to fulfil this duty.
- **Accountability Versus Systemic Failures:** Ethically, it is important to discern individual responsibility from systemic issues. Blaming solely the individual may overlook broader problems that need addressing.
- **Professional Integrity and Honesty:** Dr Miller should acknowledge the error and participate in transparent communication with the patient's family, upholding the duty of candour.
- **Support and Well-being of Healthcare Professionals:** Ethical practice includes recognizing the limits of one's ability to provide safe care and seeking support when overwhelmed.
- **Justice and Fairness:** Holding only Dr Miller accountable may be unjust if systemic factors significantly contributed to the error.

## Clinical issues

- **Patient Safety and Quality of Care:** Medication errors can have devastating consequences, especially in vulnerable populations like paediatric patients.
- **Clinical Governance and Reporting Systems:** The incident indicates potential failures in institutional systems designed to prevent errors, such as double-checking prescriptions and electronic alerts.
- **Workforce Management:** Staff shortages and excessive workload increase the likelihood of errors, affecting overall patient care.

- **Education and Training:** Junior doctors require adequate supervision, mentoring and support to develop competence and resilience.
- **Interprofessional Communication:** Clear communication among the healthcare team is essential to identify and rectify potential errors promptly.

## Potential implications

- The institution should conduct a thorough review to identify systemic failures and implement changes, such as improved staffing ratios, better IT systems and support mechanisms for overworked staff.
- While individuals must be accountable for their actions, there should be recognition of systemic factors, promoting a just culture rather than a blame culture.
- Providing psychological support and professional guidance to Dr Miller is essential for his well-being and future practice.
- This case underscores the need for healthcare policies that address staffing and systemic issues to prevent similar incidents.
- Open and honest dialogue with Emily's family, including an apology and explanation, is ethically and legally required.

## Case 6.6: Disagreement on terminal diagnosis disclosure

### Scenario summary

Dr Rachel Adams, an oncologist at a UK hospital, diagnoses her patient, Mr Ahmed, with advanced-stage pancreatic cancer. Mr Ahmed is a 55-year-old gentleman who has been experiencing abdominal discomfort but believes it to be a minor issue. His family—particularly his wife and adult children—request that Dr Adams withhold the diagnosis from Mr Ahmed. They fear that learning about his condition will cause him significant distress and possibly worsen his health. They insist that she manage his care without revealing the true nature of his illness.

### Legal aspects related to the case

- **Patient Autonomy and Consent:** Under UK law and GMC guidelines, patients have the right to be informed about their diagnosis and treatment options to make autonomous decisions regarding their care (*Montgomery v. Lanarkshire Health Board* (2015) UKSC 11). The GMC's Good Medical Practice (2024) emphasizes the doctor's duty to respect patient autonomy by providing all relevant information.
- **Duty of Confidentiality:** Doctors have a legal duty of confidentiality to their patients, protecting personal information from unauthorized disclosure (*Data Protection Act* 2018; common law duty of confidentiality). This duty is owed to the patient, not to third parties, including family members.

- **Capacity and Mental Competence:** If Mr Ahmed is deemed to have mental capacity as per the *Mental Capacity Act* 2005, he has the legal right to be informed about his diagnosis. A patient must be assumed to have capacity unless evidence suggests otherwise.

### Ethical issues raised

- **Respect for Patient Autonomy:** Dr Adams has an ethical obligation to respect Mr Ahmed's autonomy by providing him with truthful information about his health, enabling informed decision-making.
- **Beneficence and Nonmaleficence:** While the family aims to protect Mr Ahmed from potential distress (nonmaleficence), withholding information may prevent beneficial interventions or personal preparations (beneficence).
- **Truth-Telling and Honesty:** Honesty is a fundamental ethical principle in medicine. Deceiving or withholding the truth from Mr Ahmed could damage the trust inherent in the doctor–patient relationship.
- **Cultural Sensitivity:** The family's request may stem from cultural beliefs regarding illness disclosure. Dr Adams should navigate this sensitively, acknowledging their perspective while upholding ethical standards.

### Clinical issues

- **Effective Communication:** Delivering bad news requires skilful communication to support Mr Ahmed emotionally and provide clear, compassionate information.
- **Informed Consent for Treatment:** Without disclosing the diagnosis, obtaining valid informed consent for treatments becomes ethically and legally problematic.
- **Patient Participation in Care:** Mr Ahmed's involvement in decision-making is crucial for adherence to treatment plans and aligning care with his values and preferences.
- **Psychological Support:** Awareness of his diagnosis allows Mr Ahmed to access appropriate psychological and palliative care services.

### Potential implications

- Dr Adams should prioritize informing Mr Ahmed and respecting his autonomy and legal rights as per GMC guidance and ethical obligations.
- Confirm Mr Ahmed's capacity to understand the information. If he lacks capacity, decisions should be made in his best interests, possibly involving an independent mental capacity advocate.
- Withholding the diagnosis without Mr Ahmed's consent may infringe on his right to make informed decisions about his treatment and end-of-life planning.
- Hold a respectful discussion with the family to explain the importance of honesty in patient care and explore their

concerns. Emphasize that supporting Mr Ahmed together can be beneficial.

- Acknowledge cultural factors influencing the family's request. Involve culturally appropriate support services or interpreters if necessary.

## Case 6.7: Crossing professional boundaries with a vulnerable patient

### Scenario summary

Dr Michael Thompson, a general practitioner (GP), has been treating Sarah, a 30-year-old female with a history of depression and anxiety. Over several months, Dr Thompson provided regular consultations and support as Sarah navigates personal challenges, including the recent loss of her job and a difficult breakup. Sarah is vulnerable and relies heavily on Dr Thompson for emotional support. Gradually, Dr Thompson begins to develop personal feelings for Sarah and starts engaging in conversations that extend beyond professional boundaries. He shares personal details about his life and suggests meeting socially outside the clinical setting.

### Legal aspects related to the case

- **Maintaining Professional Boundaries:** The GMC's Good Medical Practice (2024) explicitly states that doctors must not use their professional position to pursue a sexual or improper emotional relationship with a patient or someone close to them.
- **GMC's Maintaining personal and professional boundaries (2024):** The document provides detailed guidance, emphasizing that any form of sexualized behaviour with a current patient is unacceptable and can result in fitness to practise proceedings.
- **Professional Misconduct:** Developing a personal relationship with a patient may lead to allegations of professional misconduct.
- *Sexual Offences Act* **2003:** While the Act primarily addresses sexual offences, engaging in a sexual relationship with a patient who is vulnerable due to mental health issues could raise legal concerns, particularly if undue influence or coercion is perceived.
- **Duty of Care and Negligence:** Entering a personal relationship may compromise Dr Thompson's ability to provide objective medical care, potentially constituting a breach of his duty of care. If harm results from the compromised care, Dr Thompson could be legally liable for negligence.

### Ethical issues raised

- **Abuse of Power and Trust:** The doctor–patient relationship involves a significant power differential. Exploiting this by pursuing a personal relationship violates ethical principles.

Such behaviour undermines the trust that is fundamental to the therapeutic relationship.
- **Nonmaleficence and Beneficence:** The relationship may harm Sarah emotionally and psychologically, especially given her vulnerability. Dr Thompson's personal interests conflict with his duty to prioritize Sarah's well-being.
- **Professional Integrity:** Crossing professional boundaries compromises the integrity and reputation of the medical profession. Maintaining clear professional roles protects patients and upholds ethical standards.
- **Patient Autonomy and Consent:** Sarah's ability to consent to a personal relationship may be impaired by her mental health and the power dynamics involved. There is a risk that she may feel pressured or unable to refuse advances due to her dependency on her doctor.

### Clinical issues

- **Compromised Care:** Dr Thompson's personal feelings may cloud his clinical judgement, leading to suboptimal care. If the relationship ends poorly, Sarah may avoid seeking necessary medical attention.
- **Patient Dependency:** The blurred boundaries may exacerbate Sarah's dependency, hindering her recovery and autonomy.

### Potential implications

- Dr Thompson must recognize the unethical nature of his actions and immediately cease any nonprofessional contact with Sarah.
- Dr Thompson should consult a trusted senior colleague, mentor or professional body (e.g. a medical defence organization) for confidential advice. If required, being honest in any investigation demonstrates integrity.
- He should engage in self-reflection to understand why boundaries were crossed and how to prevent future occurrences. Personal therapy may be beneficial in addressing underlying issues contributing to his behaviour.
- Arranging for Sarah to see another GP ensures she continues to receive appropriate care without compromised boundaries. Sarah should not be made to feel at fault for the situation.
- Upholding ethical standards reinforces public confidence in the medical profession.

## Case 6.8: Unlocked computer terminal exposes celebrity patient's medical records to unauthorized staff access

### Scenario summary

Dr Sarah Chen, a resident doctor at a large teaching hospital, discovers that her colleague, Dr Tom Wilson, has accidentally left a computer terminal unlocked in a shared office space. During this time, several administrative staff members viewed the medical records of Mr James Roberts, a well-known television presenter receiving treatment for substance abuse. The breach comes to light when details of Mr Roberts' condition are overheard being discussed in the hospital cafeteria.

## Legal aspects related to the case

- **Data Protection Act 2018:** Forms the cornerstone of information governance, requiring personal health data to be processed according to strict principles of lawfulness, fairness and transparency. Organizations must implement robust security measures, with serious breaches requiring notification to the Information Commissioner's Office within 72 hours.
- **General Medical Council's Good Medical Practice (2024):** Provides specific guidance on doctors' obligations regarding patient privacy. These requirements extend beyond direct clinical care, encompassing all aspects of information handling. Doctors must ensure they maintain appropriate security measures, including password protection and proper record management. Doctors have a duty to report any breaches of confidentiality promptly to the appropriate authority within their organization.
- **Common Law Duty of Confidentiality**: Established through cases such as *Attorney General v. Guardian Newspapers Ltd* (1988), creates a fundamental obligation to protect information shared in confidence. This duty continues even after a patient's death and can only be breached with explicit consent or if there is a legal requirement to do so. The *Human Rights Act* 1998, particularly Article 8, reinforces these protections by establishing privacy as a fundamental right, requiring any interference to be proportionate and legally justified.
- **Caldicott Principles (2020 Revision):** These principles guide the handling of patient-identifiable information, emphasizing accountability and the need to justify the purpose of data usage.

## Ethical issues raised

- **Professional Responsibility:** This extends beyond individual actions to creating a culture of privacy awareness. Healthcare professionals must balance the need for accessible medical records with security measures. This becomes particularly challenging in shared working environments where multiple staff members may need access to patient information. The incident raises questions about the collective responsibility of healthcare teams in maintaining confidentiality standards.
- **Institutional Trust:** The breach's impact on institutional trust cannot be understated. Public confidence in healthcare services relies heavily on the expectation of confidentiality.

Celebrity cases often attract media attention, potentially causing widespread damage to public trust.
- **Professional Relationships:** Medical professionals face the challenging balance between maintaining collegiate relationships and fulfilling their duty to report concerns. This case highlights the importance of creating an environment where staff feel supported in raising concerns about colleagues' practices while maintaining professional relationships.

## Clinical issues

- **Impact on Patient Care:** Patients receiving treatment for sensitive conditions like substance abuse particularly require confidence in confidentiality. When this trust is broken, patients may withhold crucial information or avoid seeking necessary treatment altogether.
- **System Security:** Considerations must extend beyond technical measures to include human factors. While automatic logout settings and role-based access controls are important, staff awareness and behaviour play crucial roles in maintaining security. Regular audit trails and monitoring systems help identify potential vulnerabilities before they lead to breaches.

## Potential implications

- Immediately secure the computer system, ensuring no further unauthorized access can occur. Patient communication must be handled with sensitivity, providing honest disclosure of the breach while maintaining professional composure. Regulatory reporting requirements must be fulfilled, ensuring appropriate authorities are notified within required timeframes.
- Organizations must demonstrate their commitment to privacy through both preventive measures and appropriate responses to breaches. This includes notifying the ICO within the required 72-hour window, providing details of the breach and planned remediation steps.
- Rebuilding therapeutic relationships after such breaches requires careful handling and a clear demonstration of improved practices.
- Failure to protect confidentiality can result in fitness to practice proceedings, potentially affecting a doctor's registration.

## Case 6.9: Ethics of gift acceptance and doctor–patient relationship

### Scenario summary

Dr James Smith, a consultant oncologist in a UK hospital, has been treating Mrs Anna Thompson, a 65-year-old patient with advanced breast cancer. Through his dedicated care and support,

Mrs Thompson's quality of life has significantly improved, and she expresses immense gratitude towards Dr Smith. After a particularly positive consultation, Mrs Thompson presents Dr Smith with a substantial gift: an expensive wristwatch valued at several thousand pounds. She insists that he accept it as a token of her appreciation for the care he has provided.

## Legal aspects related to the case

- **General Medical Council's Good Medical Practice (2024)**: States that doctors must not accept gifts or inducements that may affect, or be seen to affect, the way they treat or refer patients. Accepting substantial gifts may raise questions about the doctor's professional integrity and could be considered a conflict of interest.
- **Hospital Policy:** Many NHS Trusts have policies regarding accepting gifts and hospitality, often requiring staff to declare gifts over a certain value or prohibiting acceptance of significant gifts altogether.
- **Bribery Act 2010:** Under the *Bribery Act* 2010, accepting gifts could potentially be construed as bribery if it is intended to influence the doctor's behaviour or if there is a perception of impropriety.
- **Taxation Laws:** Gifts over a certain value may have tax implications for both the giver and the receiver. Failure to declare such gifts could lead to legal issues with the tax authorities.

## Ethical issues raised

- **Conflict of Interest:** Accepting a substantial gift may create a perceived or actual conflict of interest, potentially influencing Dr Smith's clinical judgement.
- **Professional Boundaries:** Maintaining appropriate boundaries between doctors and patients is essential to preserve the therapeutic relationship. Receiving expensive gifts can blur these boundaries and alter the dynamics of the relationship.
- **Equity and Fairness:** Accepting a significant gift from one patient may lead to perceptions of favouritism, undermining the principle of treating all patients equally.
- **Duty to Maintain Trust:** The medical profession relies on public trust. Accepting substantial gifts could damage this trust if perceived as unethical or unprofessional behaviour.

## Clinical issues

- **Impact on Doctor–Patient Relationship:** Accepting the
- gift may change the nature of the relationship, potentially impacting professional objectivity. Declining the gift may risk upsetting the patient and affecting her engagement in care.
- **Patient's Well-being:** Mrs Thompson may feel rejected or embarrassed if the gift is refused without appropriate

communication. It is important to ensure that any actions taken do not adversely affect her mental and emotional well-being.
- **Documentation and Transparency:** Proper documentation of the offer and any actions taken is necessary. Transparency is crucial to prevent misunderstandings or accusations of misconduct.

## Potential implications

- Declining the gift must be handled sensitively to avoid causing offence or distress. Dr Smith should express gratitude for Mrs Thompson's gesture but explain, in a sensitive and compassionate manner, that he cannot accept such an expensive gift due to professional obligations.
- Suggest alternative ways for Mrs Thompson to express her gratitude, such as a thank-you letter, feedback to the hospital or a donation to a relevant charity or hospital fund.
- Document the incident and any advice received to maintain transparency.

# Case 6.10: Treating a familiar patient

## Scenario summary

Dr Emily Harris, a GP, is approached by her sister, Anna, who is experiencing symptoms of anxiety and insomnia due to work-related stress. Anna asks Dr Harris to write her a prescription for a mild anxiolytic to help manage her symptoms. She insists that it is a simple request and does not want to see another doctor or go through the formal consultation process. Dr Harris feels torn between wanting to help her sister promptly and her professional obligation to maintain appropriate boundaries and follow proper medical procedures.

## Legal aspects related to the case

- **GMC Guidance on Treating Family and Friends:** The GMC's Good Medical Practice (2024) explicitly advises doctors to 'wherever possible, avoid providing medical care to yourself or anyone with whom you have a close personal relationship' (Paragraph 16). This is to ensure objectivity and to prevent personal relationships from affecting professional judgement.
- **Misuse of Drugs Regulations 2001**: Certain medications, including some anxiolytics, are controlled substances. Prescribing these medications requires careful assessment and adherence to legal protocols.
- **Controlled Drugs (Supervision of Management and Use) Regulations 2013:** Mandates that prescriptions for controlled substances must be based on a proper medical assessment and issued in the context of a bona fide practitioner-patient relationship.

## Ethical issues raised

- **Professional Boundaries:** Personal relationships may impair Dr Harris's objectivity, leading to biased decision-making or overlooking important clinical considerations. Crossing professional boundaries can undermine trust in the medical profession and set a precedent for future boundary violations.

- **Autonomy and Consent**: Anna may not receive complete information about treatment options, risks and benefits, limiting her ability to make an informed choice. Dual roles may compromise the privacy of health information, especially in family dynamics.

## Clinical issues

- **Patient Safety:** Prescribing without proper assessment increases the risk of adverse effects and interactions with other medications. Prescribing anxiolytics carries a risk of dependency. Without proper monitoring, this risk increases.
- **Lack of Documentation:** Failure to document the consultation and prescription may lead to gaps in Anna's medical records, affecting future care.
- **Continuity of Care:** Anna may miss out on referrals to specialists or support services that could provide long-term benefits. Ongoing assessment of treatment effectiveness and side effects may be neglected.

## Potential implications

- Prescribing medication to a family member without adequate assessment may be considered unprofessional conduct, potentially leading to investigations by the GMC.
- Failure to maintain proper records or to act within prescribing guidelines could result in legal action, professional sanctions or even criminal charges if misuse of controlled substances is involved.
- Dr Harris should politely decline to prescribe medication to Anna, explaining the professional reasons and emphasizing the importance of proper medical care.
- Emphasize the difference between being a sister and a healthcare provider and the importance of keeping these roles separate to protect both the personal relationship and professional integrity.

## Case 6.11: Social media post compromises patient privacy

### Scenario summary

Dr Emily Turner, a resident doctor working in a hospital, completes a challenging shift during which she treats a patient involved in a high-profile accident. Feeling the need to share her experiences, Dr Turner posts on her private social media account about the case. In her post, she includes specific details about the patient's injuries, the treatment provided and the circumstances of the accident. Although she does not mention the patient's name, the combination of details makes the patient easily identifiable to those aware of the incident.

## Legal aspects related to the case

- **Common Law Duty of Confidentiality:** Doctors have a legal obligation to maintain patient confidentiality, protecting personal information acquired during the course of professional duties. Sharing identifiable patient information without consent is a breach of this duty.
- **Data Protection Act 2018 and GDPR:** Personal data must be processed lawfully, fairly and transparently. Posting patient information on social media may constitute unlawful processing of personal data. The ICO can impose significant fines for breaches of data protection laws.
- **GMC Guidance on Confidentiality (2017):** Confidentiality is central to trust between doctors and patients. Doctors must ensure that patients are informed about how their information will be used. Disclosure without consent is permissible only under specific circumstances, such as when required by law or in the public interest.
- **Doctors' Use of Social Media (GMC, 2024):** Doctors must maintain patient confidentiality and be cautious about sharing information online. Even with privacy settings, information posted online may become public.

## Ethical issues raised

- **Patient Confidentiality and Trust:** Maintaining confidentiality is a fundamental ethical duty, vital for patient trust and the integrity of the doctor–patient relationship. Breaching confidentiality can harm the patient, both emotionally and socially, and erode public trust in the medical profession.
- **Professionalism and Boundaries:** Professional conduct extends beyond the workplace, including online activities. Sharing sensitive information on social media blurs the boundaries between personal and professional life.
- **Respect for Patient Autonomy and Dignity:** Patients have the right to control how their personal health information is shared. Unauthorized disclosure disrespects the patient's autonomy and may cause distress or stigma.
- Impact on Professional Reputation: Unprofessional online behaviour reflects poorly on the individual doctor and the profession as a whole. This may lead to a loss of credibility among colleagues and the public.
- **Duty to Report and Peer Responsibility:** Colleagues who become aware of such breaches have an ethical obligation to address the issue, following appropriate channels

## Clinical issues

- **Impact on Patient Care:** The patient may lose trust in healthcare providers, leading to reluctance in sharing necessary information or seeking care. This has the potential for strained relationships between patients and the healthcare team.

- **Institutional Reputation:** The hospital's reputation may be damaged, affecting patient confidence in the institution's ability to protect confidentiality.

## Potential implications

- Dr Turner should promptly delete the post and reflect on the implications of her actions. Consider informing the patient about the breach and offering a sincere apology, in line with the professional duty of candour.
- Dr Turner should contact her medical defence organization for legal and professional advice.
- The hospital may need to conduct an internal investigation to assess the breach and implement corrective measures.

## Case 6.12: Medical student's fear of reporting suspicion of impaired surgeon due to potential career repercussions

### Scenario summary

Michael, a final-year medical student, is scrubbed in for a major cardiac surgery under the supervision of Mr Richard Harris, a renowned consultant surgeon. Just before the operation, Michael notices a strong smell of alcohol on Mr Harris's breath and observes that his speech is slightly slurred. Concerned that the consultant may be under the influence of alcohol, Michael is unsure what to do. He fears that raising the issue could jeopardize his career prospects, especially since Mr Harris is highly respected and influential in the surgical department.

### Legal aspects related to the case

- **GMC's Good Medical Practice (2024):** States that patient safety must be the first concern of doctors and medical students. Doctors must take prompt action if they believe patient safety, dignity or comfort is being compromised.
- **Health and Safety Legislation:** Under the *Health and Safety at Work Act* 1974, employers must ensure the health and safety of patients and staff. Performing surgery while impaired contravenes legal obligations to provide safe care.
- **Fitness to Practise:** The GMC can take action against doctors whose fitness to practise is impaired due to alcohol misuse. Working under the influence of alcohol breaches professional standards and can lead to disciplinary action, including suspension or erasure from the medical register.
- **Public Interest Disclosure Act 1998 (PIDA):** Protects workers who disclose information about malpractice or safety risks from detrimental treatment or unfair dismissal. Michael is protected when raising concerns in the public interest, even as a medical student.
- **Hospital Policies:** Hospitals typically have clear policies for reporting concerns about colleague impairment. Michael

should follow the established procedures to report his observations.
- **Negligence and Duty to Report:** Failure to act on concerns about a colleague's impairment may expose individuals and the institution to legal liability if patient harm results.
- **Criminal Law:** It is a criminal offence for a healthcare professional to endanger patient safety through negligent acts or omissions.

### Ethical issues raised

- **Patient Safety and Nonmaleficence:** The primary ethical obligation is to prevent harm to the patient (nonmaleficence). Allowing an impaired surgeon to operate poses a significant risk of harm.
- **Professional Responsibility and Integrity:** Medical students and doctors have an ethical duty to uphold professional standards and act when these are compromised. Ignoring the issue undermines personal and professional integrity. GMC emphasizes the responsibility to protect patients by taking appropriate action.
- **Confidentiality and Respect:** Concerns should be raised discreetly and respectfully, ensuring the consultant's confidentiality is maintained during initial reporting.

### Clinical issues

- **Risk of Surgical Errors:** Impairment due to alcohol increases the likelihood of mistakes during surgery, potentially leading to adverse patient outcomes. Reliance on individuals to report concerns is critical for patient safety.
- **Team Dynamics and Communication:** The functioning of the surgical team may be compromised if the consultant is impaired. Other team members may also be placed in difficult positions.
- **Patient Trust and Confidence:** If the patient or public becomes aware of the incident, it could undermine trust in healthcare professionals and the institution.

### Potential implications

- Michael may fear negative repercussions, including damage to his reputation or career prospects. Balancing personal risks against ethical duties presents a moral dilemma.
- Upholding the principle that patient safety supersedes all other considerations.
- According to GMC guidelines (2024), Michael should raise his concerns with an appropriate person. If comfortable, he could discreetly speak to Mr Harris, expressing his concerns. Alternatively, he could report to a senior member of the surgical team, clinical supervisor or the hospital's designated officer for raising concerns (often called a Freedom to Speak Up Guardian).

- Immediate action may be taken to prevent Mr Harris from performing the surgery, thus protecting the patient.
- The consultant may be offered support, such as referral to occupational health or assistance programs.

## Case 6.13: Social media conduct and fitness to practise concerns

### Scenario summary

Emma Williams, a final-year medical student at a prestigious UK university, maintains a popular social media presence with thousands of followers across various platforms. She frequently posts about her life, including her experiences in medical school and during clinical placements. Recently, several of Emma's posts have raised concerns among her peers and faculty members.

Emma has shared humorous anecdotes about patients, sometimes using demeaning language and stereotypes. While she does not mention names, the details are sufficient for individuals familiar with the cases to identify the patients.

Photos and videos depict Emma engaging in excessive alcohol consumption, partying in ways that could be considered reckless and wearing her medical student uniform in inappropriate settings.

### Legal aspects related to the case

- **GMC's Good Medical Practice (2024):** Sets out the standards expected of doctors and medical students. Medical students must uphold the reputation of the profession by ensuring their conduct justifies patients' trust. There is a duty to protect patient information. Sharing identifiable patient details without consent breaches confidentiality obligations.
- **GMC's Doctors' Use of Social Media (2024):** Provides supplementary guidance. Even when anonymized, sharing details that could identify a patient is prohibited. Doctors and medical students should not share content that may undermine public confidence in the profession.
- **Data Protection Act 2018 and UK GDPR:** The Act defines personal data as any information relating to an identified or identifiable individual. Emma's posts containing diagnostic images and case details may constitute personal data. Sharing personal data requires a lawful basis, such as patient consent, which Emma does not have. Breaches can result in substantial fines and legal action against both the individual and the institution.
- **Common Law Duty of Confidentiality:** Patients have a right to expect that information shared in confidence will not be disclosed without their consent. Emma's disclosures breach this duty.
- **University Regulations and Fitness to Practise Procedures:** Universities have policies aligned with the GMC's standards. Breaching these policies can lead to disciplinary action, including suspension or expulsion.

### Ethical issues raised

- **Confidentiality and Trust:** Sharing patient details without consent violates ethical principles and erodes trust between patients and healthcare professionals. Patients may hesitate to share information or seek care if they fear their privacy will be compromised.
- **Professionalism and Public Confidence:** Emma's unprofessional posts reflect negatively on her commitment to ethical practice. Such behaviours can diminish public confidence in the medical profession as a whole.
- **Accountability and Responsibility:** Medical students are accountable for their actions both within and outside clinical settings. Fellow students and staff have an ethical obligation to address unprofessional behaviours to protect patients and uphold standards.
- **Respect and Dignity:** Derogatory comments about patients fail to respect their inherent dignity and rights.

### Clinical issues

- **Implications for Patient Care:** Patients who become aware of such breaches may lose trust in healthcare providers, affecting the therapeutic relationship. Fear of privacy violations may deter individuals from seeking necessary medical assistance.
- **Educational Environment:** As a senior student, Emma's behaviour may influence junior students, normalizing unprofessional conduct. The situation highlights the need for enhanced education on professionalism and ethics in medical curricula.
- **Support for the Student:** Emma's behaviour may indicate underlying personal challenges. Assessing her well-being is important. Providing guidance and support can help Emma understand the impact of her actions and encourage positive changes.

### Potential implications

- This case underscores the critical importance of maintaining professional conduct both online and offline. Medical students are held to high standards due to the trust placed in them by patients and society.
- Breaching patient confidentiality and displaying unprofessional behaviour on social media not only jeopardizes individual careers but also has wider implications for public confidence in the medical profession.
- Educational institutions play a vital role in setting clear expectations and providing the necessary training and support to students. Early intervention and education on the ethical use of social media can prevent such incidents.
- For Emma, a combination of disciplinary action, support and remediation may be necessary to address the issues and guide her towards fulfilling the responsibilities of a future clinician.

- Medical students should recognize that their actions, even in personal spaces like social media, are reflective of their professionalism. They must adhere to ethical guidelines to protect patient confidentiality, uphold the dignity of individuals and maintain the trust that is essential to the practice of medicine.

## CONSENT, CAPACITY AND THE DOCTOR–PATIENT RELATIONSHIP

## Case 6.14: Failure to inform the patient of rare risks

### Scenario summary

Dr Richard Bennett, a consultant orthopaedic surgeon at a leading UK hospital, is scheduled to perform spinal surgery on Mr David Clarke, a 38-year-old patient suffering from chronic lower back pain due to a herniated lumbar disc. During the preoperative consultation, Dr Bennett discusses the procedure—lumbar microdiscectomy—including common risks such as infection, bleeding and anaesthetic complications. However, he does not mention the rare but serious risk of cauda equina syndrome (CES), which occurs in approximately 0.1% of such surgeries and can lead to permanent neurological deficits, including paralysis and incontinence.

Believing he has been fully informed, Mr Clarke consents to the surgery. Unfortunately, during the operation, complications arise, and Mr Clarke develops CES postoperatively. As a result, he suffers from chronic pain, mobility issues and loss of bladder and bowel control, significantly impacting his quality of life and ability to work.

Mr Clarke asserts that had he been aware of the risk of CES, he would have preferred to explore conservative treatment options, such as physiotherapy or pain management, before consenting to surgery.

### Legal aspects related to the case

- *Montgomery v. Lanarkshire Health Board* (2015) UKSC 11: This landmark case transformed the legal standard for informed consent in the United Kingdom. The Supreme Court held that doctors have a duty to take reasonable care to ensure that patients are aware of any material risks involved in a proposed treatment. Doctors must also inform patients of reasonable alternatives.
- **Duty of Care and Disclosure**: Dr Bennett had a legal obligation to disclose all material risks associated with the surgery. A material risk is one to which a reasonable person in the patient's position would likely attach significance or a risk that the doctor knows—or should reasonably know—would likely be significant to that particular patient.

- **Breach of Duty**: By not informing Mr Clarke of the rare but serious risk of CES, Dr Bennett breached his duty of care as established in Montgomery. The test for determining negligence is whether the doctor failed to provide information that a reasonable person in the patient's position would want to know.
- **Causation and Harm**: Mr Clarke must demonstrate that the lack of disclosure caused him harm. This involves showing that, had he been informed of the risk, he would not have consented to the surgery at that time and thus would have avoided the injury.
- **Bolam Test Limitations**: The Bolam test, which protect doctors if their conduct align with a responsible body of medical opinion, is not solely applicable in cases of informed consent post-Montgomery. The court in Montgomery moved towards a patient-centred approach rather than a practitioner-centred one.
- **GMC Guidance on Consent (2024)**: The GMC emphasizes the necessity of shared decision-making, where doctors must provide patients with the information they want or need to make decisions about their care.
- **Informed Consent Documentation**: A signed consent form alone is not conclusive proof of informed consent. Adequate documentation of the consent discussion is essential but does not replace the need for actual disclosure and understanding.

### Ethical issues raised

- **Autonomy**: Dr Bennett failed to respect Mr Clarke's autonomy by withholding information necessary for making an informed decision about his own healthcare. Ethical practice necessitates considering the patient's values, circumstances and preferences. Dr Bennett did not explore Mr Clarke's concerns or what risks he might find significant.
- **Beneficence and Nonmaleficence**: The ethical principle of beneficence compels doctors to act in the best interests of the patient, while nonmaleficence requires avoiding harm. By not disclosing the risk, Dr Bennett compromised these principles, as the patient could not weigh the benefits and harms properly.
- **Trust and Transparency**: Trust is foundational in the doctor–patient relationship. Failure to disclose material risks breaches this trust and can lead to a breakdown in the therapeutic relationship.
- **Paternalism Versus Patient-Centred Care**: Dr Bennett's decision reflects a paternalistic approach, where the doctor makes decisions on behalf of the patient without full disclosure. Modern ethics advocate for patient-centred care and shared decision-making.

### Clinical issues

- **Effective Communication**: Clear, jargon-free communication about potential risks, benefits and alternatives is essential. Dr Bennett's omission indicates a failure in effective communication.

- **Risk of Cauda Equina Syndrome**: CES is a serious complication with life-altering consequences. Even though it is rare, the severity warrants disclosure.
- **Alternative Treatments**: Nonsurgical options, such as physiotherapy, pain management programmes or less invasive interventions, should have been discussed as reasonable alternatives.
- **Consent Process**: The process should be more than obtaining a signature; it should ensure the patient's understanding and voluntary agreement.
- **Patient-Centred Care**: Tailoring discussions to the individual patient's needs and concerns is crucial. Understanding Mr Clarke's preferences may have influenced the decision-making process.

## Potential implications
- **Legal Outcomes**: Dr Bennett and the hospital may face legal liability for negligence, potentially resulting in substantial compensation to Mr Clarke for damages suffered.
- **Professional Consequences**: Clinically, the case emphasizes effective communication and thorough documentation as integral to patient care. The potential implications span legal, professional and institutional realms.
- **Patient Trust and Public Confidence**: Such cases can erode public trust in the medical profession. Restoring confidence requires a commitment to transparency, accountability and improved patient care.

## Case 6.15: A 15-year-old refuses a necessary treatment despite parental consent

### Scenario summary
Grace, a 15-year-old with a chronic but manageable heart condition, has been advised by her cardiologist to undergo a relatively low risk but necessary procedure to prevent further complications. Grace's parents fully understand the situation and consent to the procedure. However, Grace refuses, stating she wants to 'wait and see' if her condition actually worsens and feels 'overwhelmed' by hospitals.

### Legal aspects related to the case
- **Children Act 1989 (amended 2004)**: Defines a 'child' as anyone under 18. Protects the welfare of minors and allows courts to override refusals of potentially life-saving treatment when it is in the child's best interests.
- **Gillick Competence (Gillick v. West Norfolk and Wisbech Area Health Authority (1986))**: If a person under 16 (and by extension, those 16 or 17 as well) demonstrates sufficient understanding and intelligence to comprehend the nature and consequences of the proposed treatment, they may

legally make their own healthcare decisions. Though Grace is 15, if she is assessed as Gillick competent, her capacity to consent or refuse is taken seriously in law.
- **Refusals of Treatment by Minors**: Under English law, where a refusal may lead to serious harm or death, courts have historically overridden a child's refusal (*NHS Trust v. X* (2021)). Even if a 15-year-old is deemed Gillick competent and capable of refusing treatment, a court may still intervene if it considers the refusal not to be in the child's best interests.
- **Parental Responsibility:** A person with parental responsibility can consent on behalf of a child who lacks competence. However, the child's own competently made decision can take precedence over parental views if the child is deemed Gillick competent.
- **Age of Legal Capacity (Scotland) Act 1991:** In Scotland, under-16s may consent to treatment if they have the capacity, assessed similarly to Gillick in England and Wales. The child's refusal still can be overridden when facing serious risk of harm.

### Ethical issues raised
- **Autonomy Versus Beneficence:** Typically, respecting patient autonomy is a core ethical principle. However, as Grace is a minor, any possible autonomy must be evaluated in the light of her maturity and understanding, while balancing beneficence (acting in her best interests).
- **Best Interests:** Healthcare professionals have a duty to focus on Grace's best interests, taking into account her physical health, emotional well-being and social circumstances. If her refusal poses a serious risk, there is an ethical rationale to override it in order to protect her from fatal or severe harm.
- **Capacity and Competence:** Determining whether Grace is Gillick competent is central. Even if she can understand and weigh the options, courts and clinicians must question whether she is mature enough to grasp long-term consequences.
- **Parental Role Versus Child's Wishes:** Grace's parents have consented, but the child's capable refusal poses a conflict. Ethically, one must explore whether Grace's refusal is the result of undue influence, fear, misunderstanding or truly autonomous choice.
- **Impact on Trust:** Overriding Grace's refusal might undermine her trust in healthcare professionals, but failing to treat her may lead to physical harm. Clinicians should balance preserving trust, respecting her views and securing her well-being.

### Clinical issues
- **Urgency and Necessity of Treatment:** The condition is manageable but potentially serious; clinicians need to assess how immediate the risk is if the procedure is not performed.

- **Assessing Her Competence:** Clinicians must determine if Grace fully comprehends the nature of the treatment, its benefits and risks and potential outcomes of refusal. This may require a specific mental capacity-style assessment for under-16s (the Gillick test).
- **Communication and Support:** A structured, empathetic and thorough discussion is critical. Grace's statement of feeling overwhelmed suggests anxiety or fear that might be mitigable through counselling, child-friendly explanations or the involvement of a trusted advocate.
- **Involving Multidisciplinary Teams (MDTs):** A psychologist, social worker or child mental health team could help ascertain whether Grace's refusal is based on a well-reasoned stance or emotional distress.

## Potential implications

- **Possible Court Intervention:** If Grace's refusal persists and her life or long-term health is in jeopardy, the hospital or parents may seek a court order to proceed.
- **Strained Relationships:** Overriding Grace's wishes without sensitive handling can damage the therapeutic relationship and her trust in healthcare. Long-term patient engagement might suffer if she feels her autonomy was dismissed.
- **Emotional and Psychological Impact:** Grace's mental well-being is a priority. If she feels coerced, there could be emotional repercussions. Alternatively, if left untreated, the evolving physical complications can lead to distress and future regret.

## Case 6.16: A 14-year-old requests contraception without her parent's knowledge

### Scenario summary

Fiona, a 14-year-old, comes to the GP surgery alone and requests contraception. She specifically asks that her parents not be informed. Fiona states she is in a relationship with someone her own age and wants to be safe and responsible. However, she is anxious about possible parental disapproval and insists on strict confidentiality.

### Legal aspects related to the case

- **Gillick competence:** In England and Wales, under-16s can consent to medical advice or treatment if they demonstrate sufficient understanding and intelligence (Gillick competence). A health professional must be satisfied that Fiona understands the nature, purpose and possible consequences of contraception, including risks and alternatives.
- **Fraser Guidelines:** These guidelines specifically address contraceptive advice to under-16s:

- The health professional must be satisfied the young person understands the advice.
- The health professional must be unable to persuade the young person to involve a parent or guardian.
- The young person is likely to begin, or to continue having, sexual intercourse regardless of advice or provision of contraception.
- The young person's physical or mental health (or both) is likely to suffer if they do not receive contraceptive advice or treatment.
- It is in the young person's best interests to receive contraceptive advice or treatment without parental knowledge or consent.
- **Sexual Offences Act 2003:** Provides that a doctor prescribing contraception to a competent person under 16 will not be found guilty of aiding or abetting a sexual offence, provided the Fraser Guidelines are followed. However, if Fiona were under 13, it would be a separate legal duty to consider safeguarding actions because a child under 13 cannot legally consent to sexual activity.
- **Children Act 1989 (amended 2004):** Reinforces the responsibility to act in the best interests of the child. If there are safeguarding concerns, doctors should consider whether Fiona is at risk of abuse or coercion.
- **Confidentiality:** Healthcare professionals must maintain confidentiality unless there is a substantial risk of serious harm or other safeguarding concerns.

### Ethical issues raised

- **Autonomy Versus Protection of a Minor:** The principle of respecting patient autonomy normally includes granting competent minors confidentiality. Yet, there is a competing ethical duty to protect children from harm.
- **Best Interests and Potential Harm:** Provision of contraception could be viewed as acting in Fiona's best interests if it prevents unintended pregnancy or harm. However, ongoing sexual activity at 14 may raise safeguarding questions.
- **Confidentiality and Trust:** If confidentiality is breached without strong justification, Fiona may no longer seek future help or advice. Healthcare professionals must balance confidentiality with the duty to protect a minor from sexual exploitation or abuse.

### Clinical issues

- **Wider Support Network:** Discussing the potential benefits of involving a trusted adult—whether a parent, guardian or another family member—while also respecting Fiona's right to confidentiality, if she meets Fraser Guidelines criteria.
- **Assessing Competence:** The GP must evaluate Fiona's maturity, understand the physical and emotional

implications of sexual activity and the potential risks and benefits of contraception.

- **Ensuring Safe, Effective Care:** If Fiona is competent and not at risk, prescribing contraception could mitigate health risks, including unwanted pregnancy. The GP should also address sexually transmitted infections, recommending appropriate testing and barrier protection.
- **Safeguarding Responsibilities:** The clinician must explore Fiona's circumstances. If there are any indicators of sexual exploitation, abuse or significant risk, the doctor must follow local safeguarding protocols.

## Potential implications

- **Safeguarding Concerns:** If Fiona's situation suggests any form of exploitation or abuse, healthcare professionals must intervene effectively, potentially involving social services or other authorities.
- **Impact on the Therapeutic Relationship:** Properly managing confidentiality can build trust and encourage Fiona to continue seeking medical guidance. Conversely, breaching confidentiality without clear justification could erode her confidence in healthcare services.
- **Long-term Outcomes:** Providing appropriate contraceptive and emotional support can protect Fiona's health and well-being. However, any misjudgement—such as missing signs of exploitation or dismissing her concerns—could have serious personal and legal consequences.

## Case 6.17: Patient with dementia makes a decision about their care that seems 'irrational'

### Scenario summary

Mr Roberts, an 82-year-old with a long-standing diagnosis of mild-to-moderate dementia, has been admitted for management of pneumonia. His medical team recommends a course of intravenous antibiotics, which is considered standard and potentially life-saving. However, Mr Roberts emphatically refuses all antibiotic treatment, stating, 'I've lived long enough and I hate hospitals'. Despite his children's pleas and the clinical team's advice, he persists in his refusal. His decision appears to lack logical consistency, yet he can articulate his reasons—even if somewhat muddled.

### Legal aspects related to the case

- **Mental Capacity Act 2005 (MCA):** Applies to individuals aged 16 and over in England and Wales. It assumes everyone has capacity unless proved otherwise. Using the four key criteria in the MCA, the healthcare team must assess Mr Roberts's capacity to consent to or refuse treatment. These criteria are: understand, retain, weigh up and communicate. 'Unwise decisions' do not, in themselves, mean a lack of

capacity. Mr Roberts's refusal may be viewed as irrational by his family, but this does not automatically render him incapable.
- **Best Interests (MCA Principle):** If Mr Roberts is found to lack capacity, clinicians must treat him in his best interests—taking into account his past and present wishes, beliefs and values, as well as input from those close to him (his children). The 'least restrictive' option should be chosen to preserve Mr Roberts's autonomy wherever possible.
- **Adults with Incapacity (Scotland) Act 2000 (if in Scotland):** Similar principles apply if Mr Roberts is in Scotland. Decisions on behalf of an incapacitated adult must reflect the benefit to the adult, the least restrictive option and the adult's previously expressed wishes, among other considerations.
- **Common Law: Duty of Care:** Clinicians are obliged to act lawfully, respecting autonomy where capacity is present and to ensure Mr Roberts receives necessary care if he is deemed incapable.

### Ethical issues raised

- **Autonomy Versus Paternalism:** If Mr Roberts retains capacity, respecting his choice—even if it appears irrational—is ethically required, unless compelling evidence of coercion exists. Overriding a capacitous adult's dissent undermines autonomy.
- **Beneficence and Nonmaleficence:** The clinical team wants to act in his best interests (beneficence), but forcibly treating him against his will (if he has the capacity) could cause him significant distress (nonmaleficence).
- **Capacity and 'Unwise Decisions':** Ethical analysis underscores that a 'bad' or 'irrational' decision alone does not mean a lack of capacity. The team must carefully evaluate comprehension, reasoning and ability to appreciate consequences.

### Clinical issues

- **Assessing Capacity Thoroughly:** The immediate priority is to conduct a formal capacity assessment. Clinicians should explore the nature of Mr Roberts's refusal—does he understand the benefits, risks and likely outcomes of not taking antibiotics?
- **Dementia and Fluctuating Capacity:** Dementia can be variable. Mr Roberts's ability to make decisions may change throughout the day. A 'snapshot' assessment might be misleading if not repeated under optimal conditions (when he is at his most lucid).
- **Communication Strategies:** Using clear, simple language and possibly involving a specialist nurse or dementia liaison team can improve Mr Roberts's comprehension. Environmental modifications (a quiet room, familiar objects or family presence) may aid decision-making.
- **Potential for Coexisting Delirium:** In an acute setting like pneumonia, Mr Roberts's cognitive status could be worsened

by infection or dehydration, posing a risk of delirium rather than sole dementia-related confusion. Addressing acute illness might improve his decision-making capacity.

## Potential implications

- Mr Roberts's situation encapsulates a core challenge in geriatric medicine: balancing respect for an older patient's autonomy with the imperative to protect him from harm, particularly when dementia is present.
- A formal capacity assessment, clear communication and sensitivity to his values are crucial. While his choice may appear irrational, healthcare professionals must carefully observe the legal framework and the ethical obligation to respect capacitous refusals of treatment.
- Discussing advanced care planning, possibly including an Advance Decision to Refuse can help avoid such dilemmas in the future if cognitive decline persists.

## Case 6.18: A patient's family requests that medication be administered covertly

### Scenario summary

Mrs Patel, a 78-year-old female, has had progressively declining cognitive function and has recently been diagnosed with moderate dementia. She has a history of type 2 diabetes and hypertension, both of which require regular medication. Over the past month, Mrs Patel has become increasingly suspicious of her treatment, refusing medication and claiming it is 'poison'. Concerned that her health will deteriorate rapidly without her essential medications, Mrs Patel's family asks the clinical team to administer her medication covertly (hidden in food or drink). They argue that this is the only way to ensure compliance.

### Legal aspects related to the case

- **Mental Capacity Act 2005 (MCA)**: Applies to adults aged 16 and over in England and Wales. It requires an assessment of Mrs Patel's capacity to decide whether or not to take her medications. If she lacks capacity, decisions must be made in her 'best interests'. Under the MCA, a person is considered to have capacity unless proven otherwise. The fact that Mrs Patel has dementia does not automatically mean she lacks the capacity for this specific decision.
- **Best Interests**: If Mrs Patel is found to lack capacity, any action taken must be in her best interests, considering her past and present wishes, feelings, beliefs and values. The potential benefits and burdens of covert administration must be weighed carefully. Healthcare professionals should consider the MCA's principle of the 'least restrictive' option—covert medication is often regarded as a last resort when all other less coercive strategies have failed.

- **Adults with Incapacity (Scotland) Act 2000**: If situated in Scotland, similar principles apply: the action taken should benefit the adult, use the least restrictive approach, involve the adult's wishes where possible, consult relevant others and encourage existing skills and capabilities.
- **Common Law and Duty of Care**: Clinicians have a duty to safeguard patients and ensure appropriate treatment if it is clinically necessary. However, covert medication may amount to a breach of autonomy and, if improperly used, could be considered battery or trespass to the person.
- **The Care Quality Commission**: England and other professional bodies have published guidance emphasizing thorough capacity assessments, multidisciplinary reviews and best interests meetings before deciding on covert medication.

### Ethical issues raised

- **Autonomy Versus Beneficence**: If Mrs Patel lacks capacity, the principle of beneficence (acting in her best interests) might support covert administration to meet her healthcare needs. However, deception undermines autonomy and, if she has any capacity, it may violate her right to choose or refuse.
- **Respect for Persons and Dignity**: Covert medication can be seen as disrespectful and a violation of dignity if not supported by a robust best interests rationale. It can also erode trust if discovered later.
- **Capacity and Informed Refusal**: A thorough capacity assessment is essential. Even if Mrs Patel's decision appears irrational, she may retain the capacity to refuse. The ethical question is whether her refusal results from a lack of understanding (due to dementia) or a genuine, autonomous choice.

### Clinical issues

- **Assessing Mrs Patel's Decision-Making Capacity**: Dementia may impair her comprehension, but a fluctuating capacity is common. A dedicated assessment, possibly at different times of day or in a calmer environment, may help determine if she truly understands the nature and consequences of refusing medication.
- **Evaluating Alternatives to Covert Medication**: Before resorting to covert methods, clinicians should explore other options such as simpler explanations, frequent reassurance, changes in dosage timing or liquid formulations. A mental health liaison or geriatric psychiatry consultant may suggest behavioural strategies that uphold Mrs Patel's dignity.
- **Multidisciplinary Involvement**: A best interests meeting with doctors, nurses, pharmacists, possibly a dietician and family members can facilitate a more holistic approach, ensuring no one viewpoint dominates. Such collaboration can reveal suitable compromises or creative solutions.

- **Continuous Review of the Therapeutic Plan**: If covert medication is initiated, an ongoing review mechanism is crucial. Mrs Patel's capacity could change, and her response to the covert approach may vary. Regular reassessments ensure covert administration remains justified and proportionate.
- **Safeguarding Concerns**: If the family's motivations were questionable (e.g. financial or abusive), healthcare professionals must be vigilant. Even well-intentioned family requests require scrutiny under safeguarding protocols.

## Potential implications

- Administering medication covertly must only be considered after thorough capacity assessments, multidisciplinary discussion and an informed best interests decision, ensuring less restrictive approaches have been tried and found wanting.
- The family's request stems from concern for Mrs Patel's health. However, healthcare providers must act primarily in Mrs Patel's interests, ensuring that any decision aligns with her previously expressed values and the legal framework, rather than simply acquiescing to family demands.
- If Mrs Patel later discovers staff were hiding medication from her, it can severely damage her trust in healthcare providers. This could exacerbate her refusal of future care.

# Case 6.19: Disagreement about the best course of treatment for an incapacitated patient

## Scenario summary

Mr Thompson, a 70-year-old male with advanced Parkinson disease and a recent severe stroke, finds himself in the high-dependency unit. He cannot meaningfully communicate, and clinicians assess that he lacks the mental capacity to decide on his own medical management. The attending consultant believes that further invasive intervention (a surgical procedure) may be futile and proposes moving towards palliative care. However, Mr Thompson's adult children want 'everything done', insisting that surgery could provide additional time for family support and possible improvement.

## Legal aspects related to the case

- **Mental Capacity Act 2005 (MCA):** Applies to individuals aged 16 and above who lack capacity. It presumes a person has capacity unless proven otherwise. In Mr Thompson's case, his incapacity must be assessed specifically for treatment decisions. If he lacks capacity, any interventions (or withdrawal of interventions) must align with his 'best interests'. The clinical team should consider his previously expressed values, beliefs and any advance statements if available.

- **Best Interests Standard:** Under the MCA, decision-makers must weigh clinical benefits, burdens and Mr Thompson's likely wishes or feelings. Consulting with those close to the patient—his children—is vital. However, their preference, while important, is not the only or final determinant. 'Best interests' does not simply mean 'whatever the family wants'. It involves a holistic assessment, including quality of life and any advanced directive Mr Thompson might have made.
- **Court of Protection:** If disagreements persist and cannot be resolved, the case can be referred to the Court of Protection in England and Wales. The court may determine what is in Mr Thompson's best interests, providing a legal basis for a treatment plan.
- *Adults with Incapacity (Scotland) Act 2000:* If the scenario took place in Scotland, similar principles apply. Benefit to the adult, least restrictive option and consultation with relevant parties are mandatory.

## Ethical issues raised

- **Autonomy (by Proxy) Versus Clinical Judgement:** Although Mr Thompson cannot decide for himself, respecting his 'autonomy' means considering any known prior statements or wishes. The family's input may reflect their interpretation of his values but could conflict with the healthcare team's view of clinical futility.
- **Beneficence and Nonmaleficence:** The doctor's recommendation aims to provide the most benefit while avoiding harm (e.g. invasive, painful procedures with limited prospect of true recovery). Family members, however, may focus on extending life, even if the likely outcome is prolonged suffering.
- **Duty of Care:** Clinicians must act in the patient's best interests, rather than solely follow family directives. Balancing empathy for the family's emotional distress with professional responsibility to prevent futile measures can be challenging.

## Clinical issues

- **Emotional and Psychological Dimensions:** The children's insistence could stem from grief or guilt, rather than a realistic understanding of outcomes. Ethically, the team must communicate compassionately, ensuring they neither dismiss the family's fears nor provide false hope.
- **Capacity Assessment and Communication:** A formal capacity evaluation ensures clarity about Mr Thompson's inability to decide. Relevant experts (e.g. a psychiatrist, geriatrician or stroke specialist) may confirm his cognitive and communicative limitations. Clear documentation is essential.
- **Exploring Mr Thompson's Prior Wishes:** Any previous Advance Decision to Refuse or informal statements about end-of-life preferences are crucial. For instance, if he had

stated he would never want life-prolonging interventions in a vegetative state, these should guide management.

- **Psychological Support for the Family:** The family may benefit from a palliative care or psychology team to help them process grief and adjust expectations. Consistent communication minimizes family distress and conflict with the clinical team.

## Potential implications

- Conflicts can cause moral distress for the medical team and exacerbate the family's anguish. Clear communication and empathy are key to minimizing harm and resentment on both sides.
- When a patient lacks capacity and the doctor's clinical judgement conflicts with the family's wishes, a best interests framework is imperative. Adequate communication, exploration of any prior patient statements, multidisciplinary discussions and, if needed, legal recourse all serve to protect the patient's welfare and uphold ethical medical practice.

# Case 6.20: A doctor suspects an adult patient is being abused but the patient refuses to allow disclosure

## Scenario summary

Rachel, a 40-year-old with a history of mild anxiety, presents to her GP with repeated bruising on her arms and episodic head-aches. On gentle questioning, Rachel provides vague explanations that do not fully account for her injuries. Over multiple visits, the GP becomes increasingly convinced that Rachel may be experiencing domestic abuse. When asked if she feels unsafe or would like help from social services or the police, Rachel insists that she is 'fine' and refuses to allow any disclosure, fearing retaliation or family embarrassment. She emphasizes that she wants everything to remain confidential.

## Legal aspects related to the case

- **Common Law Duty of Confidentiality:** In English law, healthcare professionals owe a duty of confidentiality to their patients. Disclosing personal information without consent can breach this duty unless specific exceptions apply (e.g. imminent risk of serious harm).
- **Capacity:** Rachel's capacity to make her own decisions is presumed unless there is evidence to the contrary. As long as she is competent and not under duress that compromises her decision-making, her refusal generally must be respected.
- **Safeguarding Adults (Care Act, 2014):** Statutory guidance imposes a duty on public bodies, including NHS agencies, to protect adults at risk. However, if the adult is deemed to have capacity and refuses, forced disclosure can be problematic

unless the risk extends to children, vulnerable adults or society at large.

## Ethical issues raised

- **Autonomy Versus Beneficence:** Respect for Rachel's right to self-determination (autonomy) must be balanced against the physician's desire to prevent harm (beneficence). She has the capacity and explicitly refuses disclosure.
- **Confidentiality and Trust:** Maintaining patient confidentiality underpins trust. If the GP breaches confidentiality prematurely, Rachel may disengage from healthcare, worsening her vulnerability.
- **Duty to Protect and Nonmaleficence:** The GP has a duty to act if Rachel is in imminent danger or if others could be harmed. Yet the abrupt breach of confidentiality can exacerbate the risk of harm or dissolve the therapeutic alliance.

## Clinical issues

- **Capacity Assessment:** Confirming that Rachel understands her circumstances, potential risks and possible assistance. If she comprehends these factors and can communicate a decision, she is typically deemed to have capacity despite making choices that appear risky.
- **Continuing Support:** Building rapport, offering follow-up appointments and providing information on local support services (domestic abuse helplines, safe houses) without forcing disclosure to authorities can help preserve trust.
- **Monitoring for Escalation:** Documenting injuries, the patient's statements and any signs of increasing severity is essential. Repeated episodes of worsening harm might justify closer consideration of breaching confidentiality if risk escalates.
- **Emotional and Mental Health Implications:** Rachel's anxiety or fear may be interwoven with her abusive context. A referral to mental health services (with her consent) could provide additional support and help identify any changes in capacity or willingness to disclose over time.

## Potential implications

- If the clinician believes Rachel or others (e.g. children in the same household) are in imminent danger of significant harm, disclosure without consent could be defended under public interest. If the risk is not sufficiently grave or immediate, however, common law confidentiality remains a strong obligation.
- Even if Rachel appears to have the capacity, it is possible she is under coercion. Ethical practice requires a sensitive exploration of whether her refusal truly reflects her free, informed decision.
- Maintaining open communication can eventually enable Rachel to accept help. By ensuring repeated consultations,

the GP might find a future window for safe disclosure or patient-led intervention.

## Case 6.21: Credible threat to a third party

### Scenario summary

Dr McAllister is a consultant psychiatrist working in an acute mental health unit in the United Kingdom. She is treating Samuel, a 32-year-old patient detained under Section 3 of the *Mental Health Act* 1983 (amended 2007) for treatment of a significant psychotic illness. During one of their therapy sessions, Samuel discloses disturbing details suggesting that he intends to harm a specific individual upon discharge—someone he believes wronged him in the past. He reiterates his plan several times, providing enough detail to indicate a credible threat.

### Legal aspects related to the case

- **Mental Health Act 1983 (amended 2007):** Enables Dr McAllister to detain and treat Samuel against his will if he poses a risk to himself or others. Permits disclosing confidential information if it is necessary to protect others from serious harm, aligning with the principle that public safety can outweigh confidentiality.
- **W v. Egdell (1989):** This case established that breaching confidentiality may be justified in the public interest, particularly when a patient poses a significant danger to others.
- **Common Law Duty of Confidentiality:** Doctors generally owe a duty of confidentiality to their patients. However, this duty is not absolute and may be overridden when there is an imminent risk of serious harm to others.
- **Human Rights Act 1998 (Article 8, European Convention on Human Rights):** Protects the right to respect private life. A breach of confidentiality must be proportionate and justified, particularly when it comes to preventing crime or protecting the public.
- **GMC Guidance—Confidentiality (2017, 2024) and Good Medical Practice (2024):** Allows disclosure without consent only in exceptional circumstances where colleagues or the public may be at risk of serious harm.

### Ethical issues raised

- **Confidentiality Versus Public Safety:** Balancing respect for Samuel's privacy against a moral and professional obligation to prevent harm to others.
- **Duty of Care:** Dr McAllister's responsibility includes both caring for Samuel and safeguarding society from dangerous behaviours.
- **Autonomy and Beneficence:** Samuel's autonomy (particularly in decision-making) is limited by his detention.

Ensuring his best interests may conflict with the imperative to avert harm he might cause.
- **Trust in the Therapeutic Relationship:** Breaking confidentiality could compromise trust and therapeutic rapport. However, preserving life and preventing harm may take precedence when the risk is serious and imminent.

### Clinical issues

- **Assessment of Risk:** Dr McAllister needs to evaluate Samuel's mental state, the credibility of his threat and whether he has the capacity to act on it. This involves a meticulous risk assessment approach, possibly with input from MDTs.
- **Therapeutic Management:** Adjusting treatment, such as medication or psychotherapy, to address potentially violent or antisocial features. Collaboration with forensic psychiatry might be necessary if the level of risk is high.

### Potential implications

- Breaching confidentiality might erode Samuel's trust in the mental health team, hampering therapeutic progress. However, appropriate intervention could prevent him from criminal activity and further deterioration.
- Timely disclosure of a credible threat to relevant authorities can avert harm. This might involve cooperation with police, court orders or additional restraint under the *Mental Health Act*.
- The case illustrates the delicate balance between individual patient rights and safeguarding the public. It reaffirms the need for clarity on when doctors can or must breach confidentiality.

## Case 6.22: A patient with anorexia nervosa refuses life-saving treatment

### Scenario summary

A 22-year-old patient, Alice, presents with severe anorexia nervosa. Her body mass index (BMI) is dangerously low at 13 kg/m², and she exhibits multiple physical signs of organ compromise. Despite medical advice that nasogastric feeding and intensive psychiatric support are urgently needed to prevent imminent cardiac failure, Alice is steadfastly refusing treatment. She expresses fear of weight gain and insists that her body is 'too large already'.

### Legal aspects related to the case

- **Capacity and Consent:** In UK law, consent is valid only if it is (1) voluntary, (2) based on sufficient information and (3) given by a competent patient. The *Mental Capacity Act* 2005 (MCA) (applicable in England and Wales) states someone lacks capacity if they are unable to understand, retain, weigh relevant information or communicate their decision. A patient refusing life-saving treatment may still have capacity if all four elements are met. However, the Re C test (also cited in case law) acknowledges an individual may be capable of making even a grave or seemingly 'unwise' decision, provided their mental capacity remains intact.

- **Mental Health Act 1983:** Anorexia nervosa is recognized as a mental disorder. If Alice is deemed to have impaired capacity or poses a significant risk to her own life, compulsory admission under the *Mental Health Act* could be considered for assessment and treatment. This enables treatment against her will if she is at severe risk and lacks capacity or if her decision-making is significantly impaired by her psychiatric condition.
- **Best Interests and Common Law:** Where an adult lacks the capacity for a specific treatment decision, healthcare professionals may proceed under the common law principle of 'best interests' (in England and Wales, also explicitly set out in the MCA). If Alice is found incapacitated, life-saving nutrition can be given to safeguard her life in her best interests, reflecting not only medical but also social and psychological factors.
- **Potential Deprivation of Liberty:** Intensive treatment (e.g. nasogastric feeding in a locked inpatient unit) might amount to a deprivation of liberty if Alice is under continuous supervision and not free to leave. This must be lawfully authorized—currently via Deprivation of Liberty Safeguards for adults 18+ in appropriate settings or Liberty Protection Safeguards once fully implemented.

## Ethical issues raised

- **Autonomy Versus Beneficence**: Respecting Alice's autonomy—her right to refuse treatment even if it leads to a life-threatening outcome—conflicts with the medical duty to act in her best interests (beneficence). If she retains capacity, her autonomy generally prevails. Yet, if her decision-making is significantly affected by her illness, beneficence and the duty to preserve life may take precedence.
- **Capacity and 'Unwise Decisions':** The *Mental Capacity Act* 2005 emphasizes that making an unwise decision (such as refusing life-saving therapy) does not in itself prove a lack of capacity. Clinicians must carefully assess whether her anorexia is impairing her ability to understand or weigh information.
- **Nonmaleficence and Duty of Care:** Clinicians must avoid causing harm, and a refusal of treatment in anorexia nervosa can lead to severe harm or death. Balancing respect for Alice's autonomy with avoiding harm places the team in a challenging moral position.

## Clinical issues

- **Medical Complications of Anorexia:** Alice's severely low BMI places her at risk of electrolyte imbalances, cardiac arrhythmias and multiorgan failure. Immediate intervention is often necessary to prevent mortality.
- **Psychiatric Assessment:** Diagnosing and assessing for comorbidities such as depression, anxiety or delusional thinking is crucial. Comorbid psychiatric conditions can further impair capacity. A specialist in eating disorders and psychiatry is typically required to assess the severity of Alice's anorexia and her decision-making capacity comprehensively.
- **MDT Involvement:** Treatment often involves dietitians, psychiatrists, psychologists, nursing staff and social workers. Coordinated care is essential for monitoring refeeding risks, such as refeeding syndrome, which can cause shifts in fluids and electrolytes leading to further cardiac complications.
- **Possibility of Measures:** If Alice is found to lack capacity or be under severe mental distress preventing valid refusal, a short-term use of legal frameworks (MHA 1983 or MCA 2005) may be needed to initiate life-saving treatment.

## Potential implications

- In especially contentious cases, courts can be asked for a declaration on the lawfulness of treatment—especially where refusal may lead to fatal outcomes. This provides clarity and ensures proper safeguarding for both the patient and the medical team.
- Healthcare professionals have a responsibility to uphold the best interests of vulnerable individuals while respecting the principle of autonomy. This scenario highlights the need for robust capacity assessments and reflective ethical reasoning.
- By carefully assessing capacity, considering legal frameworks (particularly the *Mental Capacity Act* 2005 and the *Mental Health Act* 1983) and weighing ethical obligations, a balanced approach can be formulated for Alice's case. Properly documenting each step—capacity evaluations, the patient's stated reasons for refusal and MDT input—remains integral to finding a lawful and ethically justifiable course of action.

## BEGINNING AND END OF LIFE

# Case 6.23: A doctor is asked to withdraw life-sustaining treatment from a patient in a persistent vegetative state

## Scenario summary

Dr Roberts, a consultant in an intensive care unit (ICU), is overseeing the care of Mr Green, a 45-year-old patient who sustained severe hypoxic brain injury after a cardiac arrest. Following months of assessment, multiple clinical teams have concluded that Mr Green meets the criteria for a persistent vegetative state

(PVS). He is dependent on artificial nutrition and hydration and has no meaningful interaction with his surroundings. Mr Green's family is divided: his spouse and adult daughter believe continuing life-sustaining treatment prolongs suffering and wish to withdraw feeding. His brother feels strongly that withdrawing treatment is morally equivalent to murder.

## Legal aspects related to the case

- **Capacity and Best Interests:** Since Mr Green lacks capacity (per the *Mental Capacity Act* 2005), decisions must be made in his best interests. In cases where the patient is in a PVS, the courts (particularly the Court of Protection in England and Wales) may be involved if there is disagreement or uncertainty.
- **Withdrawing and Withholding Treatment:** *Airedale NHS Trust v. Bland* (1993) is a landmark legal case that established that withdrawing life-sustaining treatment (such as artificial nutrition and hydration) from a patient in a persistent vegetative state is lawful, provided it is not in the patient's best interests to continue. The House of Lords concluded that artificial nutrition and hydration constitute medical treatment, and its withdrawal can be lawful if prolonging life no longer confers any benefit to the patient.
- **Acts and Omissions Doctrine:** English law draws a key distinction between actively causing a patient's death (an act) and allowing a patient to die by withdrawing futile treatment (an omission). In Bland, the court ruled that discontinuing artificial nutrition and hydration was seen as an omission rather than a positive act.
- **Role of the Courts:** Since the case of *An NHS Trust v. Y* (2018) UKSC 46, it is no longer mandatory to seek court approval before withdrawing clinically assisted nutrition and hydration (CANH) from patients in a prolonged disorder of consciousness if the clinical team and the family agree that it is not in the patient's best interests to continue. However, if there is disagreement or doubt, an application to the Court of Protection should still be made.

## Ethical issues raised

- **Best Interests and Quality of Life:** Clinicians and family must consider whether continuation of treatment offers any benefit to Mr Green or merely prolongs a state with no conscious awareness. Determining best interests often involves balancing respect for life with the recognition that life support may no longer be beneficial.
- **Autonomy:** Mr Green cannot exercise his autonomy, so an MDT and the family must represent his (previously expressed) values and wishes if known. If he created an Advance Decision (living will) or had previously shared views on such circumstances, that would heavily guide the decision.

- **Nonmaleficence and Beneficence:** Continuing futile treatment may cause unnecessary distress to the family and impose significant burdens—emotional, financial and resource based—without improving Mr Green's condition. Clinicians must weigh whether continuing treatment does more harm than good.
- **Emotional and Moral Conflict for Healthcare Providers:** Many doctors and nurses experience moral distress when withdrawing treatment, especially where family members disagree or fear that ceasing artificial nutrition and hydration is akin to ending a life prematurely. Demonstrating compassion while remaining professionally objective is an ethical obligation.

## Clinical issues

- **Diagnosis and Prognosis:** Confirming a PVS diagnosis is complex and requires repeated, robust neurological assessments. Input from neurology, neurosurgery and critical care consultants can ensure confidence in the diagnosis.
- **Burden of Treatment:** Artificial nutrition and hydration in a PVS patient can cause complications (e.g. infections, aspiration risk and procedural complications of feeding tubes). Clinicians must consider whether the burdens outweigh any perceived benefits.
- **The Role of an MDT:** Palliative care teams, specialist nurses and psychologists can help address the patient's and family's needs. Clear communication of clinical findings helps the family understand the extremely low likelihood of recovery.
- **Family Communication and Support:** Disagreements, such as those between Mr Green's spouse/daughter and his brother, require sensitive mediation. The clinical team should provide consistent updates, involve hospital chaplaincy or counsellors as needed and explore all viewpoints with empathy.

## Potential implications

- Cases like these reinforce the principles set out in *Airedale NHS Trust v. Bland*, confirming that withdrawal of futile life-sustaining treatment can be lawful if done in the patient's best interests. A need for legal clarification might arise if family disputes remain unresolved.
  -Since the *An NHS Trust v. Y* ruling, which has simplified the process for withdrawing CANH in certain cases but also placed greater emphasis on the agreement between the clinical team and the family.
- Even with legal and ethical justification, the decision to withdraw treatment can lead to significant guilt, bereavement issues or family conflict. Long-term psychological support may be vital.
- Although not the central consideration for the individual patient, prolonged ICU stays for patients in a PVS can have

wider resource implications. Transparent decision-making ensures that resources are channelled effectively without compromising individual patient care.

# Case 6.24: A patient's family requests active euthanasia to end their relative's suffering

## Scenario summary

Mr Green is a 78-year-old patient with advanced motor neurone disease (MND). He is bed-bound, receiving artificial feeding and appears to be in severe discomfort despite regular analgesia and palliative measures. His capacity to make decisions is currently unclear due to his fluctuating consciousness and compromised communication. Deeply concerned by the physical and emotional stress they witness daily, Mr Green's family approached the GP with a request for active euthanasia. They insist that ending his life would be the most humane action.

## Legal aspects related to the case

- **Current Legal Position in the United Kingdom:** Active euthanasia is currently illegal. If a doctor deliberately takes action to end a patient's life, even with the best intentions, it can be considered murder or manslaughter under the common law framework. There is no statutory exemption permitting active euthanasia currently.
- **R v. Cox (1992):** A key case where a doctor administered a lethal injection to end a patient's life and was convicted of attempted murder. This underscores that actively hastening death is legally impermissible.
- *Airedale NHS Trust v. Bland* (1993): Although this case focused on withdrawal of treatment rather than active euthanasia, it clarified that legally withdrawing or withholding futile treatment (an omission) is distinct from taking positive steps to end a person's life (an act).
- **Doctrine of Double Effect:** Increasing opioid doses for palliative purposes is lawful (*R v. Bodkin Adams*) if the primary intention is symptom control and not to kill. However, the family's request is for active euthanasia, which would not be protected by the doctrine of double effect. The law currently makes no provision to legitimize an active measure whose aim is to end life.

## Ethical issues raised

- **Autonomy and Consent:** If Mr Green retained capacity and autonomously requested assistance to end his life, the team would still face the legal prohibition of euthanasia. Given that his capacity is uncertain, the family's request alone cannot serve as a lawful or ethical basis for active euthanasia.
- **Beneficence Versus Nonmaleficence:** The family believes it is an act of kindness or beneficence to end Mr Green's

suffering. However, from a medical ethics standpoint, intentionally ending life conflicts with nonmaleficence, which obligates doctors to do no harm.
- **Role of Suffering and Compassion:** There is a strong emotional drive to respond to the patient's suffering. Nevertheless, legal and professional guidance indicate that providing optimal palliative care, including adequate pain relief and psychosocial support, is the ethically accepted approach rather than ending life by direct action.
- **Respect for the Law and Professional Integrity:** Doctors have a moral and professional duty to practise within legal limits. Engaging in active euthanasia would risk severe legal and professional sanctions, undermining public trust in the profession and violating the GMC's guidance.

## Clinical issues

- **Palliative Care Optimization:** One of the key clinical duties is to ensure Mr Green's pain and other distressing symptoms are managed as effectively as possible. This might involve reassessment by specialist palliative care teams, considering higher doses or alternative methods of pain relief and addressing any treatable complications exacerbating his suffering (e.g. infection, constipation, anxiety).
- **Assessment of Mental Capacity:** Clarifying whether Mr Green has capacity to make his own decisions is pivotal. If he does, discussing his wishes about care, including possible refusal of life-sustaining treatments, becomes central. If he lacks capacity, then decisions must be made in his best interests, always remaining within the law (which excludes active euthanasia).
- **Family Communication and Support:** The family's distress suggests an urgent need for clear, empathetic communication about what can be done to manage Mr Green's pain and meet his needs. Eliciting the family's concerns, clarifying the limits of lawful practice and offering psychosocial support may reduce the impetus for requesting euthanasia.
- **Multidisciplinary Approach:** Input from consultants in palliative medicine, nursing staff, chaplaincy or spiritual care and counsellors may provide a holistic response to patient and family suffering. The team should also ensure nurses and junior doctors similarly understand the legal and ethical boundaries.

## Potential implications

- Failure to respond empathically and adequately to Mr Green's pain may deepen family anguish, causing conflict and mistrust. Conversely, if the family see that all lawful avenues for pain and symptom control are being used, they may feel supported, even if they cannot obtain the active euthanasia they initially wanted.

- Acceding to a request for active euthanasia could result in criminal charges, GMC sanctions and serious legal consequences. Supporting Mr Green within legal means preserves professional integrity and patient safety.
- Such cases highlight the ongoing debate around end-of-life laws. Robust discussions and ethical reflection may inform future reviews of palliative care practices and potential legislative developments in end-of-life care.

There is ongoing debate about assisted dying in the United Kingdom, including recent developments such as the Assisted Dying Bill introduced in the House of Lords in 2024.

## Case 6.25: A doctor and a patient's family disagree about whether to implement a DNACPR order

### Scenario summary
Dr Patel, a consultant in General Medicine, is caring for Mr Jordan, an 82-year-old patient with advanced heart failure and multiple comorbidities. Mr Jordan's overall condition has deteriorated significantly to the point where Dr Patel believes that attempting cardiopulmonary resuscitation (CPR) would be futile and potentially harmful. The family, however, strongly objects to a 'Do Not Attempt Cardiopulmonary Resuscitation' (DNACPR) order. They argue that all possible measures, including CPR, should be tried if Mr Jordan's heart or breathing stops.

### Legal aspects related to the case
- **Right to Refuse or Withdraw Treatment:** UK law recognizes that an adult with mental capacity can refuse life-sustaining treatment, even if that refusal may result in death (*Re B* (2002)). However, when the patient lacks capacity, the clinical team must decide in the patient's best interests.
- **No Right to Demand Futile Treatment:** As established in *R (Burke) v. GMC* (2005), patients (or their families speaking on their behalf) cannot demand treatments that are not clinically appropriate or are judged to be futile.
- **Guidance on DNACPR Decisions:** The case of *R (on the application of Tracey) v. Cambridge University Hospital NHS Trust* (2014) emphasizes the importance of involving patients (wherever possible) and/or their families in DNACPR discussions unless there is a compelling reason not to do so. A DNACPR decision must be communicated clearly and sensitively.
- **Best Interests:** In cases where the patient no longer has the capacity, the *Mental Capacity Act* 2005 requires healthcare professionals to act in the patient's best interests, considering clinical judgement, the patient's previously expressed wishes (if known) and input from those close to the patient.
- **GMC and British Medical Association (BMA) Guidance:** Both the GMC and the BMA provide guidance that CPR should not be offered when it is unlikely to succeed or when its burdens outweigh its benefits. Clinicians must still discuss reasoning with the patient (if competent) or the family, taking care to explain the rationale for DNACPR decisions without implying abandonment.

### Ethical issues raised
- **Autonomy and Capacity:** If Mr Jordan lacks decision-making capacity, the decision shifts to determining his best interests while respecting any previously expressed wishes. If he has capacity, he can refuse or accept DNACPR, though he cannot insist on clinically inappropriate treatment.
- **Beneficence Versus Nonmaleficence:** Dr Patel aims to avoid harm by not subjecting Mr Jordan to a traumatic, painful and likely unsuccessful CPR attempt. Balancing the potential benefit against the risk of suffering is central to this ethical concern.
- **Duty of Care and Trust:** Families may perceive the decision for DNACPR as a withdrawal of care, leading to a breakdown in trust. The doctor must communicate compassionately, ensuring the family understands that comfort care and all other supportive measures continue.
- **Conflicts with Family Wishes:** When families insist upon interventions the medical team deems futile, conflicts can arise. The ethical principle of respecting the patient's and family's perspectives must be weighed against the professional duty to practise evidence-based medicine and avoid causing harm.
- **Emotional and Cultural Factors:** Cultural views, religious beliefs or emotional distress can heavily influence family wishes. Sensitivity to these factors is ethically important, even if the ultimate clinical decision remains unchanged.

### Clinical issues
- **Assessing Futility:** Clinically, Dr Patel must evaluate whether CPR stands a realistic chance of success, considering Mr Jordan's advanced heart failure and comorbidities. The likelihood of meaningful recovery, postresuscitation quality of life and risk of harm are key factors in determining futility.
- **Communication and Advance Care Planning:** Early, clear and empathetic communication can avert later disputes. If possible, discussions about Mr Jordan's prognosis and DNACPR should have started before the crisis point.
- **Ongoing Treatment and Care:** A DNACPR order does not mean stopping all care. Mr Jordan should still receive appropriate medical, nursing and palliative interventions, including symptom control, analgesia and comfort measures. The team must ensure the family understands that DNACPR refers only to refraining from CPR in the event of cardiac or respiratory arrest.

- **Multidisciplinary Input:** In such complex cases, involving palliative care teams, senior nursing staff and possibly a clinical ethics committee can help guide the decision-making process and support robust, compassionate discussions.

## Potential implications

- Unresolved conflict can cause significant emotional strain for everyone involved. Healthcare professionals may experience moral distress if they feel pressured to provide futile care.
- While families often seek any possible avenue to prolong a loved one's life, the healthcare team has a duty to weigh the potential benefit of an intervention against its burdens or harms.
- By following legal requirements, robust guidance from the GMC and BMA and a compassionate, transparent approach, doctors can strive to ensure that end-of-life decisions are ethically and legally sound.

## Case 6.26: A terminally ill patient requests information about assisted suicide

### Scenario summary

Mr Robinson, a 67-year-old patient with advanced and incurable MND, has reached a point where his quality of life has deteriorated significantly. Despite optimum palliative measures, his pain and breathlessness persist and he experiences profound fatigue and distress. During a routine consultation with his GP, Dr Patel, Mr Robinson expresses the wish to explore options that might hasten his death. He specifically asks about 'assisted suicide' and wonders whether anything can be arranged to help him end his life.

### Legal aspects related to the case

- **Suicide Act 1961:** Under the Act, suicide itself is no longer a criminal offence in England and Wales. However, assisting or encouraging another person's suicide remains illegal. The amending *Coroners and Justice Act* 2009 reiterates that any assistance or encouragement may attract criminal liability. Thus doctors risk prosecution if their involvement is deemed to have 'encouraged or assisted' the patient's suicide.
- **Pretty v. The United Kingdom (2002):** Established there is no 'right to die' under Article 2 (European Convention on Human Rights). Article 8 rights (private life) were held to be 'qualified', meaning the state's interest in safeguarding life can override an individual's wish to secure assistance in dying.
- **R v. Cox (1992):** Demonstrates that actively hastening a patient's death is subject to criminal prosecution.
- **GMC's Good Medical Practice (2024):** Doctors must practise within the law. Although they may discuss a patient's concerns and give objective information, they cannot facilitate, prescribe or actively assist in suicide.

### Ethical issues raised

- **Autonomy:** Mr Robinson is expressing a clear wish to consider an option that is currently illegal in the United Kingdom. Clinicians have an ethical duty to recognize his autonomy and to explore the reasons behind his request. Even though the law prohibits direct assistance, understanding his desire to die and addressing his suffering remain essential.
- **Beneficence and Nonmaleficence:** Doctors aim to act in the patient's best interests (beneficence) and avoid harm (nonmaleficence). While supporting a patient's wish to end suffering may appear compassionate, active assistance towards suicide breaches the law and the principle of 'do no harm' in the UK's current legal framework.
- **Sanctity of Life and the Slippery Slope:** Some argue that helping to end life fundamentally undermines the intrinsic value placed on human life. Others fear it may open the door to normalizing euthanasia or assisted dying in broader contexts.

### Clinical issues

- **Palliative Care and Symptom Control:** The scenario highlights the importance of optimizing palliative treatment: ensuring that Mr Robinson's pain, nausea, breathlessness and psychological/spiritual needs are adequately addressed. Under-treated symptoms may precipitate requests for assisted dying.
- **Assessing Mental Capacity and Psychological Distress:** Patients with terminal illnesses can become depressed or hopeless. Identifying and managing treatable causes of low mood or anxiety is crucial. A psychiatric assessment may be indicated if there is any concern about impaired capacity or underlying depression driving the request.
- **Patient–Doctor Communication:** The clinician must respond empathetically, acknowledging Mr Robinson's suffering while explaining legal limitations. Open communication can maintain trust and encourage the patient to consider comprehensive palliative options (e.g. hospice care, specialist palliative nursing).

### Potential implications

- When a terminally ill patient like Mr Robinson requests information regarding assisted suicide, doctors face complex ethical, legal and clinical challenges. Ensuring optimal palliative care, conducting a robust capacity assessment and maintaining empathetic communication are key.
- While the law in the United Kingdom currently prohibits physician-assisted suicide, a patient-centred approach—

offering full support for symptom control and psychological distress—remains paramount. There is ongoing debate about assisted dying in the United Kingdom, including recent developments such as the Assisted Dying Bill introduced in the House of Lords in 2204.

# Case 6.27: Deaf parents request preimplantation genetic diagnosis for embryo selection

## Scenario summary

A married couple, both of whom were born deaf, attend a fertility clinic requesting in vitro fertilization (IVF) with preimplantation genetic diagnosis (PGD). Their specific request is to select an embryo shown to carry the gene responsible for hereditary deafness (so that the child is born deaf). They view deafness as an integral part of their identity and culture rather than as a disease. Clinic staff are uncertain how to proceed, knowing that selecting a particular genetic trait raises complex ethical, legal and clinical questions and that it also may have wider implications for future practice.

## Legal aspects related to the case

- **Human Fertilisation and Embryology Acts (1990 & 2008):** The Human Fertilisation and Embryology Authority (HFEA) regulates the creation, storage and use of embryos. Any PGD procedure must be licensed under these Acts. The law focuses on preventing 'serious genetic conditions'. Selecting embryos to avoid serious disabilities or severe inherited diseases is generally permitted. However, there is no straightforward statutory provision permitting or endorsing the deliberate selection of an embryo predicted to have a disability (such as hereditary deafness). Sex selection for nonmedical reasons (i.e. personal preference) is prohibited. By analogy, choosing any genetic trait purely for personal or cultural preference remains contentious and is not clearly sanctioned by the legislation.
- **Clinic Licensing and Regulation:** Clinics must operate within HFEA guidelines, which require valid written consent, appropriate counselling and adherence to licence conditions. If the request contravenes HFEA rules, the clinic could face regulatory action.

## Ethical issues raised

- **Autonomy Versus Nonmaleficence:** The parents argue for their reproductive autonomy and cultural identity, viewing deafness as a characteristic rather than a disability. Clinicians, however, may struggle with whether deliberately selecting an embryo predicted to be deaf is in the future child's best interests.

- **Definition of 'Disability':** The Human Fertilisation and Embryology legislation and related guidance often refer to 'serious disability'. Some consider deafness disabling; others see it as a distinct culture (Deaf culture). This conceptual difference fuels substantial ethical debate.
- **Beneficence and Potential Harm:** Clinicians must act in a child's best interests. Some will query whether choosing a gene for deafness denies the child a sense of hearing, which could be regarded as harmful. Deaf parents may counter that their child will share in their community, language (British Sign Language) and cultural identity.
- **Justice and Social Implications:** Permitting selection for particular traits (especially traits commonly seen as disabilities) has broader societal ramifications. It blurs lines between avoiding serious disease (e.g. life-limiting conditions) and selecting other genetic characteristics—such as physical attributes. This could open the door to 'designer babies' arguments.

## Clinical issues

- **Counselling and Informed Consent:** The couple should thoroughly understand the medical aspects of IVF and PGD, including success rates and risks and also the broader ethical, social and legal context—particularly that selecting an embryo predicted to have deafness is legally and ethically controversial. Counselling is also required to explore how the resulting child might experience both the Deaf community and mainstream (hearing) environments.
- **Determining 'Eligibility' for PGD:** The clinic's standard pathway for PGD is often centred on preventing serious genetic diseases. Selecting an embryo precisely because it carries a 'disability' is atypical. Clinicians might face dilemmas about whether offering such a procedure aligns with standard practice or their own professional guidance.

## Potential implications

- This case of Deaf parents seeking a child who shares their deafness raises pivotal questions about the scope of parental autonomy, the definition of disability and the boundaries of genetic selection.
- Legally, there is no direct permission within UK statutes to select for a known disability, and the Human Fertilisation and Embryology framework appears primarily designed to reduce the risk of serious disease.
- Ethically, the scenario highlights debates about deafness as a difference rather than a disease, respect for Deaf culture and duties to secure a child's best interests.
- Clinically, fertility teams must navigate complex counselling, potential disputes among staff and patients and ambiguity in existing regulatory frameworks.

## Case 6.28: A female seeks a late-term abortion due to a diagnosis of a serious foetal anomaly

### Scenario summary

A 32-year-old pregnant female attends the antenatal clinic at 28 weeks' gestation. Recent investigations, including detailed ultrasound and genetic testing, confirm a severe foetal anomaly likely to result in profound physical and mental disability if the pregnancy continues. Having consulted several healthcare professionals, she requests a termination of pregnancy. The partner supports her decision.

### Legal aspects related to the case

- **Abortion Act 1967 (amended by the Human Fertilisation and Embryology Act 1990):** In England, Wales and Scotland, abortion is generally permitted up to 24 weeks if continuing the pregnancy poses a greater risk to the female's physical or mental health than termination. However, the law allows termination at any gestational stage if there is a 'substantial risk of the child being born severely physically or mentally handicapped' (s.1(1)(d) Abortion Act 1967).
- **Infant Life (Preservation) Act 1929:** Criminalises the destruction of a 'child capable of being born alive', but this does not apply if termination is carried out in good faith to preserve the mother's life or prevent grave permanent harm. Serious foetal anomaly can also fall under the exemption clause.
- **Offences Against the Person Act 1861:** Under ss.58–59, obtaining or providing abortion outside the framework of the *Abortion Act* 1967 remains a criminal offence. In this scenario, the proposed termination must be carefully documented, with medical agreement by two doctors that the statutory grounds are met.
- **Capacity and Decision-Making:** If the female has the capacity (as defined by the *Mental Capacity Act* 2005 in England and Wales), only her informed consent is required for the procedure to proceed. Partners, family members or the foetus itself do not hold legal decision-making powers in this context (*Paton v. British Pregnancy Advisory Service Trustees*, 1979).

### Ethical issues raised

- **Status of the Foetus and Late-Term Considerations:** The foetus is not a legal person, yet it gains moral significance as gestation advances. Even though the law permits abortion after the 24-week mark in cases of serious foetal anomaly, many clinicians experience ethical unease relating to the higher degrees of foetal development at this stage.
- **Balancing Autonomy and Beneficence:** Respecting the female's autonomy is paramount. She has the right to choose whether to continue the pregnancy, particularly when facing substantial foetal abnormalities. Clinicians also have a duty of beneficence—preventing harm by acknowledging the likelihood of severe disability and potential distress.
- **Conscientious Objection and Professional Duties:** Healthcare professionals opposed to providing late-term abortions on moral or religious grounds must still ensure continuity of care. Failing to refer can jeopardize the female's rights, contravening professional standards (General Medical Council, 2024).

### Clinical issues

- **Complexity of Late-Term Procedures:** Beyond 24 weeks, terminations involve increased medical and surgical complexity. Procedures such as medical induction of labour or, in rare circumstances, surgical termination demand specialist expertise to minimize risks to the female's health.
- **Assessing Maternal Well-Being:** The psychological burden can be significant. Females may require additional mental health or counselling support both before and after the procedure. The clinical team should ensure robust emotional and psychosocial care.

### Potential implications

- While the law provides scope for late-term abortion in cases of serious foetal anomaly, each situation demands thorough evaluation, clear communications, appropriate referral or shared care arrangements and unwavering compassion towards the female and her family.

## Case 6.29: A pregnant female refuses a medically recommended treatment that could prevent harm to her foetus

### Scenario summary

Ruth is 28 weeks' pregnant, and her obstetrician, Dr Morgan, has strongly recommended a particular medical intervention to address a treatable complication that poses significant risks to the foetus if left untreated. Despite understanding the information provided, Ruth firmly declines. The care team becomes concerned about the foetus, believing the intervention is time sensitive and critical for preventing potential harm. Ruth, however, insists on exercising her right to refuse treatment, referencing her personal values and distress about the procedure's risks to her own health. Conflicts arise among the healthcare team, Ruth's partner (who wants her to accept the treatment for the sake of the foetus) and Ruth herself.

### Legal aspects related to the case

- **Maternal Autonomy and Capacity:** In the United Kingdom, an adult with the capacity has the right to refuse treatment, even if refusal may harm or endanger the life of the foetus.

The *Mental Capacity Act* 2005 confirms that if a patient (in this case, Ruth) understands the information about the consequences, can retain and weigh up this information and communicate a decision, her refusal must be respected.

- **Legal Status of the Foetus:** Under English law, as highlighted in *Paton v. British Pregnancy Advisory Service Trustees* (1979) and *Re F (In Utero)* (1988), a foetus is not a separate legal person until it is born and has a separate existence from its mother. Hence, no injunction can be placed on Ruth to force her to undergo treatment purely for foetal benefit.
- **Legal Status of the Father:** The father has no legal right to compel treatment. The courts have consistently held that the pregnant female's autonomy takes legal precedence over foetal interests.

## Ethical issues raised

- **Respect for Autonomy:** Central to this scenario is Ruth's right to make informed decisions about her own body. Even where the medical team believes the foetus could be severely harmed, the principle of respect for autonomy dictates that a capacious adult should determine her own treatment choices.
- **Beneficence and Nonmaleficence:** Clinicians wish to act in the best interests of both Ruth and the foetus, aiming to prevent avoidable harm. However, forcibly administering treatment against a competent adult's wishes could itself cause harm (physical and psychological) and would breach professional and ethical standards.
- **Foetal Interests:** Although the foetus may be at risk, ethical debate persists around whether and how to balance maternal autonomy with potential foetal harm. From one standpoint, the foetus has moral significance, but in law, its interests cannot override those of a competent mother.
- **Conflict of Interests (Mother vs. Clinicians vs. Partner):** Ruth's partner, motivated by concern for the foetus, disagrees with her refusal. Clinicians may feel moral distress in appearing to place the foetus at risk. Balancing these tensions while adhering to ethical and legal principles is often challenging.

## Clinical issues

- **Assessment of Capacity and Understanding:** Before fully accepting Ruth's refusal, the clinical team must ensure she genuinely understands the benefits, risks and alternatives. A formal capacity assessment may be prudent if there is any concern about her ability to decide.
- **Possible Alternative Management Plans:** An MDT (obstetrics, midwifery, possibly mental health if required) should explore alternative strategies to mitigate the risk to the foetus, provided these respect Ruth's wishes. This may include increased foetal monitoring and discussing less invasive options or palliative measures if complications worsen.

- **Emotional and Psychological Support:** Ruth may benefit from counselling to help process her concerns. The healthcare team should also be attentive to heightened anxiety, stress or fear that might be influencing her refusal and provide appropriate support services.

## Potential implications

- Ruth's case illustrates the complex interplay between respecting adult autonomy, protecting foetal interests and navigating ethical obligations in obstetric care. While clinicians may feel a profound duty to safeguard foetal well-being, the law in England and Wales affirms that a competent pregnant female can refuse treatment.
- Upholding Ruth's autonomy is paramount, provided she has the capacity and is properly informed. Through empathetic communication, thorough support and meticulous documentation, clinicians can ethically respect Ruth's wishes and maintain professional standards.

# Case 6.30: A family insists on life-sustaining treatment for a patient despite the medical team deeming it futile

## Scenario summary

Mrs Green, an 84-year-old female with advanced heart failure and multiple comorbidities, is admitted to the intensive care unit (ICU). After several weeks of mechanical ventilation and repeated organ support measures, her clinical condition deteriorates further. The medical team concludes that continuing aggressive treatment is futile and not in Mrs Green's best interests. However, her adult children insist that 'all possible measures' be continued indefinitely. They believe withdrawing the ventilator and other life-sustaining interventions would be morally equivalent to 'giving up on her'.

## Legal aspects related to the case

- **Withholding and Withdrawing Life-Sustaining Treatment:** Under UK law, clinicians are not obliged to provide treatments deemed futile or not in the patient's best interests (*Airedale NHS Trust v. Bland* (1993)). A patient with capacity may refuse life-sustaining treatment, even if doing so will result in death (*Re B* (2002)). However, the patient (or relatives on their behalf if the patient lacks capacity) cannot demand treatment that clinicians judge to be of no benefit (*R (Burke) v. GMC (2005)*).
- **Best Interests and Mental Capacity:** If Mrs Green lacks capacity, decisions must adhere to the *Mental Capacity Act* 2005. The Act requires healthcare professionals to consider

the patient's best interests, including any previously expressed wishes, beliefs and values. Family members and those close to the patient should be consulted, but their request does not override clinicians' professional judgement if the proposed intervention confers no real prospect of benefit.

- **Do Not Attempt Cardiopulmonary Resuscitation (DNACPR) and Futility:** A DNACPR may be implemented if resuscitation is deemed futile or against previously known wishes. The case of *R (on the application of Tracey) v. Cambridge University Hospital NHS Trust* (2014) highlights the importance of open communication about DNACPR decisions, but it does not grant families an automatic right to insist on futile interventions.
- **Acts and Omissions Doctrine:** UK courts have upheld that withdrawing futile medical treatment (an omission) is legally distinct from actively hastening death (an act). Stopping ventilatory support when it no longer serves the patient's best interests is not regarded as unlawful killing.

## Ethical issues raised

- **Autonomy Versus Surrogate Decision-Making:** If Mrs Green lacks decision-making capacity, then her prior expressed wishes (if known) carry ethical weight. Family members are surrogate decision-makers by virtue of their relationship, but they cannot impose demands that conflict with Mrs Green's best interests or medical reality.
- **Beneficence and Nonmaleficence:** The healthcare team's duty is to act in Mrs Green's best interests (beneficence) while avoiding interventions likely to cause harm or prolong suffering (nonmaleficence). Persisting with painful or distressing treatments that offer no meaningful recovery can be detrimental to patient welfare.
- **Futility and Resource Allocation:** Prolonging futile care can raise questions about justice and resource allocation. Although resource considerations should not be the main driver, the potential strain on limited ICU facilities and staff time is ethically relevant.

## Clinical issues

- **Communication and Compassion:** Tension often stems from inadequate discussion or misinformation about the patient's prognosis. The family's insistence may reflect fear, grief or guilt. Clear, empathetic communication is ethically imperative to help the family understand why continued invasive measures may not benefit their loved one.
- **Determination of Futility:** Clinicians should base their judgement on medical evidence, prognosis and likelihood of achieving outcomes meaningful for Mrs Green. Repeated specialist assessments (e.g. cardiology, palliative care input) support consensus about futility.

- **Transition to Palliative Care:** Shifting care goals towards comfort measures, symptom control and psychosocial support helps prioritize quality of life. Early palliative involvement can ease suffering and guide the family through end-of-life decisions.

## Potential implications

- By integrating clear legal foundations, robust ethical reasoning and compassionate clinical practice, healthcare teams can justify and implement the withdrawal of futile interventions.
- Ultimately, ensuring the patient's best interests and quality of life (or quality of death) is paramount—even when family members struggle to accept the reality of the situation.

## Case 6.31: A family refuses to allow organ donation from a deceased relative despite their being registered on the organ donor register

### Scenario summary

Mrs Wilson, a 56-year-old female with a long-standing commitment to organ donation, dies unexpectedly in hospital. She was registered on the NHS Organ Donor Register. However, at the time of her death, her grieving family strongly refuses permission for organ donation, citing personal reasons and spiritual beliefs. They insist that, despite Mrs Wilson's documented wishes, no organs should be retrieved. The medical team must decide how to proceed, balancing the deceased's explicit commitment to donation against the family's refusal.

### Legal aspects related to the case

- **Human Tissue Act 2004 and Relevant Updates:** Created the legal framework for organ donation in England, Wales and Northern Ireland (with parallel legislation in Scotland). It establishes the principle that consent (or authorization, in Scotland) is essential for the removal, storage and use of organs. The Act also created the Human Tissue Authority, responsible for ensuring compliance with regulations surrounding organ procurement.
- **Organ Donation (Deemed Consent) Act 2019 (England):** England (and Wales, via the *Human Transplantation (Wales) Act* 2013) has adopted an 'opt-out' system ('deemed consent'). In principle, if a person did not opt out during life, they are considered willing to donate their organs. However, the law also states that no organs will be retrieved if the family strongly objects. In practice, NHS Blood and Transplant policy is to honour a family's refusal, even if the deceased was on the organ donor register.

- **Role of the Family's Views:** Legally, the expressed wish of the deceased to donate organs (by registration or explicit written consent) is authoritative. However, hospitals and transplant coordinators usually seek a family's affirmation to proceed. If a family withholds cooperation, the retrieval team may be unable to proceed, despite the legal right stemming from the deceased's registration.

## Ethical issues raised

- **Autonomy of the Deceased Versus Family Wishes:** From an ethical standpoint, respecting the autonomous choice of the deceased (who clearly registered as a donor) is paramount. Yet, the family's emotions and beliefs must also be acknowledged, particularly during acute bereavement. The tension arises when respecting the deceased's autonomy conflicts with preserving the family's well-being.
- **Beneficence and Saving Lives:** Organ donation can provide life-saving or life-enhancing transplants to waiting recipients. Denial of consent potentially means lost opportunities for those on transplant lists.
- **Nonmaleficence and Grief:** Proceeding with donation against the family's explicit wishes could exacerbate their distress, potentially causing long-term psychological harm.
- **Justice and Fair Allocation:** Organs are a scarce resource. The principle of justice supports maximizing donation where lawful and respecting the donor's stated intent. Allowing family veto may reduce the pool of organs available, impacting fairness in distribution and outcomes for patients requiring transplants.

## Clinical issues

- **Timing and Practicalities of Donation:** Organ retrieval must occur promptly after circulatory or brainstem death, especially if mechanical ventilation is maintaining organ viability. Any refusal or delay from the family may render organs unsuitable for transplantation. Clinicians and transplant coordinators are under tight time constraints; attempts to resolve conflicts must be swift yet sensitive.
- **Communication Strategies:** Sensitive, clear and empathetic communication with the family is crucial. Clinicians need to explore the reasons behind refusal, clarify the deceased's documented wishes and address any misconceptions about donation.

## Potential implications

- This scenario underscores the need for clinicians to act as advocates for both the deceased's autonomous wishes and the emotional well-being of the bereaved.
- Legally, the hospital may have grounds to proceed with a donation under the deeming provisions, but ethically and practically, family refusals are rarely challenged.

- Effective communication, empathetic engagement and recognition of cultural and emotional factors remain vital.
- Ultimately, the case illustrates the delicate balance between genuine respect for the donor's intentions and sensitivity to grieving relatives.

## Case 6.32: Parents refuse to vaccinate their child due to fears about side effects

### Scenario summary

Mr and Mrs Lawrence bring their 6-month-old daughter, Emma, to the GP surgery for a routine check-up. During the consultation, the GP notices Emma has missed her primary immunizations. Mrs Lawrence explained she is concerned about the possible adverse effects of vaccines. Mr Lawrence would like to have the vaccine. Despite reassurance and information about the recommended immunization schedule, including the safety and rarity of serious side effects, Mrs Lawrence remains firmly opposed to vaccinating Emma.

### Legal aspects related to the case

- **Parental Responsibility:** The *Children Act* 1989 sets out who has parental responsibility for a child. Mothers automatically have parental responsibility for their children. A father usually has parental responsibility if he is: married to the child's mother, listed on the birth certificate (after a certain date, depending on which part of the United Kingdom the child was born in), has a court order confirming parental responsibility
- **Child's Best Interests:** In the United Kingdom, parents generally have the right to make healthcare decisions on behalf of their children, provided these decisions do not place the child at serious risk of harm. If a healthcare professional believes the refusal of a recommended vaccine places the child or others at unacceptable risk, they could raise the case with the courts, although in practice this is rare for routine immunizations.
- **Public Health Legislation:** In the United Kingdom, vaccination is voluntary. No law mandates child immunization or penalizes parents for refusing it. However, certain communicable diseases are statutorily notifiable (such as measles). A measles outbreak can prompt broader public health measures, but it does not automatically override parental refusal of vaccination.

- **Parental disagreement:** Although the consent of one person with parental responsibility is usually sufficient (Section 2(7) of the *Children Act* 1989), if one parent agrees to immunization but the other disagrees, the immunization should not be carried out unless both parents can agree to immunization or there is a specific court approval that the immunization is in the best interests of the child.

## Ethical issues raised

- **Balancing Autonomy and Harm Principle:** Parents' independence in raising their children competes with the societal interest in reducing the spread of infectious diseases. Mill's harm principle suggests that intervention can be justified to prevent harm to others, particularly vulnerable people.
- **Child's Best Interests:** Emma is not yet competent to make her own health decisions; her welfare should guide decision-making. Clinicians must weigh the small but genuine risks of vaccination against the potentially large individual and public health benefits.
- **Duty Not to Infect and Herd Immunity:** Refusing vaccination reduces community immunity, particularly endangering vulnerable individuals (e.g. those who are immunocompromised). Ethically, some argue there is a shared responsibility to protect the broader community, while others prioritize parental autonomy.

## Clinical issues

- **Communicable Disease Risks:** Without vaccination, Emma may be at increased risk of contracting vaccine-preventable diseases such as measles, mumps and rubella. Clinicians face the challenge of maintaining a good therapeutic relationship with the family while emphasizing medical evidence about vaccine effectiveness and safety.
- **Addressing Misinformation and Fear:** The GP must offer accurate information to counter myths about vaccine side effects. Ongoing respectful dialogue and fact-based reassurance often help parents gradually understand vaccine benefits.
- **Wider Public Health Considerations:** Healthcare teams should remain alert for any signs of outbreaks in the community. They may also need to liaise with local public health officials if there are concerns about serious infectious disease risks.

## Potential implications

- This scenario illustrates the ethical, legal and clinical intricacies of childhood vaccination refusal.
- While the United Kingdom does not mandate immunization by law, healthcare professionals must carefully balance

parental autonomy with the best interests of the child and the broader public utility of vaccination.

## Case 6.33: A healthcare worker refuses the flu vaccine, citing personal beliefs

### Scenario summary

Adam is a healthcare worker in a busy NHS ward. Prior to the upcoming winter flu season, his employer arranges for staff influenza vaccinations on-site. Adam, however, declines the vaccine, citing personal beliefs about bodily autonomy and concerns about vaccine safety. His supervisor and colleagues worry that patients—particularly those who are older, immunocompromised or have chronic conditions—may be put at increased risk of infection. A discussion arises over whether Adam's refusal has any legal or professional ramifications and how best to reconcile patient safety with Adam's autonomy.

### Legal aspects related to the case

- **Health and Safety at Work Considerations:** NHS employers and healthcare environments must ensure a safe workplace for staff and patients. Although there is no absolute legal requirement in the United Kingdom for healthcare workers to receive the flu vaccine, the employer has an overarching duty under Health and Safety legislation to reduce foreseeable risks.
- **NHS Constitution and Employer Policies:** The NHS Constitution emphasizes providing high-quality care for all. Many NHS trusts strongly encourage staff vaccination to protect vulnerable patients. While staff can refuse, they may face redeployment or restrictions if their refusal poses a demonstrable risk.
- **Common Law Duty of Care and Negligence:** A question arises whether failing to take 'reasonable precautions'—including vaccination—could breach a duty of care, especially in settings with vulnerable patients. Although no direct statutory mandate exists for flu vaccination, a serious outbreak linked to staff refusal may prompt negligence claims if harm occurs and it can be shown that refusal was an avoidable risk.
- **Human Rights and Equality Considerations:** Employees have rights regarding personal beliefs and religious expression. However, under the *Equality Act* 2010, 'belief' must meet specific criteria (e.g. being genuinely held and more than an opinion). Employers must balance these rights with the legitimate aim of protecting public health.
- **The COVID-19 Parallel:** The temporary policy on mandatory COVID-19 vaccination for health and social care workers in England (ultimately withdrawn) contrasts with this scenario. Although the flu vaccine is not mandated, the

proportionality and necessity arguments that arose in COVID-19 debates highlight the tension between individual rights and population health—echoing the same legal and policy frameworks.

## Ethical issues raised

- **Autonomy Versus Public Good:** Refusing a flu jab reflects individual autonomy over one's body. Yet, from a public health standpoint, Mill's harm principle might justify efforts to encourage or even require vaccination if unvaccinated staff heighten risks to patients.
- **Beneficence and Nonmaleficence:** Healthcare professionals have an ethical duty to benefit patients and minimize harm. Adam's choice may place vulnerable individuals at risk, raising the question of whether he is meeting his professional obligation to act in patients' best interests.
- **Justice and Fairness:** Not vaccinating may shift disproportionate risk onto patients who have limited ability to protect themselves, or onto vaccinated colleagues who, in effect, 'carry' the group immunity in Adam's place. This 'free-rider dilemma' creates a question of equitable burden sharing.
- **Professionalism and Trust:** Public confidence in healthcare hinges on staff adhering to recognized standards of best practice, including recommended vaccinations. Adam's refusal could undermine trust in the healthcare system if patients perceive he is not taking all reasonable measures to protect them.

## Clinical issues

- **Infection Control:** Influenza can spread rapidly in clinical settings, raising morbidity and mortality for high-risk patients. Outbreaks can strain limited hospital resources and disrupt care.
- **Staff Health and Workforce Capacity:** If Adam contracts flu, there is a potential for significant staff shortage. Illness among staff leads to extra pressure on colleagues, which can compromise the overall quality of care.
- **Supporting Informed Decision-Making:** In line with the chapter's emphasis on education and transparent discussion, Adam may benefit from factual information about flu vaccine efficacy, side-effect profiles and the broader public health rationale. Misgivings based on misconception are often reduced by open, respectful dialogue.

## Potential implications

- Whereas mandatory vaccination can seem coercive and conflict with personal autonomy, public health ethics often emphasize proportional, evidence-based measures and the principle of least infringement.

- Transparent decision-making, clear justification and offering alternatives—such as redeployment or additional PPE (Personal Protective Equpiment)—may be key to addressing cases like Adam's without outright compulsion.

## Case 6.34: A patient with a highly contagious disease refuses to be quarantined

### Scenario summary

Mike, a 40-year-old professional, has been diagnosed with a highly contagious notifiable disease (e.g. an infectious pathogen designated under the Health Protection (Notification) Regulations 2010). Mike's symptoms are stabilized, but his clinicians strongly recommend isolation or quarantine to protect public health. Mike refuses, stating he has 'personal matters to attend to' and claiming, 'No one can force me to stay at home'. Despite repeated explanations of the serious risk to others, Mike remains unwilling to comply with quarantine advice.

### Legal aspects related to the case

- **Notifiable Diseases and Notification Duties:** Under the Health Protection (Notification) Regulations 2010, doctors in England have a legal duty to notify the local authority (proper officers) if they suspect a notifiable disease. While Adam's consent is not required for notification, this step is crucial to enable public health measures.
- **Confidentiality and its Limits:** Ordinarily, patient consent is required before disclosing personal information. However, in public health emergencies or for controlling infectious disease outbreaks, patient confidentiality may be overridden due to the significant risks posed to others (see also the principle that 'reasonable clinical suspicion' is sufficient to notify).
- **Balancing Individual Liberties with Public Protection:** The principle of individual autonomy is strong in UK law and ethics, but it can be curtailed when there is a substantial threat to others' health. The overall legal framework allows proportionate restrictions on liberty to manage infectious disease risks.
- **Potential Consequences of Noncompliance:** Should Adam actively expose others to a harmful pathogen, there is a possibility (depending on circumstances) of charges under older legislation such as the Offences Against the *Person Act 1861* (for reckless transmission), although this has more commonly applied to diseases such as HIV.

### Ethical issues raised

- **Conflict Between Autonomy and Public Good:** A central tension in public health ethics. Adam's autonomy conflicts with the need to protect the wider population from infection risk. Mill's harm principle underpins the argument that the state can intervene to prevent harm to others.

- **Proportionality and Least Infringement:** Childress's conditions (effectiveness, proportionality, necessity, least infringement and public justification) guide the ethical justification for restricting liberty. If quarantine is deemed essential and proportionate to contain a major outbreak, curtailing Adam's liberty may be ethically defensible.
- **Transparency and Reciprocity:** According to Upshur's principles, if Mike is imposed upon (for example, told to remain confined), it is ethically important that the state or health authorities provide clear communication, support and possibly compensation for any inconveniences or financial losses.
- **Duty Not to Infect:** The notion of a moral duty not to infect others applies. Ethically, though not universally agreed in all facets, many would argue that Mike has a responsibility to limit the risk he poses to the community.

## Clinical issues

- **Infectious Disease Control:** Public health priorities include preventing outbreaks. Contact tracing, surveillance and provision of supportive treatment are essential clinical measures. Mike's noncompliance jeopardizes these efforts.
- **Patient Engagement and Education:** Clinicians face the challenge of relaying the seriousness of the disease to Adam and seeking voluntary cooperation. Education about the potential complications of the disease for Mike himself and for those around him is central to effective control.
- **Support for the Patient's Practical Needs:** Mike may have practical or financial anxieties about quarantine. Addressing work, family or financial worries can promote cooperation. Ensuring he is heard and supported might increase his willingness to self-isolate.
- **Multidisciplinary Collaboration:** This situation calls for close cooperation between the clinical team, public health authorities and possibly social services to manage Mike's care, enforce necessary isolation measures and minimize negative impacts on his personal circumstances.

## Potential implications

- If Mike continues to refuse quarantine, there could be an outbreak leading to avoidable morbidity or mortality. Public trust in healthcare may be undermined if the system appears unable to contain easily identifiable threats.
- The case highlights the perennial debate about how far individual rights extend in situations of public health emergencies. Excessively coercive measures might erode trust in health services, whereas insufficient control could cause harm to large numbers of people.

## Case 6.35: A doctor must choose between two patients who need a life-saving treatment, but only one is available

### Scenario summary

Dr Patel, a consultant is nearing the end of her night shift when she is called to the intensive care unit (ICU). Two critically ill patients, Malcolm (aged 75) and Ruby (aged 30), both require an urgent, life-saving intervention (a specialist ventilatory device in extremely short supply). Due to equipment shortages and high demand, there is only one device available.

Malcolm has chronic obstructive pulmonary disease, diabetes and limited mobility. His condition has deteriorated drastically, and the consultant expects that, although the specialized ventilation might help him survive this crisis, his longer-term prognosis is poor. Ruby, a mother of young children, has suddenly become critically ill following an acute infectious complication. Her chances of making a recovery with the ventilatory device seem better, but resource allocation must consider multiple factors, not only the likelihood of immediate benefit.

### Legal aspects related to the case

- **NHS Resource Allocation and 'Rationing':** Although no specific statute dictates how an individual doctor must allocate a scarce, life-saving resource in an emergency, the NHS Constitution emphasizes fairness and equitable access. However, it offers limited detailed guidance for on-the-spot clinical rationing decisions such as this.
- **Common Law Duty of Care:** Under UK common law, Dr Patel owes a duty of care to both patients. She must arrive at a decision using reasonable care and skill in line with accepted medical standards.
- **Potential Human Rights Considerations:** The *Human Rights Act* 1998 incorporates the European Convention on Human Rights into UK law. Article 2 (the right to life) might be engaged, though it does not oblige the state to provide every possible treatment. Article 14 (protection from discrimination) could prompt scrutiny if any unjustified bias is suspected in deciding which patient should receive treatment.
- **Ethical and Policy Frameworks (NICE/NHS Trust Protocols):** While not legally binding in the sense of the statute, guidelines from NICE (National Institute for Health and Care Excellence) and local trust policies on critical care prioritization can become relevant if a decision is challenged. Adhering to established protocols helps demonstrate transparent, evidence-based reasoning. NICE has published guidance on the ethical principles for resource allocation during the COVID-19 pandemic (2021, 2024).

## Ethical issues raised

- **Distributive Justice and Fairness:** This scenario exemplifies distributive justice—how to distribute limited medical resources fairly. Should Dr Patel allocate the ventilator based on the likelihood of survival, younger age, quality of life or another value-based criterion? The idea of a 'postcode lottery' or 'bed lottery' in healthcare is heightened when only a single resource is available.
- **Utilitarian Versus Deontological Perspectives:** A utilitarian approach (maximizing overall benefit or total 'good') might favour Ruby, who appears to have better prospects for recovery, yielding a higher chance of longer and healthier life (more quality-adjusted life years (QALYs)). A deontological approach might examine universal principles: is it 'morally right' to prioritize one patient's life over another and would each patient accept being denied care under the same circumstances?
- **Double Jeopardy Critique (QALYs):** Using quality-of-life calculations can penalize older or chronically ill patients like Malcolm, effectively placing them at a 'double disadvantage' (already unwell and then further down the priority list). This creates a moral controversy over whether it is fair to prioritize younger or healthier patients for resource-intensive treatments.

## Clinical issues

- **Severity of Illness and Prognostic Uncertainty:** Clinicians use triage tools (e.g. physiological scoring and expert judgement) to estimate the likelihood of survival and potential for recovery. Yet any prognosis has uncertainties; Dr Patel might inadvertently misjudge the benefit each patient would gain. Clinical guidelines for critical care bed allocations often encourage factoring in 'frailty scores' or 'comorbidity level', as well as potential reversibility of illness.
- **Emotional Burden and Potential for Moral Injury:** The psychological toll on Dr Patel and her team could be significant. Being forced to make stark life-or-death triage decisions can lead to moral distress and burnout. Subsequent interactions with both families—supporting one in potential recovery while breaking bad news to the other—require high levels of compassion, communication and empathy.

## Potential implications

- Dr Patel's dilemma underscores the profound intersection of legal frameworks, ethical principles and clinical realities when resources are scarce.
- If rationing decisions systematically favour those with certain social or clinical advantages, health inequalities may widen. Policy-makers and clinicians must evaluate how ample or limited resources affect different segments of the population, ensuring everyone has fair access to life-saving care.
- While no universal formula can perfectly resolve every clash between moral duty and pragmatic constraint, transparent decision-making, consistent with accepted professional guidelines and robust ethical reasoning, helps safeguard patient trust, professional integrity and fairness in the NHS.

---

## Notice to readers

# SELF-ASSESSMENT

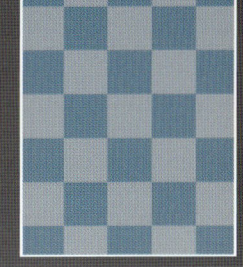

# MLA Single Best Answer (SBA) questions

## Chapter 1  Introduction

### 1.  Prescribing medicines

A 50-year-old patient who is normally well has returned from a holiday in Spain with a cough productive of green sputum that started 4 days ago. They ache all over and have a slightly sore throat and intermittent headache with no breathlessness or other red flag features. They say their spouse had similar symptoms first and is now recovered. Their clinical examination is normal, apart from a hoarse voice and nasal congestion. The doctor makes a working diagnosis of influenza infection, explains the likely course of illness and provides safety netting advice. The patient requests a prescription to treat their condition and is upset to have waited 6 hours in the accident and emergency department and go home without an antibiotic. The doctor politely explains their duty to only provide appropriate treatments.

**Which of the following best explains the doctor's response?**

A.  Facilitating patient choice
B.  Following deontological principles
C.  Following utilitarian principles
D.  Ignoring the patient's right to treatment
E.  Practising shared decision-making

### 2.  Ethics of interpersonal communication

A patient finds out shortly after giving birth that her father carries the gene for an autosomal dominant inherited condition. She does not tell her sister, who was born to the same father and is now also pregnant, about the genetic risk. Some years later, the patient brings a case for wrongful birth, saying she would have sought tests and termination of pregnancy if she had been told by doctors about the genetic risk soon enough. Weighing up the case, the judge comments on an apparent inconsistency in the way the patient says she would have managed the situation for herself and how she actually handled the situation by not sharing information with her sister.

**Which of the following traditions most clearly underpins the judge's comments about communication from the patient to her sister?**

A.  Kantian
B.  Religious
C.  Rights
D.  Utilitarian
E.  Virtue

### 3.  Clinical negligence

A 50-year-old male with a history of heart disease arrives at the emergency department at 3:00 a.m. complaining of severe chest pain and radiating left arm numbness. The registrar performs an ECG (electrocardiogram) but misinterprets it as showing minor irregularities. As a result, they diagnose the patient with indigestion and send him home with antacids. The patient suffers a heart attack later that night and is rushed back to the hospital in critical condition.

**Which of the following best explains this as a clinical negligence event?**

A.  Indigestion was masking the heart problems.
B.  The patient should have insisted on further investigations as he was competent.
C.  The pre-existing heart condition should not have been missed.
D.  The registrar misinterpreted the ECG.
E.  The registrar worked a long shift that night.

### 4.  Clinical negligence

A 75-year-old patient is admitted to the hospital with an infective exacerbation of chronic obstructive pulmonary disease. They have a past medical history of a cholecystectomy, gout and revision of a total knee replacement. The first total knee replacement failed very quickly, and the patient is thinking of bringing a clinical negligence case against the surgeon.

**Which of the following is required to support the patient's potential negligence case?**

A.  There was no duty of care.
B.  Doctors had a legal obligation to give emergency treatment at any time required.
C.  The medical interventions given are later judged by the court to have been 'responsible'.
D.  The standard of care given must have been below the standard expected of an ordinary clinician in that role.
E.  A breach in the duty of care did not cause the patient harm.

### 5.  Human rights

A general practitioner forgets to check about the family history of BRCA gene mutation in a patient who has come to consult about a breast lump. He calls the patient's landline and leaves a voicemail asking her to call back specifying he would like to know more information about the family history regarding the consultation she attended 2 days ago. He does not say what the consultation was about. The voicemail is picked up by her cleaner as the patient works away regularly and asks the cleaner to communicate about posts and telephone messages.

**Which of the following from the Human Rights Act best explains this as a breach of patient confidentiality?**

A. Article 2: The right to life.

B. Article 3: Prohibition of torture, inhuman and degrading treatment.

C. Article 8: Right to respect for private and family life.

D. Article 12: Right to marry and found a family.

E. Article 14: Right to protection from discrimination.

6. **Duty of care**

A Foundation Year 1 doctor has not received their contract in time for their first shift due to an administration error. However, as there is a severe staff shortage they are instructed to commence work while the paperwork is completed.

**Which of the following best explains why the Foundation Year 1 doctor still owes a duty of care to patients?**

A. Consequentialist principles require that all doctors owe a duty of care.

B. A duty of care owed to patients is statutory.

C. General Medical Council's good medical practice requires doctors to owe a duty of care to all citizens.

D. Not owing a duty of care will lead to negligence.

E. Patient autonomy means no doctor can escape the duty of care.

# Chapter 2 Professionalism

1. **Complaints and clinical errors**

A 72-year-old male with bilateral carpal tunnel syndrome is on the waiting list for surgical release and struggling with night pain despite taking gabapentin 600 mg three times daily. A medical colleague has previously told him the dosage can be increased to 900 mg three times daily if required, and the patient telephones to check if this is still okay. During the telephone consultation, the doctor notices he has chronic kidney disease stage 3b and decides to calculate the creatinine clearance, before agreeing with the previously suggested dose increase. After the phone call, the doctor double-checks the creatinine clearance calculation and realizes further gabapentin dose increases are inappropriate given the degree of renal impairment. The doctor phones the patient back, apologizing for the error and agreeing to a new plan to stop gabapentin and try an alternative drug – pregabalin.

**What best describes the course of action taken?**

A. Clinical audit

B. Expressing the duty of candour

C. Prescribing error

D. Reporting a near miss

E. Significant event analysis

2. **Patient safety and working relationships**

You are a junior doctor and are housemates and friends with a fellow junior doctor colleague. He often works beyond his contracted hours and you know the relationship with his girlfriend has become strained. Over the past few months he has increasingly appeared exhausted and sometimes quite dishevelled and spends a lot of time alone in his room when he is at home. One morning when you are both getting ready and are about to leave for work, you notice a strong smell of alcohol about him.

**What is the most appropriate next step you should take?**

A. Advise him to book an urgent appointment with his general practitioner.

B. Advise him to book an urgent appointment with Occupational Health.

C. Advise him to book an urgent appointment with the Practitioner Health Programme.

D. Phone the Ward Manager or Consultant he is working with to prevent harm to patients this morning.

E. Talk to him, encouraging him not to work this morning and to seek appropriate help.

3. **Driving advice**

A 45-year-old female Consultant Rheumatologist attends an appointment with her general practitioner due to intermittent visual loss. She is stressed at work as her department is understaffed, and there has been recent strike action leading to further workload increases, and at home she has three children who she takes to school each morning in the car. Physical examination is normal. The general practitioner considers the possibility of a stress-related illness and explains that transient ischaemic attack (TIA) also needs to be considered in the differential diagnosis. The patient agrees to be referred to the TIA clinic to be seen the next day as is usual practice.

**What else does the general practitioner need to do?**

A. Ask the patient to report the possible TIA to the Driver and Vehicle Licensing Authority.

B. Insist the patient does not drive her car until further advice from the neurologist tomorrow.

C. Report the possible TIA to the Driver and Vehicle Licensing Authority.

D. Speak to the practice manager, because they happen to be married to the Clinical Lead for Rheumatology in the local hospital.

E. Tell the patient to inform her car insurance company.

4. **Professional boundaries**

You have been working in the elderly medicine ward for several months as a junior doctor, and your longest staying patient, 96 years old, has recovered from a chest infection and gained enough strength to be discharged to an intermediate care bed for ongoing rehabilitation. You have seen her almost every day for over 2 months because you hardly have a day off, and on the much-awaited day of her discharge she hands you an envelope with a thank you card and £25 cash in it. She says she hopes you will find time to get a well-earned break from work and maybe even go out with someone nice. She recommends one of your colleagues.

**What should you do next?**

A. Say thank you for the card and cash and tell her you will ask your colleague for a date.

B. Say thank you for the card and say you appreciate her kindness but will need to decline the gift of cash.

C. Say thank you for the card and say you can only accept £10 in cash.

D. Say thank you for the card and take the cash but donate it to the hospital charity.

E. Say thank you for the card and take the cash but give it to the administrator to put aside for ward expenses.

5. **Professional boundaries**

A 55-year-old general practitioner works 5 days a week in the clinic and 1 day a week from home and develops a dry cough lasting for 5 weeks. He has had a similar cough before and it settled with omeprazole taken for a month, so it was put down to gastro-oesophageal reflux disease made worse by stress. He is generally well and exercises regularly. He asks a medical colleague in the surgery to prescribe omeprazole 20 mg on a private prescription.

**What should the general practitioner's medical colleague do?**

A. Advise him to make an appointment with his own doctor.

B. Report him to the General Medical Council.

C. Tell him that omeprazole can be bought over the counter.

D. Tell him to write himself a prescription.

E. Walk off and ignore him at the next practice meeting.

6. **Social media conduct**

Dr J regularly posts humorous content on TikTok featuring herself lip-syncing to popular music while wearing her scrubs. During one video, she appears to mock a specific condition, referencing an exaggerated physical symptom in a 'comical' way. Shortly after, several of her patients express their discomfort and disappointment online with the portrayal of their experience in her TikTok post.

**What is the most likely ethical concern arising from the actions of Dr J?**

A. Dr J has acted acceptably as free speech applies to all professions.

B. Dr J has breached trust with colleagues by publicly mocking a medical condition.

C. Dr J has compromised her professional image by engaging in frivolous behaviour.

D. Dr J has compromised trust with her patients by trivializing their condition.

E. Dr J has violated patient confidentiality by revealing identifiable information.

7. **Confidentiality**

Dr D has been treating patient P with a long-term illness for several years. After the patient dies, their niece N approaches Dr D asking to see the medical records of deceased patient P. Niece N explains that she wants to understand patient P's health and illness to better manage her own health risks.

**Which of the following is the most appropriate next step?**

A. Dr D can release records as long as any information related to mental health or substance abuse is removed.

B. Dr D can release records only if patient P had explicitly authorized access in their written living will.

C. Dr D should assess niece N's relationship with patient P and the potential benefit of information sharing before deciding.

D. Dr D should immediately release all records to niece N as the family has a right to access the deceased patient information.

E. Dr D should refuse to release any records, as confidentiality remains absolute even after death.

8. **Quality improvement**

A medical practice is aiming to improve the quality of care for patients with diabetes and makes this an area of focus in a quality improvement project. They identify that a significant proportion of patients with diabetes miss their follow-up appointments.

**Which of the following is the most sustainable measure to improve patient attendance?**

A. Conduct educational sessions with patients about the importance of follow-up care.

B. Implement a reminder system with automated phone calls and text messages.

C. Offer same-day appointments for patients who miss their scheduled appointments.

D. Partner with local community organizations to provide transportation for appointments.

E. Provide financial incentives for patients who attend all follow-up appointments.

9. **Human factors and health technology**

A new medication dispensing system with barcode scanning technology has been implemented in your hospital. While usage statistics show a decrease in medication errors, nurses report increased stress and time pressure—feeling rushed during medication administration.

**How can human factors principles be applied to improve the experience of the nursing staff?**

A. Focus on increasing the efficiency of the barcode scanning technology itself.

B. Implement stricter disciplinary measures for any medication errors made with the new system.

C. Introduce an additional dispensing system.

D. Introduce financial incentives for nurses who achieve high medication administration accuracy.

E. Reduce the number of steps in the barcode scanning process.

## Chapter 3  Doctors, patients and society

### 1.  Mental capacity

A 50-year-old comes to see the consultant physician concerned about her mother's care plan. Her mother is 75 years old and has had a recent diagnosis of Alzheimer disease. The daughter asks to discuss the plan in detail and requests access to her mother's medical notes. **What is the most appropriate next step in this situation?**

A. Call the patient and ask if she is comfortable with the daughter seeing her notes and proceed based on her response.

B. Explain to the daughter the importance of respecting her mother's privacy and suggest a family meeting to discuss the care plan together.

C. Grant the daughter full access to her mother's medical notes without further discussion.

D. Refer the daughter to a social worker to discuss concerns about her mother's care.

E. Review the care plan with the daughter alone, providing general information without disclosing specific details.

### 2.  Consent

A 38-year-old female patient has been recommended to consider a hysterectomy for severe menorrhagia because she remains symptomatic after trying all other appropriate treatments. She comes to the preoperative assessment clinic with her husband, who speaks English well while her understanding of and speech in English is limited. The clinic is already running an hour late after a power cut. **How should the consultant proceed to obtain informed consent?**

A. Defer the consent consultation to a later time as this is not an emergency.

B. Thank her husband for his support and check if the patient is happy for him to interpret.

C. Thank her husband for his support and arrange a professional interpreter.

D. Take consent directly from the patient.

E. Ask the Senior Registrar to come to the clinic to help.

### 3.  Medical emergencies

A 25-year-old patient is brought to the emergency department of an English hospital by ambulance as a major trauma patient following a car crash and is unconscious on arrival. A team of paramedics, nurses and doctors attend to stabilize the patient using the ABCDE approach, although the prognosis is bleak. **On what basis is assessment and treatment provided?**

A. A valid advance decision.

B. Common law best interests.

C. Potential for organ donation.

D. Presumption of capacity.

E. The patient's parents are now present.

### 4.  Children

A 15-year-old female books an appointment and presents to her general practitioner asking for oral contraception. She has no significant medical conditions and does not want her parents to know about the consultation. She attends mainstream school and met her boyfriend, who lives nearby, when she was on her way home from school one day. **What is the ethico-legal basis that necessitates the general practitioner finding out more about the boyfriend and their relationship?**

A. Assessment of Gillick competence.

B. Deprivation of Liberty Safeguards.

C. Her boyfriend may be vulnerable.

D. Safeguarding vulnerable people.

E. The Fraser Guidelines.

### 5.  Older people

A general practitioner is asked to visit an 83-year-old housebound widow who has a new cough. Her son, who lives with her and is also her sole carer, has requested the visit. Her son pleasantly greets the doctor, who notices all the windows and doors are open and it is a cold day. The kitchen smells of alcohol. Her son is registered to the same general practice and is known to have had a traumatic brain injury several years ago. He is able to function independently but is not fit for work. The patient is in bed upstairs. The doctor examines her chest and decides to prescribe oral antibiotics to treat community- acquired pneumonia. Before leaving, the doctor decides to examine the legs to look for any evidence of deep vein thrombosis. Removing the bed sheets covering the patient, severe bruising is seen on both legs in varying degrees of healing. There is no history of falls and the patient quietly says there is no need for any treatment for her legs. **What action should the doctor take next?**

A. Ask a medical colleague to attend to give a second opinion.

B. Ask the son to explain himself.

C. Maintain patient confidentiality.

D. Section the son under the Mental Health Act to prevent further harm.

E. Speak to the duty social worker asking for urgent intervention.

### 6.  Gender identity

A 24-year-old transgender female with a background of depression and anxiety, who has taken citalopram for some time, presents with self-harm behaviours. She has cut her forearms and is emotionally distressed. She tells you life is not worth living without the hormone prescriptions that will help her feel more like herself, and says her low mood and self-harm are purely borne out of frustration that the expected wait for specialist assessment is several more years. She says she has been suffering already for half her life and asks if you can do anything to speed up her referral.

**What is the most appropriate next step?**
A. Take action proportionate to the assessed suicide risk.
B. Explain she will have to wait her turn as there are other patients to consider.
C. Involve the patient's family.
D. Prescribe oestrogen to relieve patient distress.
E. Use the preferred pronouns of the patient.

# Chapter 4  The beginning and end of life

1. **Conscientious objection**
A 34-year-old female is 8 weeks' pregnant and books to see her general practitioner (GP). She has a past medical history of type 1 diabetes, has struggled with glycaemic control and is concerned that continuing with the pregnancy may further impair the management of her condition. She requests to be referred for a termination of pregnancy. The GP has a conscientious objection to abortion.
**What is the most appropriate action for the GP to take?**
A. Explain their views regarding abortion and attempt to persuade the patient to change their mind.
B. Sensitively tell the patient this is not part of their clinical practice and advise the patient to make an appointment with a colleague for this request.
C. Refer the patient to a colleague in the practice.
D. Refer the patient to gynaecology.
E. Refuse to refer the patient.

2. **Termination of pregnancy**
Ms A is a 27-year-old who has been referred for a termination of pregnancy.
**Which of the following can be accepted as grounds for a termination of pregnancy?**
A. All of the following.
B. Chromosomal abnormality at 17 weeks.
C. Grave risk to maternal health at 29 weeks.
D. Risk of harm to the mother's physical health at 9 weeks.
E. Risk of permanent harm to the mother's physical health at 18 weeks.

3. **Pregnancy**
During your Obstetrics and Gynaecology placement, you see a patient who is 13 weeks' pregnant and continuing to use illicit drugs. Afterwards your consultant asks you about the legal status of the foetus.
**Which of the following is true?**
A. A patient can be prosecuted for requesting an abortion from a general practitioner.
B. The foetus has interests that may be protected by law.
C. Any one doctor can approve a termination.
D. The foetus has some rights protected by law.
E. The foetus is a legal person.

4. **Organ donation**
You are a junior doctor working in an intensive care unit and have a patient with severe traumatic brain injury. There is concern among the doctors that the patient may be brain-dead. Before brainstem testing is carried out, the patient's mother comes to see you. She wants to know more about the new organ donation deemed consent legislation in 2019.
**Which of the following applies to opt-out organ donation legislation?**
A. Applies only in Scotland and Wales, not in England or Northern Ireland.
B. If an individual does not wish to be considered as a potential organ donor, they must opt out of being one.
C. If the individual has not opted out, the family cannot stop them from being an organ donor.
D. Includes prisoners and the mentally incompetent.
E. The family automatically gains custody of the body when a relative dies.

5. **Euthanaisa**
While working in the geriatrics ward, you are looking after Mr O with severe Parkinson disease. Mr O has repeatedly stated that he wants to die and has asked you to help him. When asked why, he states that he is tired of being in pain and wants some painkillers to help him slip away. He states that he believes that as he can make decisions about all other parts of his life, he should be allowed to decide to die too.
**Which of the following best describes the ethical argument for euthanasia Mr O is alluding to?**
A. Kantian deontology.
B. Principle of autonomy.
C. Principle of beneficence.
D. Doctrine of double effect.
E. Utilitarianism.

6. **Cardiopulmonary resuscitation**
An 85-year-old male with metastatic bowel cancer, heart failure, chronic kidney disease and a hip replacement has been admitted to the respiratory ward for pneumonia. A junior doctor goes to see him to discuss a Do Not Attempt Cardiopulmonary Resuscitation (DNACPR) decision. The patient adamantly wants full escalation of care and does not want to talk about a DNACPR any further, saying this is defeatist.
**What is the most appropriate action for the junior doctor to take next?**
A. Discuss with the consultant in charge of the patient's care.
B. Document that the patient wants a full escalation of care and leave the DNACPR blank.
C. Fill in the DNACPR anyway, without informing the patient.
D. Inform the patient that CPR is a medical decision that he cannot demand it and therefore a DNACPR decision will be put in place.
E. Try and persuade the patient's family to agree to a DNACPR decision.

## 7. Surrogacy

A couple are seen in the infertility clinic following their inability to conceive for more than 2 years. They ask the gynaecologist about the possibility of surrogacy.

**Which of the following best describes surrogacy in the United Kingdom?**

A. Altruistic surrogacy is legal.
B. Neither intended parent is required to be related to the child conceived.
C. Surrogacy is illegal.
D. Surrogate mothers can be paid.
E. The intended parents are automatically the legal parents.

## 8. Death certification

A patient on the vascular surgery ward has poorly controlled type 2 diabetes, stage 4 chronic kidney disease, gangrene of the foot secondary to peripheral neuropathy, chronic obstructive pulmonary disease (COPD) and hospital-acquired pneumonia. The patient later dies from respiratory failure.

**What is the most appropriate primary cause of death to state on the death certificate?**

A. COPD.
B. Hospital-acquired pneumonia.
C. Respiratory failure.
D. Sepsis.
E. Type 2 diabetes.

# Chapter 5 Public health

## 1. Communicable disease

A 4-year-old child is brought to the emergency department with symptoms that started 4 days ago and have worsened—these include a high fever, cough, runny nose and watery eyes. The child is now only eating and drinking small amounts and has come out in a rash today. On examination, you find a rash on the face and also on the neck and trunk, which is red-brown and slightly raised in some places. The child has had one dose of the MMR vaccine, and you make a clinical diagnosis of measles. You complete a notifiable disease form and send it to the Local Authority.

**Which of the following best justifies compromising patient confidentiality by completing the notifiable disease form?**

A. Duty not to infect.
B. Free riding.
C. Health promotion.
D. Mill's harm principle.
E. Underdetermination.

## 2. Pandemic communicable disease

In March 2020 various social 'lockdown' measures were introduced by the UK government aimed at controlling the spread of the COVID-19 virus and managing a surge in demand for health services associated with the onset of a pandemic infectious disease. 'Lockdown' created severe restrictions on daily life for people in all walks of life, including children in educational settings.

**Which ethical principle best justifies these restrictions?**

A. Equity principle.
B. Least restrictive principle.
C. Precautionary principle.
D. Reciprocity principle.
E. Transparency principle.

## 3. Screening

A 60-year-old male is invited to participate in the bowel cancer screening programme and returns a sample for faecal immunohistochemical testing. Screening is positive and he is invited to attend for a colonoscopy, which he undergoes and which does not find evidence of cancer. Before returning his screening sample he had felt well and hoped to receive reassurance by participating in the screening programme. He has now become anxious about his health.

**Which of the following best justifies inviting the male to participate in screening?**

A. Destigmatization.
B. Empowerment.
C. Means to an end.
D. Psychological distress.
E. Utilitarianism.

## 4. Utilitarianism

A husband and wife are both aged 45 years and keen climbers. They are airlifted to hospital with injuries after they both fell around 100 m, sustaining similar injuries including multiple broken ribs. The husband has a background of well-controlled type 1 diabetes mellitus since childhood, and the wife is previously well. They both develop pneumonia after a few days in the hospital and require escalation to high-dependency care; however, the hospital is already experiencing severe winter pressures and only one ventilated bed is available.

**What criticism can be made of the quality-adjusted life years approach to assessing utility here?**

A. Conflict of interest.
B. Doctrine of double effect.
C. Double jeopardy.
D. Inverse care law.
E. Profit motive.

## 5. Illness narratives

An 8-year-old with an up-to-date history of childhood immunizations and no significant past medical history attends with their parent, presenting with 2 days of nondischarging right-sided earache and fever of 37.9°C. They are generally well on examination and are somewhat dubiously prescribed amoxicillin to treat otitis media. They start to feel better within 3 days, do not experience any side effects of treatment and their parent attributes the improvement to the antibiotics.

**Which ethical tradition best describes the line of reasoning employed by the parent?**

A. Liberalism.
B. Virtue ethics.
C. Consequentialism.
D. Deontology.
E. Utilitarianism.

6. **Contact tracing**

A 16-year-old female patient presents to a general practitioner (GP) with symptoms of vaginal discharge and pain during intercourse; she confirms she has a boyfriend and is taking the combined oral contraceptive and not using any barrier contraception. A swab is taken, and chlamydia is diagnosed and treated with doxycycline 100 mg twice daily for 7 days. The GP gives the patient a leaflet about partner notification with details of the condition and advice for the boyfriend to be checked. The patient says she is too embarrassed and does not want to mention this to her boyfriend. The GP feels frustrated and really wants to ask for the phone number of the boyfriend so they can both be appropriately treated.

**What ethical underpinning best explains the concern of the GP for the boyfriend?**

A. Confidentiality.
B. Consequentialism.
C. Doctrine of double effect.
D. Social production of disease.
E. Virtue ethics.

7. **Volunteering**

A Consultant Paediatrician has been following media reports of a humanitarian crisis in another country which has led to many deaths so far and is predicted to worsen. Expert analysis from representatives of international organizations is broadcast on television, where the burden on children is highlighted and attributed to a shortage of suitably trained doctors. The TV feature ends with a request for help and a phone number. The doctor has a brief conversation with their partner about whether they should volunteer, and the partner agrees but raises concerns about safety in the crisis country and also what they would do about existing work commitments. The doctor says it will be fine and sends a quick email to their manager saying they are taking urgent leave, makes arrangements to volunteer and leaves to travel to the country in the following days.

**An advocate of which ethical tradition is most likely to defend the actions of the doctor?**

A. Autonomy.
B. Consequentialism.
C. Deontology.
D. Justice.
E. Virtue ethics.

8. **Behavioural change**

Stella is a GP partner in a city-centre practice who has become increasingly concerned about high amounts of alcohol consumption among their patients. She regularly offers lifestyle modification advice in consultations but is concerned that other doctors in the practice are not providing similar advice and that existing efforts are not leading to reduced alcohol intake in the registered population. Stella installs a television in the surgery waiting area which plays health promotion videos on loop about the harms of excess alcohol consumption and strategies to reduce this and mounts posters and places leaflets with similar messages. She is approached by several clinical and administrative colleagues and a few patients who complain these changes are excessive. She defends the actions as important to improve the health of the practice population.

**What ethical justification might Stella rely on?**

A. Consequentialism.
B. Hard paternalism.
C. Liberalism.
D. Quality and Outcomes Framework.
E. Soft paternalism.

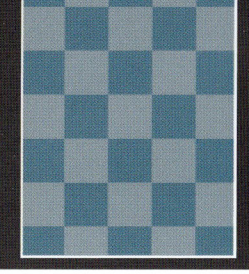

## Chapter 1 Introduction

1. B—Following deontological principles
A doctor has a duty to assess and provide appropriate treatment in a given situation; such duties are deontological in nature. Utilitarian principles are about maximizing 'good'—which is up for debate here as the patient being upset is not 'good', despite the doctor doing the right thing and also being polite. The patient choice agenda has limits and does not have an automatic right to a particular treatment based on their own assessment or opinion. This sometimes poses a challenge to the shared decision-making paradigm, and while it may be possible to provide further information and assurance to the patient which relieves her distress, some decisions are ultimately 'doctor led'.

2. A—Kantian
This case is based on *ABC v. St George's Healthcare NHS Trust & Others* (2020), and you can read a fuller account in Chapter 3. A medical negligence case was brought but it was not held to be a breach of the duty of care: the professionals had not communicated the genetic risk during pregnancy in the particular case because there was another patient to consider (the father) as well as the general erosion of public trust in the profession associated with breaking confidentiality. While answers B, C and E might all lean to some extent on the idea of 'treating others how you would like to be treated', the categorical imperative or universalisability test comes from the tradition of Immanuel Kant and is deontological. Kantian thought relies on an assumption that a person thinks and also acts rationally. In *ABC v. St George's Healthcare NHS Trust & Others* (2020), the judge also recognized the patient would have been distressed at the time of learning the information and not informing her sister. 'Utility maximizing' utilitarian calculations are altogether different (Option D).

3. D—The registrar misinterpreted the ECG
The key criteria required to determine clinical negligence is that the patient was owed a duty of care, and this duty of care was breached and the patient came to harm as a result of this. Of the options presented the one that most likely captures these criteria is option D. The reasonable standard is judged against that of an 'ordinarily competent practitioner' performing the same task or role and may be a matter of judgement for the expert witness(es).

4. D—The standard of care given must have been below the standard expectation of an ordinary clinician in that role
This is often known as the Bolam test. A is incorrect as there must be a duty of care for a negligence claim to succeed, and B is incorrect as there is no legal obligation in English law for doctors to give emergency treatment outside of a healthcare setting. C is also incorrect as the medical opinion should be 'reasonable and responsible', not just 'responsible'. E is incorrect since there must be a causative link between the two.

5. C—Article 8: Right to respect for private and family life
Article 8 best explains the rights of the person to maintain privacy in their affairs. This case describes the actions of one clinical practitioner that go against the professional codes of conduct of the medical regulator, and it should be remembered the Human Rights Act can only be used legally against the state and its organizations rather than individual practitioners. In clinical practice, be very cautious about leaving voicemails.

6. B—Duty of care owed to patients is statutory
Options A and E are incorrect as a duty of care is not core to consequentialism, and autonomy is not key to the duty of care. It is not true that Good Medical Practice means the duty of care is owed to all citizens by each doctor; it takes effect when a doctor commences care for a patient. Because of this D is also untrue. The correct answer is B as the duty of care owed is a statutory obligation as captured within the *NHS Act* (2006) and is not about the contract held by an individual employee with the healthcare organization they work in. The Foundation Year 1 doctor will have agreed in principle to commence work in the given service from a given date.

## Chapter 2 Professionalism

1. B—Expressing the duty of candour
Prescribing errors are common in medical practice, but the course of action taken here goes beyond making an error, as steps are taken both to apologize and correct it—which reflects an expression of the duty of candour. An incident like this could be reported as a near miss in an organizational reporting system (e.g. a Datix form or similar) as this may lead to educational information being shared with other prescribers about the need to calculate creatinine clearance when prescribing gabapentin to a patient with renal impairment. The magnitude of this error does not amount to a significant event. A situation like this could provide a prompt for a clinical audit to be designed

and undertaken, involving a review of whether all recent gabapentin prescriptions in the organization or department have been appropriately really adjusted. Patients usually appreciate a prompt explanation, apology and correction of clinical errors.

2. E—Talk to him, encouraging him not to work this morning and to seek appropriate help
If you have reason to believe a colleague poses a risk to patients, you must take proportionate steps to protect patient safety. Here there has been a gradual escalation of concern about a colleague and housemate, and you do not necessarily know exactly what the underlying problem is. It could be work-related stress, depression, substance misuse, something else entirely or a combination of factors—and he may or may not want to share this with you, either now or later. The question asks what you will do first: as you are at a similar stage professionally and are friends, there is no obvious power difference between you—so trying to talk to him is the best option. You will want to encourage him to make the decision not to work today and to arrange himself an appropriate assessment (any of A, B or C are reasonable in an NHS context). You may even offer to attend with him if that is possible and welcomed. Option D may become necessary if he is unwilling to receive your concerns and act on them and should trigger further mechanisms to protect patient safety in the future proportionate to the level of risk posed. This scenario illustrates a need to consider an appropriate hierarchy of steps when raising a concern—so the first step is trying to speak to your friend, before deciding whether Option D is necessary.

3. B—Insist the patient does not drive her car until further advice from the neurologist tomorrow
Where TIA is a reasonable differential diagnosis, the patient needs to be advised not to drive until further assessment by a specialist. This will undoubtedly inconvenience the patient, but that is unavoidable. Other road users need to be protected, and the doctor might sensitively help the patient to explore how to manage her transport conundrums. If the patient did drive and had a road incident after this consultation, her car insurance would potentially be invalid and this is reasonable to communicate if the patient is resistant to the advice not to drive. It is absolutely inappropriate to break confidentiality by sharing this situation with the practice manager, whose spouse happens to have some organizational management responsibility for the patient. The Driver and Vehicle Licensing Authority (DVLA) Medical Fitness to Drive document contains detailed advice relating to different medical conditions. In a case like this, it is reasonable to let the neurologist make or refute a diagnosis, so there is no immediate need for the DVLA to be informed as the patient will not be driving and posing a risk to other road users in the meantime.

4. B—Say thank you for the card and say you appreciate her kindness but will need to decline the gift of cash
Patients can be delightful sometimes, and this gift offer seems well thought out and well intentioned. However, you do not know if the professional relationship will resume at some future point—what if she returns after a few days in a 'failed discharge' situation, or her spouse or a sibling later becomes a patient?—and in any case accepting a cash gift (or voucher) is seen as an inappropriate blurring of professional boundaries. If the patient wishes to donate money to the hospital charity, she can do, and generally a receipt will be issued. You should not take the money and reappropriate it without her knowledge, as she would think you have accepted the gift, and you would have been dishonest with her.

5. A—Advise him to make an appointment with his own doctor
The doctor with the cough is potentially stressed and taking a less than ideal course of action here. Reporting him to the General Medical Council, for asking for a private prescription without a proper consultation for a drug that can be bought over the counter anyway, is a disproportionate response. Ignoring him is a form of bullying and undermining and is never appropriate. Telling him to write his own prescription is wrong, and doctors should avoid providing medical care to themself where possible and it is clearly possible to avoid it here. Even if there is a good working relationship, it would still be inadvisable to meet his request because his colleague does not know about any other medicines being taken and cannot make a defensible diagnosis. It might be worth mentioning that he could buy it over the counter, albeit perhaps at a greater cost than an NHS or private prescription; while recommending the best thing to do is get a proper assessment even if it means taking some time out of work.

6. D—Dr J has compromised trust with her patients by trivializing their condition
The key ethical concern here lies in Dr J's mockery potentially undermining the seriousness of a medical condition that she treats. Even with the intent of humour, it can impact patient trust and a sense of validation concerning their health.

7. C—Dr D should assess niece N's relationship with patient P and the potential benefit of information access before deciding
While a right to confidentiality generally persists for the patient after death, and any specific wishes the patient has made known around this prior to their death should typically be respected, there are exceptions and there is no absolute right to confidentiality. Specific individuals like close family members may have the right to access certain medical records. Healthcare professionals can make case-by-case decisions based on factors like potential public

health benefits, minimizing harm or providing benefits to survivors/family members. Therefore Dr D needs to weigh niece N's relationship with patient P, the specific information requested and the potential benefit of disclosure against the duty of confidentiality before making a decision. There is detailed information in the General Medical Council guidance on Confidentiality: good practice in handling patient information.

**8.** A—Conduct educational sessions with patients about the importance of follow-up care
Reminders and incentives may provide short-term boosts in attendance. Same-day appointments may not prove to be practical or sustainable, and arranging mass transport to appointments is also unlikely to be sustainable. Teaching patients the importance of follow-up care is more likely to increase commitment to attending follow-up appointments.

**9.** E—Reduce the number of steps in the barcode scanning process
Option E directly responds to the issues and is the best because it will also reduce cognitive load and stress experienced. The nurses are not reporting as they are unfamiliar with the system or they have unmet equipment needs, but the system itself is causing issues. Financial incentives will not deal with the underlying issues in the system and are not certain to be sustainable.

## Chapter 3  Doctors, patients and society

**1.** B—Explain to the daughter the importance of respecting her mother's privacy and suggest a family meeting to discuss the care plan together
It is a priority to respect and maximize patient participation and autonomy while still addressing the daughter's concerns. Option B achieves that. A diagnosis of Alzheimer disease does not automatically translate into a lack of autonomy or loss of mental capacity. Giving generic information may not fully address the daughter's concerns and is a little dishonest to the patient. The doctor calling the patient to ask if the daughter can see the notes may put the patient in an uncomfortable position. The daughter is likely to be concerned for her mother's welfare, but it is not clear that a social worker will be well placed to address those concerns. It is important to remember that older people with advanced cognitive impairment can become vulnerable to exploitation and that elder abuse can involve a close family member. Option B allows prioritizing the patient's privacy while also acknowledging the daughter's concerns and facilitating open communication within the family.

**2.** C—Thank her husband for his support and arrange a professional interpreter
The power cut is unfortunate, but not a good enough reason to justify deferring the consultation unless the

patient suggests this. Her husband appears supportive and this may well be the case, but you cannot be sure of the accuracy of his interpretation and the proposed clinical intervention is highly significant for the patient's future. Asking her husband to translate offers him the power to pursue his own agenda for the consultation if he so wishes, and unless you also speak the language you will be none the wiser. The patient is unable to understand English to a sufficient extent to give informed consent directly, and while recruiting additional staff to help with the clinic is a good idea which will not directly lead to the consent being obtained. The best answer is C; a professional interpreter is bound by codes of conduct, including impartiality and confidentiality.

**3.** B—Common law best interests
Presumption of capacity is one of the general principles of the Mental Capacity Act and is not relevant here because the patient lacks capacity at the time any decision needs to be made. An advance decision can only be made to refuse treatment; a patient does not have an automatic right to demand a particular treatment. Instead doctors have a professional duty to offer and/or provide treatment that is in the patient's best interests in a given circumstance. In an emergency where the patient cannot consent, this is done under common law. England now has an opt-out system for organ donation, meaning if the patient dies and has not opted out (and is not part of an excluded group: generally speaking this means people with Creutzfeldt–Jakob disease, Ebola, active cancer, HIV), then they are potentially an organ donor. Organ donation would generally only be carried through in discussion with the family. The fact some family members are present does not alter the basis for assessment and treatment.

**4.** D—Safeguarding vulnerable people
The Deprivation of Liberty Safeguards applies to a compliant but incapacitated person; the patient here is actually too young for the Mental Capacity Act to be applied, and the parlance of competence is relevant. Gillick competence is important to this consultation and corresponds to assessing sufficient maturity to consent to medical advice and treatment. The Fraser Guidelines relate specifically to contraceptive treatment and advice for those below 16 years and are also crucial here, but they do not provide the basis for the general practitioner seeking more information about her boyfriend or the relationship. It is true that her boyfriend could also be a vulnerable person, we do not know if he is older or younger or has learning disabilities for example, but the patient is also potentially vulnerable in this situation and so the best answer is D.

**5.** E—Speak to the duty social worker asking for urgent intervention
Asking the son to explain himself may be making an unfair assumption, and if it is a correct assumption it

could put a vulnerable patient at further risk by inflaming him. There is no good evidence that the son has a mental illness requiring assessment or treatment so the Mental Health Act is inappropriate. Asking a second doctor to attend is unlikely to add any further useful clinical information to the existing assessment. The patient has not strictly asked for confidentiality to be maintained about her situation. Even if she did it would be reasonable, given her vulnerability and evidence of harm having already probably occurred, to override this as a safeguarding concern in her best interests. Ideally, the duty social worker will arrange a further assessment on the day and potentially move her to safe temporary accommodation.

6. A—Take action proportionate to the assessed suicide risk
Using the preferred pronouns of the patient is a feature of personal communication and a consultation skill rather than a management plan. It may be helpful to sympathetically recognize the long waiting times for specialist services. There is no indication to involve the patient's family here, as it has not been asked for by the patient, although often it can be helpful to understand what social support the patient has. Prescribing hormones in this situation without specialist guidance goes beyond the scope of competent practice for most doctors. For any patient with self-harm, a suicide risk assessment and action proportionate to the level of risk is the appropriate management. This might vary from arranging a follow-up appointment at a suitable interval for a lower-risk situation to a referral to liaison psychiatry in the hospital setting or to the mental health crisis team in the community setting to application of the Mental Health Act or (rarely) involving the police where there is an imminent and serious threat to the patient and/or others in the community.

# Chapter 4 The beginning and end of life

1. B—Sensitively tell the patient this is not part of their clinical practice and advise the patient to make an appointment with a colleague for this request
It is assumed that the patient can make another appointment for herself, and therefore it is not necessary for the GP to arrange this. Refusing to refer the patient without explaining that she has the right to another doctor's opinion is inappropriate. As the GP conscientiously objects to abortion, it is not necessary for them to refer the patient to gynaecology, unless the situation is life threatening. Trying to persuade the patient not to have an abortion would be inappropriate, and the GP must not express judgement about a patient or their lifestyle.

2. A—All of the following
Options B, C, D and E are valid grounds for termination of pregnancy under the *Abortion Act* (1967).

3. B—The foetus has interests that may be protected by law
The foetus is not a legal person and therefore has no rights protected in law. However, it may have interests that can be protected. The *Abortion Act* (1967) generally requires two doctors to approve the decision for a termination. A request for termination made to a general practitioner is not illegal, but it is still possible that a patient can be prosecuted for seeking an illegal means of abortion.

4. B—If an individual does not wish to be considered as a potential organ donor, they must opt out of being one
The new legislation means that anyone who has not registered their decision on organ donation (either to be a donor, or to refuse to be a donor) is assumed not to have objected to being an organ donor. However, the hospital will make every effort to contact the family, and will not go ahead with donation if the family objects. Prisoners, the mentally incompetent and overseas visitors are excluded from this legislation. The body of a deceased person is not legally 'owned' by anyone and this is well established in case law; soon after death there will need to be a professional verification of death assessment, and reasonably soon afterwards a Medical Certificate of Cause of Death (MCCD) will be issued and/or referral made to the coroner. If there are no suspicious circumstances and no indications for involving the coroner, the personal representatives (executors) of the deceased have the right to determine where the body goes, how it goes, and what is ultimately done with it.

5. B—Principle of autonomy
This is a classic argument for assisted dying on the grounds of the principle of autonomy.

6. A—Discuss with the consultant in charge of the patient's care
In a case such as this, it is always best to discuss with the consultant responsible for the patient's care. In the aftermath of the Tracey case, it is generally not acceptable to not involve patients in discussions around DNACPR. However, CPR is an actively provided treatment and still remains a medical decision. As the patient has capacity, his family members cannot consent to a DNACPR on his behalf.

7. A—Altruistic surrogacy is legal
While commercial surrogacy is illegal, altruistic surrogacy is permitted and the surrogate mothers may be compensated for expenses. At least one intended parent is required to be genetically related to the child conceived, and the intended parents must petition the courts to be granted custody of the child.

8. B—Hospital-acquired pneumonia
The scenario states that the patient dies from respiratory failure. This is most likely to be as a result of pneumonia, so this would be the primary cause of death. A, D and/or E

may be secondary or contributory causes. Respiratory failure is a pathophysiological 'mode of dying' rather than a pathological cause of death, so it is inappropriate for the death certificate.

# Chapter 5  Public health

1.  D—Mill's harm principle
    A single dose of the MMR vaccine protects only 9 in 10 children, with a second dose of MMR vaccine protecting almost 100% of children. Measles infection has a fatality rate of 1 to 3 per 1000 cases, and severe pulmonary and cerebral complications can also happen, making it an important public health concern. Mill's harm principle states that interference with personal freedoms (e.g. confidentiality to a point) is justified to prevent harm to others. In this case, the 'proper officer' at the local council or local health protection team needs to be informed so any appropriate actions can be taken to reduce the risk to others and identify any individuals or groups at risk. Free riding is an argument used in favour of mandatory vaccination; taking the line that individuals who refuse vaccination are not making a contribution to a conception of 'the common good' but are still benefitting from other people in the community taking the risk of being vaccinated. A duty not to infect others is a contested principle that applies at the level of an individual making choices about how they conduct themselves when they have an infectious illness, rather than at the communal level of public health in terms of identifying and risk-managing local disease outbreaks. Health promotion usually refers to the encouragement of healthy lifestyles; health protection is a better umbrella term for the processes around notifiable diseases, but it is not an answer option here. Underdetermination is a common challenge made to the nature of scientific evidence in public health—that it can be used to support various potentially competing hypotheses. It tends to follow that the interpretation of epidemiological data is value laden. This leads to a central question about what is and should be valued.

2.  C—Precautionary principle
    The precautionary principle describes taking action to avoid a potential threat in conditions of scientific uncertainty, which was the situation when COVID-19 lockdown measures were first introduced to combat a new and incompletely understood infectious illness with early data suggesting a high case rate of severe illness and mortality. The transparency principle aspires to uphold trust in public health institutions and decision-making, and for this reason a UK public enquiry into the handling of COVID-19 was organized after the initial upheaval. The equity principle relates to fair resource allocation to factor against socioeconomic disadvantage—and as lockdown laws applied to everyone equally this is not the best answer. Lockdowns highlighted various inequalities,

including the ability of some people to continue working from home. The reciprocity principle describes the state acting to proportionately compensate people for the inconvenience of imposing public health priorities. An example was the UK COVID-19 furlough scheme, a government-sponsored payment for a proportion of usual earnings for people unable to continue working due to lockdown. It is normally preferable to start with education and discussion around public health issues before using emergency legislation: the least restrictive principle is an entirely inaccurate way to describe the lockdown of a whole society.

3.  E—Utilitarianism
    Various criteria for screening programmes exist, including those by Wilson and Junger and the NHS National Screening Committee, and are based on conceptions of 'good' as defined at a pooled population level. This is utilitarianism. The threshold for 'a positive screen' can be influenced by epidemiological data, pragmatic realities like the extent of human and physical resources that are available to follow up those who screen positive, and the public perception about a disease which can create political pressure to be seen to be doing something about high-profile conditions. Competent screening participants may feel disempowered when it comes to refusing a screening test since refusals are sometimes met by others with stigmatization. Kantian ethics takes the view that individuals should not be used as a means to an end—for example, as part of a mass population approach aimed at improving the national statistics around bowel cancer. This makes informed individual consent to participate so important, since positive screening tests can set off a series of diagnostic tests (and potentially treatments), giving rise to feelings of loss of control in a person who previously felt well and has now been made into a patient.

4.  C—Double jeopardy
    QALYs as a value system tend to favour younger and healthier people on the 'self-evident' basis that this is rational and that health is possible to objectively define. In situations of resource limitation like the one described, the wife stands to gain more QALYs from high-dependency care simply because she has no background comorbidity and because on average females currently have longer life expectancies than males. This creates an effect called double jeopardy for the husband because unchangeable circumstances in his life can adversely influence the priority assigned to him in receiving treatment for an unrelated condition under the QALY system. Profit motive can be a concern with private companies being allowed to provide state-funded health services in the UK NHS because it may generate a real or perceived tension between profit motive and patient care; in contrast, the QALY system offers a mechanism that attempts to ensure treatments for different conditions with similar cost–benefit profiles are funded equitably. Actual or perceived conflicts of interest

are important to avoid in resource allocation decisions at the macro level—where commissioners of health services must not be able to commission a service that they are also involved in providing. Conflicts of interest should not occur in bedside medicine, as doctors should avoid treating family members or anyone with whom they have a close personal relationship. The inverse care law states that health care is least available where it is most needed—that is in areas with more significant social deprivation. The doctrine of double effect is sometimes used to justify treatment decisions in end-of-life care situations, where a medicine might be prescribed with the intention of relieving a severe symptom such as pain but has the foreseeable possible side effect of hastening the death of the patient.

5.  C—Consequentialism
Consequentialist reasoning holds that the outcomes of a course of action are the ultimate basis for judging whether the action was right or wrong, and in the absence of further information the patient and parent could be forgiven for thinking here that seeking medical assessment and obtaining a prescribed treatment has led to the desirable outcome of recovery from the illness. Approached from a utilitarian perspective and applying good epidemiological evidence the doctor would not have prescribed: since eight out of 10 children like the one described with otitis media who do not take antibiotics feel better within 3 days, whereas nine out of 10 children like the one described with otitis media who do take antibiotics feel better within 3 days but three out of 10 of them experience antibiotic side effects while also driving the rise of antibiotic resistance. Deontological thinking separates the course of action from the outcome and says that an action in itself can be right or wrong independent of whether the outcome is 'good' or 'bad'. It does not apply to the reasoning of the patient and parent here; the doctor can just say they are reasonable in seeking assessment because they believe themselves and/or are believed to be ill. Virtue ethics focuses on character traits like kindness, courage, honesty and so on which are not alluded to in the description. Liberalism is the dominant political philosophy in Western nations and tends to favour state neutrality—governments tend not to enforce judgements about how a person should live and there are pluralistic ideas of what 'a good life' entails. There is a leaning towards individualism, autonomy and self-determination; however, liberalism does not confer on a patient a right to demand a particular prescription-only (or other restricted) treatment when a registered and regulated practitioner assesses that it is inappropriate.

6.  B—Consequentialism
Partner tracing is a basic feature of public health practice and recognizes there may be one or more contacts at risk of infection based on the diagnosis in an index case. This is used in communicable disease control and was undertaken in the COVID-19 pandemic initially and is

recommended in sexually transmitted infections like this. The GP wants to ensure the boyfriend is tested/treated and to prevent reinfection of the index case: this thinking is consequentialist and has the aim to reduce overall harm and suffering. However to make such a calculation on overall 'good', it is important to consider not just a single outcome (infection-free people) but other effects including how the index patient will be affected, the impact on the relationship and possible disclosure to others, as well as possible reinfection of the index patient if the boyfriend is not treated. Virtue ethics would require the GP to consider their values and beliefs—perhaps in this case being compassionate to both the patient and the boyfriend and any others involved. The doctrine of double effect applies when an action taken with a 'permissible intended outcome' also causes another outcome that is not permitted as the main intention: it does not apply here. Arguably there are multiple conflicting duties for the doctor here: towards the index patient but also to the boyfriend and the public. Partner notification is linked to a public interest duty, but it is usually argued that the duty to the patient is stronger in a case like this. Confidentiality would arguably be inappropriately breached if the GP insisted on informing the boyfriend against the patient's wishes; as the risk to him is unlikely to be accepted as a 'serious harm'. In practice, it may be better to ask the patient to present to a Sexual Health (Genito-Urinary Medicine) Clinic, where wider sexual health screening and contact tracing are embedded into the systems of daily practice. Venereal disease regulations create special considerations around confidentiality and information sharing: so be aware the patient probably has a right to request further information is not shared back to the GP in this case, if they so wish. Social production of disease, or the political economy of health, is a macro level theory of social epidemiology.

7.  E—Virtue ethics
Volunteering is a beneficent act and, while often providing some benefits to the volunteer, usually involves a high level of concern for the needs of others. Virtue ethics is the single best answer because it draws on attributes or characteristics of an individual that are valued. In the scenario described, we might infer courage and kindness among other traits. Autonomy is relevant as the consultant is an autonomous person who can choose what they do, but it does not explain why one situation is being prioritized while others are deprioritized. Consequentialism might justify leaving home and work and indeed taking risks with the hope that more 'good' results from the volunteer work. However, the scenario does not provide enough information about the upset that may be caused to the partner or the consultant's regular work, where the actions taken will abruptly reduce clinical capacity and negatively impact patients nearer to home. Deontological duties apply in many respects: particularly towards patients and colleagues who would be adversely affected by sudden changes in availability. There are also, perhaps, duties

'towards everyone;' and if this is the case, the doctor should make long-term plans to volunteer more often to meet a sense of wider duties to a globalized society, and this requires adapting day-to-day work accordingly and in an appropriate manner. Justice requires a consideration of how actions and goods are distributed and is relevant here but again does not best explain the volunteering decision when there is a need to continue to provide care for current patients. The actions taken by the doctor in the scenario, considering the potential disruption and reneging on existing commitments, could lead to disciplinary action from the employer and/or fitness to practise proceedings.

8. **E—Soft paternalism**

Stella is attempting to change the behaviour of patients in the practice but trying to use approaches that still respect their autonomy and liberal values. This is soft paternalism, where someone would like to change something and achieve an outcome—often in the face of resistance—but also do so in a way that is not coercive nor that restricts choice in a mandatory sense like hard paternalism. Liberalism is relevant but tends to oppose even soft paternalism as it can be viewed as a nudge or subtle attempt to modify behaviour which, while not appearing to directly curtail liberty, still has this as an aim and may come from a base of uneven power. Consequentialism often pertains to ethical arguments involving populations and could support Stella's decision if overall 'good' were maximized. This could ultimately be the case if there are net benefits through alcohol reduction, but there are many other aspects, such as the disutility of unhappiness from so many behavioural change messages, possible emotional and shaming consequences through repeated reminders and possibly a compromise to the uptake of other services if patients felt the general practitioner practice was an increasingly judgemental place where health promotion and behavioural change were in sharp focus. The Quality and Outcomes Framework (QOF) provides financial incentives to practices to improve several public health–related outcomes, such as obesity, smoking and blood pressure. The 2023–24 QOF included giving advice about safe alcohol consumption targeted at patients with known hypertension, but there was no practice-wide indicator. In any case, a financial incentive scheme is unlikely to be the single best answer to this question asking for an ethical justification.

# Case Index

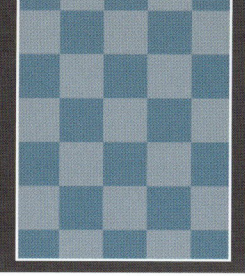

## Short clinical cases by chapter

- Case 5.8 Public Participation in Health Service Commissioning
- Case 5.9 QALYs and Double Jeopardy
- Case 5.10 Harm Reduction: Underage Sex and Illicit Drug Use

## Short clinical cases for self-directed study

- **Aintree Hospitals NHS Trust v. James (2013)**
  A case considering how doctors and the courts should decide about giving or withdrawing life-sustaining treatments in the best interests of a patient lacking capacity. These must be considered on a case-by-case basis; both the likely (or known) wishes or feelings of the individual patient and their clinical condition need to be taken into account. *Aintree University Hospitals NHS Foundation Trust (Respondent) v. James (Appellant)* [2013] UKSC 67 On appeal from [2013] EWCA Civ 65.

- **Alfie Evans**
  After admission to the hospital with a neurodegenerative condition and worsening seizures, Alfie Evans was admitted to paediatric intensive care and ventilated. MRI scans showed a progressive and fatal neurodegenerative disorder. His parents sought for Alfie to be transferred to Bambino Gesu Hospital in Rome and then potentially onwards to Munich to explore further treatment options. Alfie's treating doctors felt this would be futile and that the best option would be to palliate him and remove ventilatory support. Several courts upheld this. *Alder Hey Hospital v. Evans* [2018] EWHC 818 (Fam).

- **Babylon**
  A digital-first primary care provider that also included an artificial intelligent chatbot; it gained over 100,000 NHS patients operating as a subcontractor to an originally small GP Practice in London that had traditionally served a local population of around 5000 patients. Babylon joined the New York Stock Exchange in 2021 with a valuation of over $4 billion, lost most of its value and was delisted in 2023. The Babylon 'GP At Hand' App was sold and became part of eMed Healthcare UK Limited (UK company number 15086104) with links to eMed LLC based in the United States.

- **Ian Paterson (clinical events 1997–2011, General Medical Council erasure 2017)**
  The private practice of a breast surgeon came into question and led to convictions on 17 counts of wounding with intent to do grievous bodily harm and three counts of wounding/inflicting grievous bodily harm. Details can be found on the General Medical Council list of registered medical practitioners.

- **Kerrie Wooltorton (inquest 2009)**
  The patient took antifreeze with the intent to end her life. She presented for medical attention with a letter she had written, requesting only palliative treatments to keep her comfortable and so she would not be alone at home in the dying process. As an adult with capacity, she was allowed to refuse treatment, with the outcome being her death.

- **Lucy Letby**
  A former neonatal nurse who was convicted in 2023 of multiple counts of murder and attempted murder of infants in the course of her work at the Countess of Chester Hospital between 2015 and 2016. (Sentencing remarks are available from https://www.judiciary.uk/wp-content/uploads/2023/08/LETBY-Sentencing-Remarks.pdf and accessed on February 2024.)

- **Martha Mills**
  Martha's rule follows the outcome of the case of Martha Mills who died in 2021 aged 13 years from sepsis. She was admitted to the hospital with a pancreatic injury after falling off her bike. A 2023 coroner's ruling concluded that Martha would likely have survived if the family's concerns had been promptly responded to and Martha was moved to intensive care earlier. Since 2024 in England Martha's rule has existed for NHS hospital staff, patients, families, carers and advocates to have easier access to a second opinion from a critical care outreach team when there are concerns about a patient. (Wise, J. (2023). Martha's rule recommendations are laid out to government. *British Medical Journal*, *383*, 2565.)

- **Re A (conjoined twins) [2001] 2 WLR 480**
  Two twins, Mary and Jodie, were born conjoined. Jodie was stronger and would survive if she was surgically separated from Mary; however, Mary would die. If the twins were left conjoined they would eventually both die. The parents refused permission for the operation to go ahead. The hospital applied to the court for an order to allow separation of the twins which was granted on the grounds that it was, on balance, the approach of best interests.

- **Simon Bramhall (clinical events 2013, General Medical Council erasure 2022)**
  A liver transplant surgeon had marked his initials on the livers of patients during transplant surgery using an argon beam coagulator. This later involved the criminal courts and the Medical Practitioners Tribunal Service. Details can be found on the General Medical Council list of registered medical practitioners.

# Index

Page numbers followed by *f* indicate figures, *t* indicate tables and *b* indicate boxes.